ORGAN CULTURE

Edited by
J. ANDRÉ THOMAS
DEPARTMENT OF CELLULAR BIOLOGY AT THE SORBONNE
ACADEMY OF MEDICINE
PARIS, FRANCE

TRANSLATED BY EXPRESS TRANSLATION SERVICE

1970

ΛCADEMIC PRESS   New York and London

LIST OF CONTRIBUTORS

Numbers in parentheses indicate the pages on which the authors' contributions begin.

F. Dieterlen-Lièvre, *Institut d'Embryologie Expérimentale du C.N.R.S. et du Collège de France, Paris, France* (177)

Katy Haffen, *Institut d'Embryologie et de Tératologie Expérimentale du C.N.R.S. et du Collège de France, Paris, France* (121)

Madeleine Kieny, *Institut d'Embryologie Expérimentale du C.N.R.S. et du Collège de France, Paris, France* (71)*

Georges Le Douarin, *Institut d'Embryologie et de Tératologie Expérimentale du C.N.R.S., Paris, France* (13)†

Nicole Le Douarin (53)

Berthe Salzgeber, *Institut d'Embryologie et de Tératologie Expérimentale du C.N.R.S., Paris, France* (233)

Philippe Sengel, *Laboratoire d'Embryologie Expérimentale du Collège de France, Paris, France* (379)

Michel Sigot, *Institut d'Embryologie et de Tératologie Expérimentale du C.N.R.S. et du Collège de France, Paris, France* (343)

Emilienne Wolff, *Institut d'Embryologie Expérimentale du C.N.R.S. et du Collège de France, Paris, France* (459)

Etienne Wolff, *Institut d'Embryologie et de Tératologie Expérimentale du C.N.R.S. et du Collège de France, Paris, France* (1)

C. Ziller-Sengel, *Institut d'Embryologie et de Tératologie Expérimentale du C.N.R.S. et du Collège de France, Paris, France* (301)

* Present address: *Faculté des Sciences de Grenoble, Laboratoire de Zoologie, Domaine Universitaire, Saint-Martin-D'Heres.*

† Present address: *Laboratoire de Physiologie Animale et Cellulaire, Faculté des Sciences de Nantes, Nantes, France.*

PREFACE

This monograph is the work of Professor Etienne Wolff and his colleagues. Professor Wolff reviews the general principles of organ culture *in vitro* and indicates that the main aim is the study of autodifferentiation. He summarizes many aspects of organ culture: physiological differentiation, the action of substances that stimulate or inhibit growth, and the interactions of associated organs.

G. Le Douarin discusses the differentiation of embryonic organs in natural media. He describes the development of skeletal rudiments of the skin and its derivatives, the respiratory organs, glands, and viscera, such as the kidney and the gastrointestinal tract, and the organs of special sense. He concludes with a review of the physiological aspects of autodifferentiation *in vitro*.

This is followed by a study of differentiation in synthetic solid or liquid media. Mme M. Kieny describes the development of the genital glands, the syrinx, the skin, the uropygial gland, the thyroid, and the bone rudiments. She also discusses in detail the physiological and biochemical requirements of the tissues.

Mme K. Haffen deals with the problems of sexual differentiation and intersexuality *in vitro*. This is a comparative study of avian and mammalian embryos. She describes spontaneous sexual autodifferentiation, intersexuality and sexual inversion due to hormones, the effects of teratogenic agents, and the results of parabiosis between different species.

Mme F. Dieterlen-Lièvre analyzes the interactions between hormones, inhibitor substances, and receptor organs *in vitro*. She studies the hormonal relationships of endocrine glands during development, and gives a detailed account of the uptake of materials which have been added to the culture media, principally by bone and the mammary gland in varying physiological states.

Mme B. Salzgeber describes the culture of whole avian blastoderms, giving a detailed account of the conditions which induce precocious or delayed morphogenesis. The regulatory potential and the migrations of the germ cells are also discussed. She gives a physiological analysis of the nutritional needs of organs and whole blastoderms, and the effects of teratogens, inhibitors, and toxic materials. Finally, the challenging question of the culture of mammalian ova is outlined, together with the problems of embryogenesis.

Mme Ziller-Sengel describes organ culture in invertebrates. She is concerned with sexual differentiation, endocrinology, genetic variation, and regeneration.

M. Sigot contributes a chapter on the dissociation and reassociation of cells *in vitro*. He considers the relationships of the derivatives of the various embryonic layers in various isotypical and heterotypical experimental combinations. Cellular adhesion is discussed; various physiological and physical hypotheses for the phenomena of cellular reaggregation are also put forward.

P. Sengel discusses dissociation and reassociation of rudiments. The following subjects are described: primary induction in Amphibia, morphogenic interactions in the chick, differentiation of the skin and its derivatives, analysis of the feather germs, dermal–epidermal relationships, keratinization, the uropygial gland, tubular organs with particular reference to the experimental induction of the kidney, and, in some cases, the inductive action of substances transmissible from a distance.

Mme Emilienne Wolff concludes the work with a study of organ chimeras *in vitro* and the related study of the organ culture of malignant tumors. Many experimental combinations are obtained by associating different organs, namely heterotypical homologous organs, heterologous organs, gonads, and viscera. These combinations allow morphogenesis to be analyzed outside the normal pathways of embryogenesis.

The xenoplastic association of avian embryonic organs with tumorous explants by Professor and Mme Wolff's school has made possible the organ culture of human and other mammalian cancers. In particular, many malignant tumors may be grown with chick mesonephros. This final chapter contains a study of the nutrition of the explants considered from the following aspects: direct contact with the mesonephros which is being parasitized, the effect of extracts of the mesonephros, the passage of nutrient materials across the interposed vitelline membrane, and an analysis of long-term cultures of malignant tissue.

J. ANDRÉ THOMAS

ADDENDUM

The articles which comprise this work were written in 1963, the material having first been presented in the form of lectures, which my colleagues and myself gave as part of a course on cell biology in the Faculty of Sciences, at the invitation of Professor J. A. Thomas. The articles were published in French in 1964.

Since great advances have been made since 1963, the articles have been updated by the addition of addenda which include the most important work carried out from 1963 to 1968; some are in abridged form due to lack of space.

I should like to thank my colleagues for their generous and unselfish contributions to this work.

ETIENNE WOLFF

CONTENTS

Chapter V. The Action of Hormones and Inhibitors on Organs Cultured *in Vitro*

F. Dieterlen-Lièvre

Chapter VI. Culture and Parabiosis of Blastoderms

Berthe Salzgeber

Chapter VII. Organ Culture in the Invertebrates

C. Ziller-Sengel

Chapter VIII. *In Vitro* Reassociation of Dissociated Cells

Michel Sigot

Chapter IX. **Study of Organogenesis by Dissociation and Reassociation of Embryonic Rudiments *in Vitro***

PHILIPPE SENGEL

Chapter X. **Organ Chimeras and Organ Culture of Malignant Tumors**

EMILIENNE WOLFF

CHAPTER I

THE GENERAL PRINCIPLES
OF ORGAN CULTURE *IN VITRO*

Etienne Wolff

COLLÈGE DE FRANCE
INSTITUT D'EMBRYOLOGIE ET DE TÉRATOLOGIE EXPÉRIMENTALES DU C.N.R.S.
PARIS, FRANCE

The aim of explanting tissues *in vitro* is to study the behavior and fate of cells, tissues, or organs separated from the whole organism. More precisely, in the case of embryonic tissues, the questions are (a) do the isolated cells or groups of cells continue their proliferation and differentiation as they would in the normal organism, (b) do they behave in an aberrant fashion, and (c) is it possible to modify or reestablish their normal development by external operations?

Thus one satisfies the condition set down by Claude Bernard: "We must, as far as we can, isolate physiological occurrences outside the organism by means of experimental procedures. This isolation allows us to see and understand better the deepest associations of the phenomenon, so that their vital role may be followed later in the organism."

Two principal directions have been explored since tissues were first explanted *in vitro:* the culture of isolated cells and the culture of groups of cells of varying complexity—tissues, organs, parts of organisms, or whole organisms.

The culture of cells is called histotypical culture or, very commonly though less precisely, "tissue culture." We shall call the culture of organized material "organ culture" where tissues or organs are concerned, and "organism culture" when we are dealing with whole embryos or large parts of an organism.

The first attempts at *in vitro* explantation were made by the French anatomist Vulpian (1859) and the German embryologist Born (1897). These workers removed large pieces such as the tail from frog embryos and cultured them in ordinary water; continued growth and differentiation were observed.

These simple experiments foreshadowed organ culture. Amphibian embryos are well suited to this type of experiment, since their cells contain reserves that enable them to survive a long time in isolation. Holtfreter (1931) made use of this characteristic when he explanted embryonic rudiments *in vitro* before differentiation had occurred.

We shall not be dealing with the culture of organs that have already evolved or are adult, since these can be made to survive by means of aseptic perfusion techniques. Such techniques, first described by Carrel and Lindberg (1938), involve isolating a fully grown organ, and maintaining its nutrition and respiration by perfusion, using a pump in an aseptic circuit. Thomas (1948) brought this technique to perfection, and was able to keep alive quite heavy calf fetuses. The perfusion method has been used in many other ways, one of the most outstanding being the use of the heart-lung machine in open heart surgery.

Such techniques are very useful in physiology. Outstanding experiments have been carried out in this field by Peeters and Massart (1947) on the udder of an adult cow. Using artificial circulation, Peeters and Massart perfused an isolated mammary gland with blood, and by varying the composition of the perfusate they were able to alter the composition of the milk collected from the nipple. It is possible in this way to make milk from blood outside of the organism.

In vitro culture began developing steadily from about 1910, following the pioneer work of Carrel and Burrows, who introduced a general method for explanting tissues from amniote vertebrates. This technique is now generally known and applied. On the other hand, relatively little is heard of the experiments of the early workers. The name of Harrison is well known in this context, and the magnificent work of Jolly at the Collège de France should not be forgotten. In 1903, he kept blood globules alive outside the organism for the first time. These globules, from *Triton*, were kept alive for several months and their movements and divisions were observed. Subsequently, Jolly made many contributions to this field, especially in the *in vitro* culture of whole mammalian embryos (1936, 1938).

Two lines of research have developed since the early experiments—tissue culture and organ culture. While the former proved successful from the beginning, organ culture was not practiced for many years. Cell culture leads to the proliferation of cells independently of the organ from which they were derived. Many pure cultures of both normal and malignant cells have been obtained from a variety of cells. The cell lines selected in this way can reproduce themselves indefinitely, like bacterial cultures. The principal characteristics of these cells are their autonomy and uncontrolled proliferation. To take a specific example, a primary explant of chicken heart made by Carrel in 1910 continued to live and multiply for many years, exhibiting potential immortality. Spectacular discovery as this was, it must be remembered that these cells were only the fibroblasts that migrated from the original explant; the organized structure of the explant was lost after a few hours of culture. It was not the heart, nor a fragment of the heart that had survived, but a few cells that escaped from the organ and became disorganized on finding a favorable medium.

On the other hand, the aim of organ culture is to maintain cohesion between the cells of a tissue and between the tissues of an organ, retaining the original structure. Thus some elements must not be favored at the expense of others, so that they develop in an uncoordinated way. Workers like Thompson (Thompson *et al.*, 1914) and Maximow (1925) used techniques very like those of tissue culture. Fell used the same techniques in the successful culture of many organs, after her first work in collaboration with Strangeways (Strangeways and Fell, 1926–1928), and her pupils and colleagues pioneered many developments in organ culture between 1926 and 1950. In 1951, the present author himself developed a technique that preserved the integrity of explanted organs while avoiding the escape of cells from the explant. In this way we achieved organ cultures free from cell cultures (Et. Wolff and Haffen, 1951, 1952).

I. EXPLANTATION *IN VIVO* AND *IN VITRO*

Organ culture as defined above may consist of explantation either *in vivo* or *in vitro*. Each technique has its advantages and drawbacks. Undoubtedly, the former technique places the graft under conditions that are closer to the normal medium. Explantation *in vivo* consists of grafting a fragment of tissue or organ into the body of an adult or embryonic host, or into the accessory tissues of an embryo. The explant is perfused by the host, and is thus better nourished. An explant cultured *in vitro* usually finds itself under poorer conditions of nutrition and respiration, and once it has attained a certain volume, its further existence is grossly handicapped. This is one of the reasons that survival and growth are limited. On the other hand, *in vitro* culture has the great advantage that the explant is removed from the complex influences of the intact organism.

This may be strikingly illustrated by the following example. About 1929–1931, Holtfreter separated the presumptive regions of a *Triton* gastrula and then explanted them, using two different processes. When the precursors were grafted into the lymphatic spaces or the peritoneal cavity of a tadpole, the presumptive epidermis, neural plate, and chordamesoderm gave rise to very varied tissues, neural, epidermal, mesodermal, and so on. It was not possible to say that the different primordia had characteristic potentialities that would distinguish them. On the contrary, the cultures *in vitro* showed that the presumptive epidermis and neural plate were both incapable of producing any differentiated tissue, whilst the presumptive chordamesoderm produced practically all tissues. It seems that the host tissues in the *in vivo* experiment contained materials which had the same effects as the embryonic organizers.

Hence it is often preferable to explant tissues *in vitro* despite the limitations that are imposed by the experiment. A useful technique that has often been applied in this laboratory is that of regrafting into a living embryo an explant that commenced differentiation *in vitro* (Salzgeber, 1958; Et. Wolff and Haffen, 1961).

What problems can organ culture solve? In what way can it be usefully employed?

a. Proof of Autodifferentiation. What happens to the undifferentiated rudiment of an organ, or to an organ that is in the process of differentiation?

We have already quoted Holtfreter's results obtained by explanting presumptive regions of an amphibian gastrula. This showed a lack of differentiation of the presumptive ectoderm, with multiple differentiation of the presumptive chordamesoderm that verged on coherent organization. These results cannot be challenged, since the culture medium, Holtfreter's solution, was simply a solution of inorganic salts. However, differentiation is possible because of the yolk reserves in the explanted cells.

Nevertheless, in the case of some amphibian species, such as *Amblystoma punctatum*, Holtfreter's experimental conditions cannot remain uncriticized. Thus Barth (1941) was able to show that the presumptive ectoderm of this species can form nervous tissue in Holtfreter's solution without the intervention of any inducing agent. Holtfreter's later work (1944, 1945) showed that in this case the saline solution was slightly toxic and provoked the onset of cytolysis. The paradoxical result is explained by the fact that the altered cells probably release into the medium a substance that has inductive properties. This merely shows how much care must be taken in interpreting results, even when the experimental conditions are made as simple as possible.

If already determined but as yet undifferentiated organs are removed from chick embryos, differentiation occurs in many cases. Such organs are the skeleton (tibia, vertebrae), liver, pancreas, intestine, skin, thyroid, gonads, Mullerian ducts, lung and syrinx, and the eye. Most of these examples of differentiation are drawn from work performed in our laboratories, and will be amplified in the following chapters.

In certain cases the normal development of an organ is not differentiation but rather atrophy or regression. This is true of the mesonephros, of the Mullerian ducts in the male, and of the right gonad in the female chick embryo. It is worth noting that many of these organs (mesonephros, right female gonad) always regress when explanted *in vitro*, just as they would in the normal animal. The male Mullerian ducts regress only when they are explanted after sexual differentiation of the gonads has occurred.

Organs such as the gonads are already differentiated to a certain extent if they are removed at about the 8th day of incubation, but they have not differentiated sexually. If they are cultured on a medium that contains no hormones, they will differentiate into ovaries or testes, but this determination is not fixed since it can be altered by adding sex hormones to the culture medium.

Organs with a well-defined form, such as parts of the skeleton, attain their usual shape and form as they grow *in vitro*. Moreover, a bone such as the tibia develops the articular facets at the epiphyses in the absence of the articulating bones (femur and tarsometatarsus).

b. Physiological Differentiation of Explanted Organs. Another problem that arises concerns morphological differentiation. Do explanted organs have the same physiological functions as in the organism? Do they manufacture the same substances and the same secretions? Obviously this will depend on the conditions of the culture medium and on the nutrient materials. Will these organs develop their specific activity in the absence of all related influences, if the culture conditions are favorable? Do the liver, pancreas, thyroid, and gonads become active in the absence of the hormones that regulate their secretions in the adult? The answer is quite clear. All of these organs function spontaneously soon after commencement of the culture. Liver isolated on the 4th day of incubation stores glycogen, thyroid explanted on the 7th day produces colloid, pancreas explanted on the 5th day produces first glucagon then insulin, and gonads explanted between the 5th and 8th days secrete their hormones.

There are many ways of establishing such effects. Some of the materials produced can be revealed by specific staining (glycogen, thyroid colloid). Others are demonstrated by associating two organs *in vitro*, one being the target organ of the other. The gonads act on the Mullerian duct, the pancreas acts on the liver. Such interactions are discussed later in Subsection d. Substances that are secreted into the culture medium by the explanted organ may also be studied. The explanted organ is removed, and an organ capable of reacting to the substances is placed in the medium (as in the case of the gonads).

c. The Action of Materials That Stimulate or Inhibit Organs in the Culture. An attempt can be made to alter the normal process of development by adding a chemical compound or the extract of an organ to the culture medium in order to stimulate or inhibit the differentiation of a presumptive region. Many experiments are possible in this field. The effects of many hormones on their target organs have been studied. Young male gonads are feminized by estrogenic hormones; the Mullerian ducts are stimulated by female hormones, but undergo necrosis and autolysis under the influence of androgens; the syrinx of the drake will develop into the female type under the influence of estrogens, when it would evolve into the male type in the absence of hormones.

The skin epidermis of the chick embryo does not keratinize when an excess of vitamin A is present, whilst the mucous membranes become cornified in the absence of vitamin A (Fell and Mellanby, 1953).

Many substances have an inhibitory effect that is analogous to the effects of some hormones. Thus trypaflavine makes the medulla of both male and female gonads regress, but it has no stimulating effect on male germinal epithelium. Colchicine and narcotine selectively destroy the cortex of the female gonad. Thus these substances have an exclusive effect on one or other constituent of the gonad, either the cortex or the medulla.

Extracts of embryos with the achondroplastic creeper mutation inhibit the development of long bones explanted from normal individuals.

d. Interaction of Organs in Parabiosis in Vitro. Among the many avenues of research revealed by organ culture one has proved to be extremely fruitful, with limitless possibilities. Two organs may be cultured together to investigate their interactions. In this way it is possible to show whether any direct correlations exist between two organs. Thus the precise endocrinology of the embryo can be built up, by analyzing the correlations between certain structures, and eliminating the effect of other organs.

Suspected interactions between gonads of both sexes, between gonads and hypophysis, between thyroid and hypophysis, and between pancreas and liver have already been investigated by these methods.

Organs that are normally never related in time or space may also be cultured together. For example, parabiotic unions can be formed between organs of different ages, between embryonic and adult tissues. Two gonads of different sexes may be united, or two organs with no apparent connection, such as the thyroid and the mesonephros or the lung and the mesonephros, may be cultured together. Organs from different species may be grown on the same medium. Thus it has been possible to associate organs from such dissimilar species as chick and mouse.

Briefly, when two identical or different organs from two species come into contact, they unite and intermix their cells, which collaborate in the formation of the same structures and show remarkable affinities.

To pursue such paradoxical situations even further, we have put chick embryo tissues into a parabiotic relationship with cancerous mammalian cells, especially from human malignant tumors. Such experiments have been successful, but in this case the malignant cells multiply at the expense of the embryonic cells. The symbiosis that existed between normal cells from different species has developed into parasitism.

Such cases of parabiosis can often confirm and define relations that were previously suspected between two different organs. Unsuspected potentialities are revealed in other cases. This is far removed from the simple autodifferentiation of an isolated organ.

e. Culture in Synthetic Media. The original culture media used by the first workers contained only extracts and nutrient liquids, such as embryo extracts, plasma, and serum. The media used in this laboratory have a semisolid agar substrate in physiological saline solution, with added nutrients, glucose, and embryo extract. Experiments were carried out to determine whether the embryo extract could be replaced by specific chemical compounds, amino acids, vitamins, and so on. In this way it is possible to progress from very simple to complex media.

Substances that are necessary for survival, differentiation, and growth have been determined in this way. The simplest medium (minimum medium) that will allow limited survival is composed of the substrate with added glucose (Spratt, 1949; Et. Wolff *et al.*, 1953). The requirements for growth and differentiation may be the same or different. Differentiation is a sensitive criterion for judging the value of a medium, since it does not follow the law of "all or nothing" but rather that of more or less. In poor media, differentiation may be absent or incomplete, whilst in richer media, it may progress normally. Thus the drake syrinx is better developed, and contains more cartilage, when it is cultured on a medium that is both qualitatively and quantitatively rich in amino acids (Em. Wolff, 1957). Differentiation of the female gonad requires more amino acids than that of the male gonad (Stenger-Haffen, 1957). Also the secretions of a gland may be somewhat deficient.

The use of synthetic media is a useful means of investigating the secretion of an organ and the enzymes necessary for its development. Research of this type is still in its infancy. A new method adapted from the Warburg technique by Berman (1964) makes it possible to follow the oxygen consumption of living organ cultures *in vitro*. It is also possible to study directly certain metabolic processes.

f. Dissociation and Reassociation of the Components of an Organ. Wilson (1907) and Fauré-Fremiet (1925) were the first to study the disintegration of (sponge) tissues into isolated cells. Recently these techniques have been used on vertebrate tissues and organs in culture.

Two main directions have been followed. The cells may be separated from one another, mixed at random whatever their tissue of origin, and then allowed to reassociate (Holtfreter, Moscona). Alternatively, the constituent tissues in an embryonic rudiment may be separated (Grobstein), for example, the epithelium and the connective tissue, as in skin, mucous membranes of the digestive tract, lung, mesonephros, salivary glands, and so on.

The first method has shown that the cells of an organ or even of an organism regroup themselves by type, showing affinities between the cells of the same tissue and repulsions between cells of different tissues. Thus Townes and Holtfreter (1955) showed that when the cells from two tissues were mixed, they reconstituted the primitive organization. Thus cells from the neural tube and epidermis of amphibian embryos, when mixed together, sort themselves out to produce a neural tube lying beneath the epidermis.

The second method allows two tissues from different parts of the body and from different organs to be associated. Thus mesoderm from the foot and epidermis from the wing may be associated or vice versa. Will feathers or scales then develop? Sengel (1958), in this laboratory, showed that it is the mesoderm that determines differentiation. Similarly, the epithelium of the gizzard and the proventriculus, or the lung and the metanephros may be exchanged. It is possible to analyze the factors inducing differentiation if such experiments are carried out on very young rudiments. One of the articles in this volume is devoted to this work.

g. *Culture of Whole Organisms or Parts of Organisms.* This type of organ culture is especially applicable to the embryos of viviparous animals such as mammals. In these cases it is difficult to carry out experiments *in vivo*, particularly in the early stages. The technique may also be applied to the embryos of oviparous animals such as the blastoderms of fish and birds, where it is useful to separate them from the yolk. The nutritional needs of the embryo may be studied, by substitution of the placental or vitelline nutrition. Surgical procedures such as excisions or parabiosis that are difficult or impossible under normal circumstances may be carried out quite easily.

h. *Culture of Invertebrate Organs.* Methods similar to those used for vertebrates have recently been applied to invertebrates. They have been originated following the development of experimental embryology and the recent progress in the field of invertebrate endocrinology. The object of these investigations is to see whether embryonic rudiments and differentiating organs show autodifferentiation.

It is also desirable to demonstrate inductive actions and to define the hormonal interactions between two organs. Although these experiments have just begin in the past 3 years, many investigations have already been carried out. Thus the gonads of mollusks, insects, crustaceans, and ascidians have been cultured, as well as tissues from *Limulus*, the parapodia of annelids, and the regenerating buds of planarians.

Usually the methods have been based on those that have proved useful among the vertebrates. An agar base is used, prepared with a physiological saline solution appropriate to the animal. A nutrient liquid is incorporated into this base. These nutrients may be composed of separate chemical compounds, or a natural fluid such as an extract of chick embryos, which is often very active.

These methods have already provided important results in the field of autodifferentiation of isolated organs. They have opened up numerous promising avenues of research into the role of the endocrine organs in many groups of invertebrates.

II. CONCLUSIONS

Organ culture is one of the best methods of studying embryonic differentiation, and the conditions under which it occurs. The capacity of the rudiments for autodifferentiation and the role of inductors and endocrine secretions may be demonstrated under simple, precise conditions which cannot usually be achieved with other experimental methods. Many other problems may be studied with organ culture. Do explants acquire full function at the same time as they develop mature form? Do they produce their specific secretion *in vitro* as in the intact organism? Their effect on other organs can be found by putting them in direct contact with the latter.

In this way, suspected correlations may be verified and unknown interactions revealed. It is possible to check whether an endocrine gland acts directly or indirectly on a known effector organ, or whether the effect of an intermediate organ is necessary. Thus certain chains of correlations may be elucidated.

By putting explants into conditions that never occur naturally—in the presence of older organs or explants from other species—they can be given the opportunity to manifest latent or unknown properties. They may be broken down into their tissues and into their constituent cells to see whether the dissociated elements can reassociate and reorganize.

Innumerable problems may be attacked by these methods, problems such as those of the nutritional requirements for morphogenesis and for functional activity, the factors responsible for organization, and the substances stimulating or inhibiting the proliferation of malignant tumors.

The techniques of organ culture are today applied to a large number of vertebrate and invertebrate types, and constitute a very general method of research. It must, however, be remembered that they have their limitations, and at the present state of technical progress, one should not ask of them more than they can give—a development limited in time and space. Only cultures of malignant tumors have shown an unlimited capacity for growth. This difference between normal and cancerous tissues alone constitutes a very important result.

An explant of normal organized tissue probably cannot multiply indefinitely, but the aim is to allow explants to develop for a longer period and to a larger size. At present, there is a wide gap between the size attained by an organ in culture, and that attained in the intact organism. Such a result cannot be obtained unless the techniques of transfusion and irrigation used in adult organs can be adapted to very young organs. This would be a very valuable advance, from which a rich harvest of results could be expected. In the absence of such means, explantation *in vivo*, though inconvenient, is a useful method complementary to culture *in vitro*. It must be stressed that in cases where it is necessary to follow the differentiation of an organ it is useful to culture an explant first *in vitro* and then *in vivo*. In this way an undifferentiated or an incompletely differentiated rudiment can be allowed to develop its potential *in vitro*, and differentiate unaffected by external influences, reacting only to an organ or substance deliberately administered. The determination of an organ, whether spontaneous or provoked, is generally complete in the first few days or hours of culture. The explant can then be regrafted without inconvenience into an organism that will be its source of circulation, that is, which will provide better nutritional conditions. The prolonged development of an explant allows a better understanding and control of the determinants acquired during its period of culture. In this way, by alternation between culture *in vitro* and culture *in vivo*, we can now obtain the development of an organ or a part of an organ whose destiny was oriented *in vitro* in the course of the first phases of its embryonic life.

BIBLIOGRAPHY

1. Barth L. G.   Neural differentiation without organizer. *J. exp. Zool.*, 1941, **87**, 371–384.
2. Bermann F.   Étude manométrique du métabolisme respiratoire d'une culture d'organe embryonnaire. Peau d'embryon de Poulet cultivée sur milieu gélifié. *Arch. Sc. Physiol.*, 1964, **18**, 89–113.
3. Born G.   Ueber Verwachsungsversuche mit Amphibien Larven. *Roux' Arch. f. Entwickl.*, 1897, **4**, 517–623.
4. Carrel A. and Burrows M. T.   Culture de tissus adultes en dehors de l'organisme. *C. R. Soc. Biol.*, 1910, **69**, 293–294.
5. Carrel A. and Lindberg C.   The culture of organs. *Ham. Hamilton Medic. Books*, Londres, 1938, 221 p.
6. Fauré-Fremiet E.   Le mécanisme de la formation des complexes à partir de cellules d'éponges dissociées. *C. R. Soc. Biol.*, 1925, **93**, 618.

7. Fell H. B. and Mellanby E.   Metaplasia produced in cultures of chick ectoderm by high vitamin A. *J. Physiol.*, 1953, **119**, 470–488.

8. Holtfreter J.   Ueber die Aufzucht isolierter Teile des Amphibienkeimes. I: Methode einer Gewebezüchtung *in vivo*. *Roux' Arch. f. Entwickl.*, 1929, **117**, 421–510.

9. Holtfreter J.   Ueber die Aufzucht isolierter Teile des Amphibienkeimes. II: Züchtung von Keimen und Keimteilen in Salzlösung. *Roux' Arch. f. Entwickl.*, 1931, **124**, 404–466.

10. Holtfreter J.   Neural differentiation of ectoderm through exposure to saline solution. *J. exp. Zool.*, 1944, **95**, 307–340.

11. Holtfreter J.   Neuralization and epidermization of gastrula ectoderm. *J. exp. Zool.*, 1945, **98**, 162–209.

12. Jolly J.   Sur la durée de la vie et de la multiplication des cellules animales en dehors de l'organisme. *C. R. Soc. Biol.*, 1903, **55**, 1266–1268.

13. Jolly J. and Lieure C.   Sur la culture des œufs de Mammifères. *C. R. Soc. Biol.*, 1936, **122**, 723–726.

14. Jolly J. and Lieure C.   Recherches sur la culture des œufs de Mammifères. *Arch. Anat. micr. Morph. exp.*, 1938, **34**, 307–373.

15. Maximow A.   Tissue cultures of young mammalian embryos. *Contribs. Embryol. Carneg. Inst. Wash.*, 1925, **16**, 49–113.

16. Peeters G. and Massart L.   La perfusion de la glande mammaire isolée. *Arch. int. Pharmacod. Thér.*, 1947, **74**, 83–89.

17. Salzgeber B.   Évolution des gonades embryonnaires de Poulet greffées dans un embryon-hôte après culture *in vitro*. *C. R. Soc. Biol.*, 1958, **52**, 764–765.

18. Sengel Ph.   Recherches expérimentales sur la différenciation des germes plumaires et du pigment de la peau de l'embryon de Poulet en culture *in vitro*. *Ann. Sc. Nat. Zool.*, 1958, **20**, 431–514.

19. Spratt N. T.   Nutritional requirements of the early chick embryo. I: The utilization of carbohydrate substrates. *J. exp. Zool.*, 1949, **110**, 273–298.

20. Stenger-Haffen K.   Étude des besoins nutritifs des gonades embryonnaires d'Oiseau cultivées en milieux synthétiques. *Arch. Anat. micr. Morph. exp.*, 1957, **46**, 521–607.

21. Strangeways T. S. P. and Fell H. B.   Experimental studies on the differentiation of embryonic tissues growing *in vivo* and *in vitro*. I: The development of the undifferentiated limb bud. *Proc. Roy. Soc.*, B, 1926, **99**, 340–364.

22. Strangeways T. S. P. and Fell H. B.   Experimental studies on the differentiation of embryonic tissues growing *in vivo* and *in vitro*. II: The development of the isolated early eye of the fowl when cultivated *in vitro*. *Proc. Roy. Soc.*, B, 1927, **100**, 273–283.

23. Thomas J. A.   Nouveaux procédés de perfusion physiologique et aseptique, permettant la survie prolongée d'organes ou d'organismes pesant plusieurs kilogrammes. *J. Physiol.*, 1948, **40**, 123–146.

24. Thompson D., Elin C. E. and Cantab D. P.   Some further researches on the cultivation of tissues *in vitro*. *Proc. Roy. Soc. Med.*, 1914, **7**, 21–46.

25. Townes Ph. L. and Holtfreter J.   Directed movements and selective adhesion of embryonic amphibian cells. *J. exp. Zool.*, 1955, **128**, 53–120.

26. Vulpian M. A.   Note sur les phénomènes de développement qui se manifestent dans la queue de très jeunes embryons de Grenouille, après qu'on l'a séparée du corps par une section transversale. *C. R. Acad. Sc.*, 1859, **48**, 807–811.

27. Wilson H. V.   On some phenomena of coalescence and regeneration in sponges. *J. exp. Zool.*, 1907, **5**, 245–258.

28. Wolff Em.   La différenciation sexuelle de la syrinx de l'embryon de Canard explantée *in vitro* sur milieux chimiquement définis. *Bull. biol. Fr. Belg.*, 1957, **91**, 271–283.

29. Wolff Em. Analyse des besoins nutritifs d'organes embryonnaires, la syrinx d'Oiseau cultivée en milieu synthétique. *Arch. Anat. micr. Morph. exp.*, 1957, **46**, 407–468.
30. Wolff Et. and Haffen K. Sur la culture *in vitro* des glandes génitales des embryons d'Oiseau: obtention de la différenciation sexuelle et de l'intersexualité expérimentale des gonades explantées. *C. R. Acad. Sc.*, 1951, **233**, 439–441.
31. Wolff Et. and Haffen K. Sur une méthode de culture d'organes embryonnaires *in vitro*. *Texas Rep. Biol. Med.*, 1952, **10**, 463–472.
32. Wolff Et. and Haffen K. Sur la féminisation induite par les gonades mâles inter-sexuées chez l'embryon de Poulet. *Arch. Anat. Hist. Embryol.*, 1961, **44** suppl., 273–302.
33. Wolff Et., Haffen K., Kieny M. and Wolff Em. Essais de culture *in vitro* d'organes embryonnaires en milieux synthétiques. *J. Embryol. exp. Morph.*, 1953, **1**, 55–84.

CHAPTER II

DIFFERENTIATION
OF ORGANS IN NATURAL MEDIA

Georges Le Douarin

INSTITUT D'EMBRYOLOGIE ET DE TÉRATOLOGIE EXPÉRIMENTALE DU C.N.R.S.
PARIS, FRANCE

In vitro culture of embryonic rudiments can be carried out on various kinds of media, either natural or synthetic. The simplest natural media are composed purely of blood plasma, whereas the simplest synthetic media have a clearly defined chemical composition. In practice, the organic liquids used in the natural media are often diluted in physiological saline, Tyrode's solution, for example.

Most of the natural media that are used for the culture of embryonic organs contain embryo extract. Thus, the classical technique described by Strangeways and Fell (1926, 1927) and later refined by Fell and Robinson (1929) consists of cultivating explanted organs in a watchglass on a coagulum composed of equal parts of adult plasma and chick embryo extract diluted with saline solution. Gaillard (1951) and Martinovitch (1953) used modifications of this method. Occasionally this technique is inconvenient since the explant becomes progressively surrounded by a covering of migratory cells. Some tissues progressively liquefy the clot and asphyxiate in the resulting fluid. Chen (1954) tried to overcome these difficulties and perfected a method of culture in a liquid medium that was derived from Trowell's technique (1954). In this procedure the explants are placed on a piece of paper floating on a medium composed of dilute embryo extract and fowl serum.

The inclusion of nutrient materials in a nonnutritive substrate was advocated by Et. Wolff and Haffen (1952), who perfected a method of organ culture that is especially favorable for the growth and differentiation of embryonic rudiments. This method eliminates all parasitic cell culture from the explant, which thus preserves its organization. The dry explant is placed on the surface of the gelled medium. The proportions of nutrient materials incorporated in the medium can be varied without changing its physical properties. The composition of Wolff and Haffen's "standard" medium is given below as an example:

Agar-agar, containing 1 g of agar per 100 ml of Gey's solution   6 parts
7-Day chick embryo extract, diluted 50% with Tyrode's solution   3 parts
Tyrode's solution   3 parts
Penicillin retard (100–200 units Oxford)   1 drop

Other organic fluids from adult animals (for example, fowl plasma, horse or ox serum) can be added, or substituted for the Tyrode's solution or embryo extract, according to the needs of the explanted organ.

Among the many problems that can be explored by the techniques of explantation, that of the differentiation of embryonic rudiments has benefited considerably from culture *in vitro* on natural media. These methods not only allow the survival and cellular proliferation of isolated embryonic organs, but also in many cases, the young explanted embryonic rudiment differentiates in culture in a way more or less similar to its development *in vivo*.

The object of this review is to indicate the main results that have been obtained regarding the differentiation of vertebrate embryonic organs on natural media.* The first part will be devoted to a description of the differentiation of certain rudiments during culture *in vitro*. The problems raised by the results and the effect of modifying the culture method (variations in the medium, or physical factors) will be discussed in the second part.

I. EXAMPLES OF DIFFERENTIATION IN EMBRYONIC ORGANS

Saline solutions are the most frequent constituents of natural media. Where the cells contain nutritional reserves, as in the Amphibia, these natural media may even alone allow the survival and development of rudiments. Vulpian (1859) and Born (1897) observed that various isolated fragments of frog embryo continued to grow and differentiate for a limited time. Holtfreter (1931) showed that the different regions of the *Triton* gastrula retain their potentialities for differentiation and regulation in an isotonic solution with embryonic cells. Jolly and Lieure (1941) observed differentiation of the blood vessels in a caudal bud isolated from a tadpole. However, the continued differentiation of rudiments isolated from the organism requires the presence of nutrient materials. The natural media have been used mainly for the culture of rudiments taken from avian and mammalian embryos.

Thomson (1914) first demonstrated the *in vitro* survival and differentiation of embryonic rudiments from the chick, and referred to the growth of organs isolated from the rest of the organism as "somatic growth." Organs that grow and differentiate apart from their normal connections were termed "artificial organisms" by Fischer (1922). The term organ culture was introduced by Maximow (1925) and is used to describe those experiments in

---

* Differentiation of the sex organs will be studied in another chapter.

explantation that tend to conserve *in vitro* the organic integrity of the rudiment.

The principles of organ culture have now been defined and the techniques of explantation *in vitro* have been used by many workers in the field of experimental embryology. There is now such a great volume of results that it would be difficult to mention them all and impossible to discuss them here. Even though attention is limited to the mammals and birds, obviously the differentiation of many embryonic rudiments has been studied. The technique of organ culture is generally useful and the results obtained have solved many problems in embryology and have raised many more new and important ones.

A. Skeletal Rudiments

The rudiments of the limb skeleton were shown by Strangeways and Fell (1926) to differentiate *in vitro*. The limb bud of a chick embryo of 72–80 hours' incubation consists of a mesenchymal blastema with an ectodermal covering. On a medium consisting of fowl plasma and chick embryo extract, the limb bud formed cartilaginous elements of the limb bones in 2 days. These elements always remained purely cartilaginous, and ossification never occurred. However, 3-day old limb buds could be cultured for 28 days (Fell, 1928).

When explantation was carried out at a later stage, on the sixth day of incubation, for instance, the limb bones differentiated distinctly. Thus the tarsus and metatarsus formed in the hind foot (Momigliano Levi, 1930). Moreover, ossification commenced and progressed (Gliozzi, 1958).

After a certain stage of development it was possible to remove individual limb bones from the cartilaginous rudiment (Fell, 1928; Fell and Robinson, 1929; and others). Cartilaginous rudiments explanted after 8 days of incubation grew considerably in culture with trebling of the initial length. Morphogenesis was partially completed and the epiphyses formed and grew. Histological differentiation reached the stage where the cartilage hypertrophied, and a cuff of periosteal bone was formed in the diaphysis. There was never any formation of a bony medulla and endochondral ossification did not occur.

Similar results have been obtained with mammalian embryos by Gaillard (1951) and Niven (1931). Zaaijer (1953) explanted the cartilaginous rudiments of the metacarpus, metatarsus, and phalanges from 6–8 week human fetuses. Differentiation occurred *in vitro* during the 28 days of culture. The epiphyses grew and the cartilage cells hypertrophied in the center of the diaphysis.

While investigating the nutritional requirements of the tibia of the chick embryo Et. Wolff and Kieny (1956) and Kieny (1958) measured the amount

of growth and differentiation which occurred when rudiments explanted on
the 8th day of incubation were cultivated *in vitro* for 7 days using Wolff and
Haffen's method. At the time of explantation the tibial rudiment consisted
of a cartilaginous rod with slightly swollen ends. In the first stage of culture
the tibias flattened their surface and became translucent and shining. The
outline became regular, the small injuries that had occurred during explantation were healed, and the explant became enclosed by a thin membrane.
This "epithelialization," noted by Gaillard (1949) and Wilde (1950), is a
general characteristic of explants in organ culture (Et. Wolff, 1952) and is
essential for survival of the culture. In the days following explantation, the

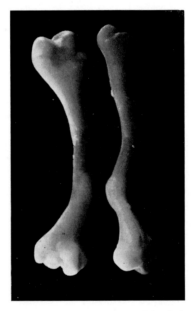

FIG. 1.   Tibias from 7-day chick embryos, cultured for 7 days on Wolff and Haffen's
standard medium (Kieny, 1958).

diaphysis elongated and the epiphyses became swollen and developed facets
(Fig. 1). Although the tibia was isolated from the rest of the organism and
in particular from neighboring bones, some morphological structures did
differentiate normally. Among these were the two condyles, the groove for
the digital extensor muscles, and the cnemial crest. Often the elongation of
the tibia caused an abnormal bend to appear in the diaphysis. This was due
to the fact that the epiphyses were fixed in the culture medium and could not
move over its surface. The bend in the diaphysis, although abnormal, was a
good indication that the rudiment had grown.

Kieny studied the increases in length, weight, and total nitrogen content. The rate of growth in length was greatest in the first 2 days of culture and then decreased progressively, becoming almost zero by the 8th day. The mean length of the rudiments was 4.45 mm at explantation and had reached 7 mm after 7 days of culture. The linear growth was less than that obtained using Fell and Robinson's medium, but on the standard medium of Wolff and Haffen there was no swarming out of the cells and the explants maintained their organic integrity, which made possible an assessment of weight increase and nitrogen retention. After 7 days of culture the mean weight of the tibia had increased from 1.5 to 2.7 mg, mainly as a result of protein synthesis. The amount of nitrogen contained in the explants increased from 55 to 91% in 7 days. At the time of explantation, the three zones of cartilage, composed of round, flattened, and hypertrophied cells, were already present. During culture the normal processes of cartilage development continued. After 7 days the zone of hypertrophied chondroblasts extended over more than half the length of the tibia. Hypertrophy of the cartilaginous cells also occurred, but to a lesser extent in the region of the epiphyses. In the diaphysis, the zone of hypertrophied cartilage was covered with a periosteal sheath of varying thickness and containing osteoblasts. There was never more than a slight periosteal ossification during culture in the standard medium, and endochondral ossification was never seen.

The method of *in vitro* culture has made possible the study of the autonomous differentiation of many skeletal rudiments.

The patella of a 9-day chick embryo developed cartilage after 3 days of culture and progressively acquired the normal triangular shape, but ossification did not occur during 20 days of culture *in vitro* (Niven, 1933). Explantation of the palatus quadratus and Meckel's cartilage from 5–6 day chick embryos (Fell and Robinson, 1930; Fell, 1931) showed that at this stage of development only the former was capable of bone formation *in vitro*. Jacobson and Fell (1941) explanted the mandibular rudiment from its presumptive tissues between the 3rd and 7th days of incubation. The results of this experiment showed that after the 4th day of incubation the presumptive region of the mandible was already determined and was independent of the rudiment of Meckel's cartilage. However, the latter played an important part in organogenesis, distending the branchial arches and thus giving the mandible its elongated form.

Fell (1939) investigated the processes governing organogenesis in the sternum of the chick embryo. In birds, the sternum is not derived from the ribs or the coracoid bone, but independently from two rudiments in the body wall, situated ventrally on either side of the midline. When these two rudiments were explanted *in vitro* in a normal position in relation to one another, they joined up and fused. After this had occurred morphological differentiation of the sternum proceeded almost normally. The keel developed, and also the posterolateral processes giving the body of the sternum its characteristic curvature. However, this curvature deformed progressively *in vitro*. Fell showed that union and fusion of the two sternal rudiments occurred as a result of an active migration of median mesenchymal cells. In fact, if the two rudiments were oriented so that their external surfaces were against the surface of the medium, they did not fuse but moved apart from one another. Chen (1952, 1953) showed that the sternal rudiment in the mouse fetus behaved in the same way. The segmentation of the sternum in mammals depends on the influence of the ribs; they inhibit the hypertrophy of the cartilage where they touch the sternum. In the absence of the ribs, the sternal rudiment shows cartilaginous hypertrophy throughout its length. This inhibitor effect is specific and is not induced by bony rudiments other than the ribs.

B. Skin and Its Derivatives

1. SKIN AND APPENDAGES

The first attempt to culture embryonic skin from birds was unsuccessful, with no major growth of the explanted feather germs (Kapel, 1929; Champy, 1933; Rossi and Borghese, 1935). Fell and Robinson's watch glass culture technique was used by several workers to study the development of skin fragments explanted at a relatively late stage of development (Gropp and Hilwig, 1954). Miszurski (1937) showed that 6-day chick embryo skin keratinized normally *in vitro*. Fell and Mellanby (1953) and Lipori (1953) obtained differentiation of feather germs in a fragment of undifferentiated skin from a 6-day embryo.

Moreover, Lipori showed that the dorsal region of the 6-day duck embryo developed pigment in a constant manner when it was cultured on Wolff and Haffen's standard medium. No pigment was present at explantation. In contrast, when the skin was explanted after 5 days of incubation, pigment formation was not constant. Lipori suggested that skin taken after 5 days of incubation did not always contain sufficient melanoblasts for the pigment to become visible. It is known that bird melanoblasts migrate from the neural crest and then multiply in the skin between 6 and $6\frac{1}{2}$ days of incubation (the migration of melanoblasts has been studied *in vitro* by Dorris, 1936, 1938). Skin from the neck of chick embryos from a pigmented stock always produces pigment when explanted at 6 days, but when explanted at 5 days the pigment production is not constant. On the other hand, Dorris (1938) and Hamilton (1940) showed that skin taken from White Leghorn chick embryos could produce pigment in culture.

The problem of the differentiation of feather germs and pigment in the skin of chick embryos cultured *in vitro* has been studied by Sengel (1956, 1957, 1958). Fragments of skin (about 2 × 1.5 mm) from 5–8½ day chick embryos were taken from some part of the dorsal midline between the base of the wings and the tail. The explants grew easily on Wolff and Haffen's standard medium, without being transplanted or washed. When skin was explanted on the 8th day of incubation epidermal keratinization began after about 6 days of culture and the cornified layer began to thicken.

During the first 24 hours of culture the skin explants retracted, but mainly in the dermis rather than the epidermis. Subsequent development of the two tissues was then different. The epidermis continued to retract until the end of the 3rd day of culture (Fig. 2). The dermis, on the other hand spread out and regained its initial size on about the 5th day of culture.

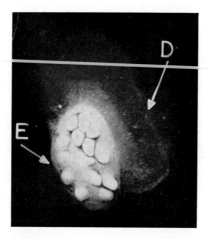

FIG. 2.   Explants of stage 1 skin after 3 days of culture on Wolff and Haffen's standard medium (Sengel, 1958). D, dermis; E, epidermis.

Sengel obtained differentiation of the feather germs on Wolff and Haffen's standard medium, when the explants were taken from embryos of at least 6½ days of incubation, that is, when the stage of skin differentiation is reached. Between 6½ and 7 days (stage 1 in the differentiation of the skin as defined by Sengel) the dorsal skin showed 0–3 rows of feather rudiments on either side of the median line (Fig. 12b). These rudiments consisted of mesenchymal condensations in the dermis, whilst the epidermis was still flat, or showed only small swellings. Explants taken at stage 1 resorbed their feather rudiments during the 1st day of culture and the piece of skin again became homogeneous. During the following days, new feather rudiments appeared, but their distribution was not as before. The first row differentiated along the median line of the explant and not along the mediodorsal edge. The other rows were arranged on either side of the median line (Fig. 3). After 3 days of culture the feather germs had begun to grow and developed normally. After 5 days the longest feather germs were 0.3 mm long. Sengel stressed the structural alteration that had occurred in stage 1 explants *in vitro*.

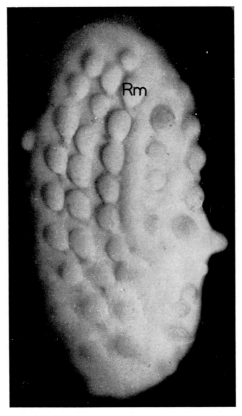

FIG. 3.   Piece of skin explanted at stage 1 (Sengel, 1958). After the reconstruction of the dermal elements, the median row (Rm) of feather germs is the best developed.

Half of the dorsal skin, either the right or the left side in relation to the midline, would reform into a symmetrical whole. The explant then developed a new bilaterally symmetrical structure.

Sengel observed that skin from White Leghorn embryos, explanted after 6–8 days of incubation and containing no differentiated melanocytes, sometimes produced pigment on the standard medium. This agreed with the observations of other workers. The melanocytes seen under these conditions were scanty and were found at the base of the feather germs. When explants were taken from embryos of the Black Alsace strain pigment always appeared after culture. In a fragment of skin explanted at the undifferentiated stage (stage 0), that is, after less than $6\frac{1}{2}$ days of incubation, the epidermis contained star-shaped melanocytes. Differentiation of the melanocytes was thus independent of the feather germs. When the skin was explanted after $6\frac{1}{2}$ days

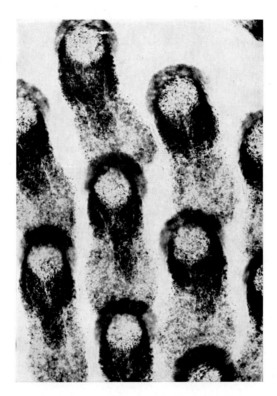

Fig. 4.   Feather germs in a piece of skin from the Black Alsace strain, after 5 days of culture on Wolff and Haffen's standard medium (Sengel, 1958).

of incubation, it continued to differentiate and produce pigment *in vitro*. The melanocytes that differentiated at the base of the feather germs were carried up by the growth of the feather germs (Fig. 4).

Less work has been carried out on the organogenesis of mammalian skin *in vitro*. Hardy (1949, 1951) and Davidson and Hardy (1952) explanted pieces of undifferentiated skin from 12-day embryo mice. These pieces differentiated in culture. The hair follicles appeared, distributed in a normal way, and they produced hairs that sometimes emerged from the skin. The pigment cells also differentiated and melanin granules were deposited in the growing hairs exactly as they would be under normal conditions.

2. TEETH

Glasstone (1938, 1952) studied the *in vitro* differentiation of the tooth germs of embryonic rats and rabbits. The tooth rudiment of the 18–20 day rat fetus consists of a papilla covered by the enamel organ. Explanted at this stage, it gave rise to odontoblasts which produced dentine. The molar tooth germs of 10-day rat and 20-day rabbit fetuses had not yet formed crests, but these formed *in vitro*. The inner enamel epithelium became invaginated into the papilla. Calcification of these rudiments also occurred in culture.

3. UROPYGIAL GLAND OF THE DUCK

The uropygial gland of the duck is the only cutaneous gland found in birds. Its development in culture *in vitro* has been studied by Gomot (1956, 1959, 1961). He cultured the dorsocaudal skin of duck embryos on Wolff and Haffen's medium and defined stages of differentiation parallel to those given by Sengel for chicken skin. Explants taken before the 8th day of incubation retracted markedly on the culture medium. They formed the rudiments of several tail feathers but the uropygial invaginations did not appear. Explants of the dorsocaudal skin of 8–10 day embryos formed feather germs and uropygial invaginations of varying depth. In explants from $10\frac{1}{2}$-day embryos the invaginations present before explantation deepened and closed. Uropygial glands from 12–18 day embryos underwent *in vitro* differentiation in fairly normal fashion.

C. Respiratory Organs

Loffredo-Sampaolo and Sampaolo (1956, 1957) and Dameron (1962) studied the *in vitro* development of chick embryo lung rudiments.

Using Wolff and Haffen's standard medium, Dameron explanted the lung rudiment from a 5-day chick embryo. At this stage, the lung consists of a small mesenchymal sac, at the center of which is an epithelial tube (Fig. 5) with 1–3 rounded fingerlike outgrowths. In the first phase of culture, the explant became flattened on the medium and the mesenchyme became transparent. After 48 hours, a few fingerlike outgrowths appeared on the epithelial tube. The mesenchyme condensed around the epithelium, especially at the proliferating areas. After culture for 5 days the mesenchyme had thinned considerably and the epithelium had grown markedly. The original dilatations had become true sacs and new fingerlike outgrowths had appeared (Fig. 6).

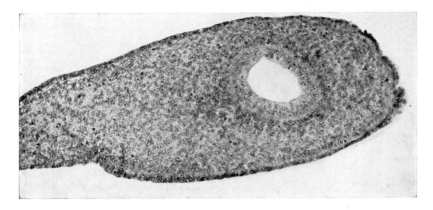

FIG. 5.   Section of 5-day chick embryo lung (Dameron, 1952).

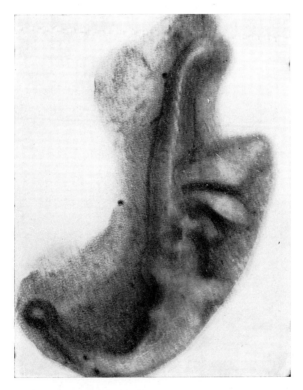

FIG. 6.   Five-day chick embryo lung cultured for 5 days (Dameron, 1962). Carmine hydrochloride preparation.

In the region of the mesobronchus the epithelial cells were tall and cylindrical; they were more flattened in the recently formed invaginations. The embryonic lung continued to develop in culture for 5 days. Dameron also noted that the best results were obtained when the explant contained abundant mesenchyme.

Many workers have studied the differentiation of mammalian embryonic lung *in vitro*. Chen (1954) showed that when the lung rudiment of the rat was explanted at the stage when the primary bronchi showed 2–3 buds, considerable differentiation occurred in the culture. The bronchi ramified in a complex manner and histological examination showed the presence of bronchi, bronchioles, and terminal buds. Similar results were obtained by Sorokin (1961) and by Sampaolo and Loffredo-Sampaolo (1958, 1959). Advanced differentiation of pulmonary structure could be seen using *in vitro* culture.

Alescio (1960) paid special attention to three aspects of pulmonary differentiation. These were the factors governing the branching of the bronchial tree, the formation of the interlobar fissures, and the histological differentiation. He worked with mouse embryos and used the hanging drop and watch glass techniques. The lung rudiments were explanted at the 12th day of pregnancy, at a stage when the primary bronchi had started to divide into lobar bronchi. Under culture conditions the primary bronchi gave rise to secondary bronchi. The latter grew and underwent dichotomous branching. This branching could continue until fourth-order bronchi had been formed. The interlobar fissures which were not apparent at the time of explantation appeared in culture, indicating that their formation was not due to any extrinsic mechanical effect. During the first 6 days of culture histological differentiation occurred as *in vivo*. The epithelium over the bronchial outgrowths formed characteristic folds over a mesenchymal stroma, the epithelium became progressively flattened in the smaller bronchi, and cartilaginous rings appeared in the trachea. These rings were neither as regular nor so numerous as they would have been *in vivo*. During the 5th and 6th days of culture the bronchioles, consisting of a single layer of epithelial cells, showed irregular cavities. The terminal parts of the bronchial tube had an appearance similar to that seen *in vivo*.

D. Glandular Organs

1. SALIVARY GLANDS

Relatively few experiments have been carried out on the differentiation of salivary glands *in vitro*. Zymbal (1932) showed that human fetal parotid gland in culture produced abundant peripheral cellular proliferation. At the same time, the center of the explant ceased differentiation and became necrotic. However, Borghese (1950) cultured fetal mouse salivary gland using Fell and Robinson's technique, and observed considerable differentiation of the rudiments. He studied the submandibular and sublingual glands of 13–16 day fetuses. On the 13th day of gestation the submandibular gland consists of the main duct with a terminal bud, while the sublingual gland is scarcely visible. Explants taken at this stage produced a variable number of acini and some intermediate ducts. Better results were obtained when the submandibular gland already showed 4–10 buds at the time of explantation. The epithelial ducts subdivided by successive dichotomous divisions. After a few days culture, a mucous secretion was seen in the submandibular gland. The mesenchymal cells became concentrically arranged around the acini and groups of acini.

At the points where two concentric systems met, there was a thickening that represented the rudiment of a septum. Borghese also noted that the submaxillary and sublingual glands developed better if they were explanted together rather than separately in their connective tissue capsule. Grobstein (1953) also observed normal differentiation of the mouse submandibular gland in culture during his study of the influence of the mesenchyme on the differentiation of the rudiment.

2. MAMMARY GLANDS

Balinsky (1949) noted some differentiation of the mammary glands during culture *in vitro*. Hardy (1950) obtained a more marked development when he cultured the ventral body wall of mouse embryos for 25 days on Fell and Robinson's medium. The mammary ducts formed *in vitro* and branched in an almost normal fashion. The rate of growth of the rudiments was slow in the initial stage of culture, but increased when the ducts started to produce outgrowths.

3. ENDOCRINE GLANDS

Certain embryonic endocrine glands differentiate during culture *in vitro*. Thyroid rudiments from 8-day chick embryos formed follicles when they were cultured using Fell and Robinson's technique (Carpenter, 1942). Tixier-Vidal (1955) observed only partial autodifferentiation of the thyroid gland when it was explanted alone, and also showed that the differentiation regressed after 3 days of culture. Dieterlen (1960) studied the degree of differentiation obtained in explants of varying age. On Wolff and Haffen's standard medium, the thyroid of a 6-day chick embryo proved difficult to culture; however, a 7-day explant survived and produced colloid. After 24 hours of culture, small intracellular droplets were observed. These became larger and more numerous, but after 5 days of culture the characteristic follicular structure had not developed. When the thyroid was explanted after 8 days of incubation, the intracellular droplets of colloid formed rapidly, and after 4–5 days of culture the explants showed characteristic thyroid follicles filled with colloid.

Chen (1954) explanted the thyroid of 20-day rat fetuses. At this stage the gland does not contain follicles in the central area. They differentiated in culture and retained their structural integrity for at least 13 days.

The pituitary of the 6-day chick embryo developed almost normally in culture (Moscona and Moscona, 1952). Cords and lobules of cells developed and after 6 days characteristic acidophile and basophile cells could be seen. The infundibulum divided into several diverticula and glial cells differentiated in it.

In 1954 Chen perfected a method of culture using a liquid medium, and observed the development of several embryonic organs under these conditions. He obtained advanced differentiation of the adrenal cortex of a 15-day rat fetus. At explantation the rat adrenal gland was composed mainly of the cortical rudiment. Underneath the fibrous capsule there was a thin layer of small cells and a central area consisting of a network of epithelial cell cords. Occasional rare chromaffin cells had begun to penetrate the gland. After 6 days of culture, the adrenal cortex had differentiated into the zona glomerulosa and the zona fasciculata, the central area of which degenerated as it would have done *in vivo*. The medulla did not differentiate, probably because the rudiment did not yet contain enough chromaffin cells.

Vidmar (1953) showed that the 4–12 day chick embryo pineal gland also differentiated in culture. Epithelial buds were formed from the original invagination in the roof of the diencephalon and these became organized and developed normally. Moszkowska (1958) cultured the pineal glands of 12–16 day chick embryos on Wolff and Haffen's standard medium. The explants differentiated, the number of epithelial cells increased, and their cytoplasm condensed. The follicles shrank progressively. After 4 days of culture many epithelial cells, ependymocytes, and hypodymocytes contained melanin granules.

4. PANCREAS

The two regions of chick embryo pancreas, that is, the acini and the islets of Langerhans, can differentiate to a certain degree in organ culture. The first experiments were carried out by Black and Comolli (1954), using Wolff and Haffen's method. Explants of pancreatic rudiments from 6-day or older chick embryos continued to differentiate. The number of acini increased and one type of islets appeared. When the rudiment was explanted from 11–14 day embryos, the number of islets increased during culture. Dieterlen-Lièvre

(1960) cultured embryonic pancreas and liver together and was able to show that only the splenic lobe of the pancreas secreted glucagon (hypoglycemic factor). Recently Drukker (1964), using Wolff and Haffen's method, cultured 6–19 day chick embryo pancreas. The 6–7 day rudiments were cultured *in toto*, the older explants being small pieces taken from the splenic and duodenal poles. Explants from the splenic lobe of 10-day embryos produced two types of structure, resembling islets, after culture for 2 days. These two types of islet differed in their cell constituents. The islets disappeared progressively when culture was continued for more than 7 days.

Chen (1954) studied the differentiation of the dorsal and ventral pancreatic rudiments explanted from 13-day rat embryos. At this stage the pancreas is composed essentially of an anastomosing network of tubules, limited by a single layer of cells. The explant remained transparent for the first 3 days of culture. Then the fragments became progressively opaque, initially at the periphery and later in the center. This opacity was due to an increase in the number of zymogen granules in the acinar cells. The islets differentiated but the α and β cells could not be distinguished. The culture could be prolonged for at least 10 days with the explants remaining healthy, the number of islets increasing and mitotic figures being visible. Golosow and Grobstein (1962) also showed differentiation of the mouse pancreas *in vitro*.

E. Kidneys

Ever since the first experiments using organ culture as defined by Wolff and Haffen, Wolff and his school have been able to obtain the survival and development of chick embryo mesonephros *in vitro* (Et. Wolff, 1952). In fact, this organ adapted very well to parabiosis *in vitro* and has been used widely in the new applications of organ culture that are described by Madame Wolff in this volume.

Calame (1961) used Wolff and Haffen's method to study the differentiation of chick embryo metanephros in organ culture. The culture medium was an enriched standard medium with foal serum replacing Tyrode's solution. The rudiment of the metanephros was taken from $5\frac{1}{2}$-day chick embryos. It consisted of a thin sheet of mesenchyme and the ureter, which extended for about one third of the length of the sheet. During the first 6 days of culture development of the rudiment could be followed by direct observation. During the 1st day the mesenchyme became flattened on the medium, and the ureter, visible because of its transparency, showed progressive growth, reaching the end of the mesenchymal sheet by the 2nd day. At this time it possessed small buds, localized in two distinct zones. These basal and distal zones were separated by a smooth segment. From the 3rd day, the ureteric buds formed primary branches with a distribution similar to that seen *in ovo*. Figure 7 is a diagrammatic representation of this development. The secondary and tertiary ramifications of the primary branches could be followed later (Fig. 8). In this way, the metanephric rudiment assumed the appearance of a bunch of grapes, the ends of the terminal branches being covered by a thick layer

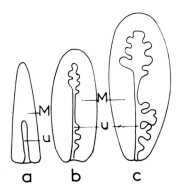

FIG. 7. Various stages of culture in the metanephros (Calame, 1961). a, At explantation; b, at the beginning of the second day of culture; c, during the third day of culture. M, metanephric mesenchyme; u, ureter.

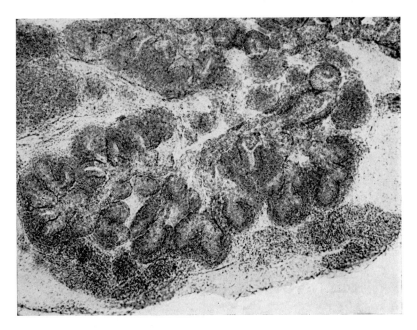

FIG. 8. Branching in the metanephros after 7 days of culture (Calame, 1961). Carmine hydrochloride preparation.

of mesenchyme. This latter differentiated into the excretory tubules. Calame observed that after the 12th day of culture differentiation did not progress further and only a few well-differentiated glomeruli were formed (Fig. 9).

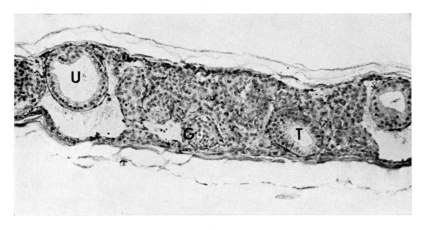

FIG. 9.   Histological section of the metanephros after 6 days of culture (Calame, 1961). G, glomerulus; T, excretory tubule; U, ureter.

F. Alimentary Canal and Liver

Many workers have cultured the intestine of the chick embryo. Pieces of intestine have been explanted at relatively late stages of development; after the 9th day (Monesi, 1960), on the 10th day (Dameron, 1961), or on the 12th (Kirrmann, 1962). In a general way, the intestine continued to differentiate *in vitro* (Fig. 10). The villi grew and attained their definitive form. An analogous result was obtained by Chlopin (1922) on rabbit embryos.

Monesi (1960) also studied the differentiation of the enterochromaffin cells *in vitro*. These cells appeared in culture when the explant was taken from 12–13 day embryos, but did not appear in explants from younger embryos. If the intestine already contained some chromaffin cells at the time of explantation, the number of cells increased noticeably in the culture.

Sigot (1961) cultivated the proventriculus of 5-day chick embryos on different natural media. At this stage the epithelial glands had not yet formed. Better differentiation was obtained if the culture medium was enriched with an extract of 12-day chick embryos from which the digestive tracts had already been removed.

Considerable movement was seen in explants of 7–9 day chick embryo liver, explanted for organ culture on Wolff and Haffen's standard medium (Wolff and Marin, 1957). The first observable phenomenon seen after the culture commenced was a rounding off of the explant. A rounded form

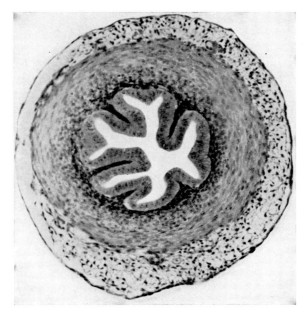

Fig. 10.   Intestine of a 12-day chick embryo, cultured for 6 days on Wolff and Haffen's standard medium (Kirrmann, 1962).

developed regardless of the initial shape. These modifications were not due to a simple retraction of the mass of hepatic cells. Carmine markers placed on the explant showed that currents were produced in the cell mass and that these persisted for some time after the mass had attained a regular shape. When several pieces were placed in contact with one another they fused intimately. Moreover, two separate explants would meet as a result of their own intrinsic movement, and would then fuse even if they had already formed their protective membranes. Moreover, liver explants could surround and engulf inert objects placed in contact with them on the culture medium. Their movements recalled ameboid movement and phagocytosis.

Borghese (1956) cultured liver from 12-day mouse embryos. Differentiation of the epithelial elements continued *in vitro*, but the hemopoietic tissue underwent considerable degeneration.

Chen (1954) used his technique for culture in a fluid medium to study the development of the different components of the liver of 13–15 day rat embryos. In this phase the liver is dark red, with the sinusoids filled with hemopoietic cells. The hepatic lobules have not yet reached their definitive position. During culture the blood cells left the explant and became dispersed in the medium. Thus the explant became paler. After 6 days of culture, the sinusoids contained a much smaller number of hemopoietic cells than they did at the time of explantation. The Kupffer cells were visible throughout the length of the sinusoids. The hepatic lobules became more regular. After 8 days some of the epithelial cells contained glycogen granules and the lumina of the bile ducts were visible. Chen continued to culture the explants for 15 days without observing any significant degeneration. However, the sinusoidal spaces and the bile ducts were abnormally dilated.

G. Sense Organs

1. EYE

The ocular rudiment of the chick embryo has been cultured *in vitro* on media composed of plasma and embryo extract (Strangeways and Fell, 1926; Dorris, 1938; Harrison, 1951, 1954). Differentiation of pigment in the external layer of the retina and the acquisition of sensory structures could be seen under these conditions. Meanwhile, the morphology of the rudiment was greatly altered.

Survival and organ development of the explanted eye rudiment was obtained using Wolff and Haffen's standard technique (Et. Wolff, 1952). This method was used by Reinbold (1954) in his study of the *in vitro* differentiation of the ocular rudiment of 3-day chick embryo. At this stage, the eye consists of the optic cup, the external layer of which contains no pigment, and the lens. During the first 5 days of culture the rudiment grew progressively. The lens remained transparent and the external layer of the retina became pigmented (Fig. 11). Reinbold noted that the pigmentation occurred mainly in the part of the explant that was exposed to air, whilst there was little pigmentation in the part in contact with the medium. When culture was prolonged for more than 5 days, the explant ceased to grow but anatomical and histological differentiation continued. A halo appeared on the circular border of the retina in front of the lens, corresponding to the iris rudiment. The sensory layer of the retina of an eye from a 3-day embryo was composed of regularly arranged rectangular cells whose long axes were arranged radially. After about 10 days of culture, marked histological differentiation could be seen. The sensory layer contained numerous cells which became arranged into a zone with external nuclei, a zone with internal nuclei, and a zone of ganglion cells. The edge of the retina nearest the pupil became thin, and the internal layer became progressively reduced to a single layer of cells that constituted the rudiment of the iris. The sclerotic did not differentiate during culture *in vitro*.

2. OTOCYST

Like the optic rudiment, the otocyst showed histological but not morphological differentiation *in vitro* when Fell and Robinson's method was used.

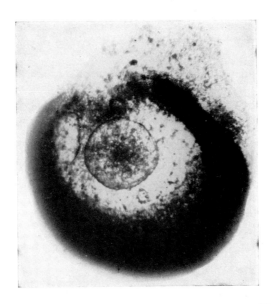

FIG. 11. Development of the optic rudiment in organ culture on Wolff and Haffen's standard medium (Et. Wolff, 1954).

Fell (1928) explanted the otocyst from 3-day chick embryos. The rudiment consisted of an oval sac limited by an undifferentiated epithelium with a small appendage that was the rudiment of the endolymphatic canal. From the 5th day of culture the explant contained sensory cells. After 8 days all of the sensory cells of the labyrinth had differentiated. It was possible to distinguish elongated cells with long cilia, characteristic of the macula acoustica, and the cells of Corti with short cilia and covered by a membrane showing the characteristics of the membrane of Corti. A few supporting cells were also present. After 14 days of culture the histological structure of the explants was very similar to that of the auditory organ of an embryo of 17 days' incubation. Meanwhile, though histogenesis had proceeded normally, organogenesis did not occur *in vitro*.

II. ANALYSIS OF THE CHARACTERISTICS OF DIFFERENTIATION *IN VITRO*

The above examples of differentiation of organs *in vitro* show that some embryonic rudiments can continue to differentiate even when isolated from the remainder of the organism. This implies that explantation occurred after the stage of determination of the rudiment and that the rudiment contained all the constituents necessary for organogenesis to proceed.

The degree of differentiation reached by the explant depends on a complex of factors, some of which depend on the nature of the rudiment while others are related to the conditions of culture.

A. The Characteristics of Autodifferentiation *in Vitro*

1. Influence of the Stage of Development Reached by the Rudiment at the Time of Explantation

The results of experiments using explantation *in vitro* are greatly influenced by the stage of development reached by the organ at the time of explantation.

In most cases it has been found that to obtain the advanced differentiation of an organ *in vitro* it is necessary to explant the rudiment only after a certain stage of development has been reached. It has often been observed that a much more advanced stage of development is reached when the embryonic rudiment is explanted at a later stage. Thus, an undifferentiated limb bud could produce cartilaginous rudiments in culture but ossification would not occur. In contrast, cartilaginous rudiments taken at a later stage could develop much further when they were isolated. Cartilaginous hypertrophy and periosteal ossification could take place.

Kieny (1958) showed that the size of the tibia at the time of explantation had a marked effect on the linear growth that subsequently occurred *in vitro*. Rudiments measuring 3.5–5 mm showed the best growth in culture. Longer tibias showed less growth, since the zone of cartilaginous hypertrophy was already well established at the time of explantation. Fewer cells were available for hypertrophy, and elongation was reduced. A tibia measuring less than 3.5 mm showed little growth during culture on Wolff and Haffen's standard medium. It is probable that this medium cannot provide all of the nutrients necessary for the maturation and differentiation of the cells of these young rudiments.

The behavior of the skin of chick embryos was also a good example of the effect of the age of the explant on the type of differentiation that occurred in culture (Sengel, 1958). Three stages in the differentiation of the skin have been defined (Fig. 12). The undifferentiated stage (stage 0) corresponds to an incubation time of $5\frac{3}{4}$–$6\frac{1}{2}$ days. It is characterized by a flat epidermis and an optically homogeneous dermis. The mediodorsal crest is still invisible. At the feather rudiment stage (stage 1, $6\frac{1}{2}$–7 days of incubation), the dermis shows three rows of feather rudiments on either side of the dorsal midline, but the epidermis remains smooth or shows only small lumps. Finally, the feather germ stage (stage 2, 7–$8\frac{1}{2}$ days of incubation) corresponds to already differentiated skin.

When cultured *in vitro* on Wolff and Haffen's medium, the behavior of the explant varied according to the age of the donor embryo. Stage 0 explants did not develop feather germs. The gross contraction of the epidermis prevented any morphogenesis from occurring. Stage 1 explants differentiated feather germs but only after a structural reorganization that involved regression of the original feather rudiments. Stage 2 explants did not undergo this remodeling of the dermis. The rudiments gradually changed into feather germs, thus retaining their initial arrangement.

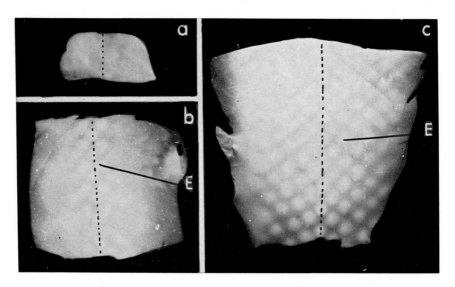

FIG. 12. Stages in the differentiation of the skin (Sengel, 1958). a, Undifferentiated stage—stage 0; b, feather rudiment stage—stage 1; c, feather germ stage—stage 2. The dotted line corresponds to the mediodorsal line of the embryo. E, feather rudiments.

Many more examples of the effect of the age of the explant on differentiation could be cited. In some cases, the explants showed no differentiation in culture when they were taken before a specific stage of development. Thus, chick somatic mesoderm from a pre-27 somite embryo could not produce cartilage when cultured on Wolff and Haffen's standard medium (Strudel, 1963).

2. THE AUTONOMOUS DEVELOPMENT OF RUDIMENTS

When an embryonic organ is explanted *in vitro* and differentiates under these conditions it expresses its histogenetic and morphogenetic potential in the absence of any influence from the remainder of the organism. Vascular connections, extrinsic innervation, and hormonal influences are all eliminated.

Even the mechanical factors that may intervene during development are eliminated by culture *in vitro*. The explanted organ is dependent only on the culture medium used and on the immediate experimental conditions. The complete suppression of certain hormones in the culture medium is obtained by the exclusion of all fluids derived from a mature individual. This is true of Wolff and Haffen's standard medium which contains an extract of 7-day chick embryo as the only nutrient.

Under these conditions the autodifferentiation of certain endocrine glands, that is, the thyroid gland shows that, after the action of the inductors during the early stages of development, morphogenesis and hormone production are not dependent on any other endocrine gland or specific stimulant.

Although the extrinsic innervation can have no effect during culture *in vitro* this is not true of the intrinsic innervation. Keuning (1944, 1948) showed that nerve cells appeared, developed neurofibrils, and anastomosed in a network in the wall of explants from the embryonic digestive tract. These explants included the esophagus, stomach, and trachea of young embryos, and were cultured by a continuous perfusion technique. Peristaltic activity of intestine cultured *in vitro* has been observed by several workers (Bisceglie, 1932; Gozzi, 1940; Dameron, 1961; Kirrmann, 1962) and the intrinsic innervation of the intestine was thought to play a part in this movement. According to De Jong and De Haan (1943), when the intestine of a 4–5 day chick embryo was explanted the contractions appeared only after the intrinsic nervous system had differentiated.

Analysis of the effect of mechanical factors using *in vitro* culture has been limited mainly to the study of the skeletal rudiments. Since the earliest explantation experiments with bone rudiments, it has been seen that the morphogenesis of each piece of skeleton is, in the main, independent of extrinsic factors. The long bone rudiments develop normally in culture and other pieces of the skeleton behave similarly, for example, the patella (Niven, 1933) or the sternum (Fell, 1939; Chen, 1952, 1953). The tibia of the 8-day chick embryo shows a morphogenesis very close to normal (Kieny, 1958).

Meanwhile, *in vitro* skeletal morphogenesis may differ from the normal for different mechanical reasons—either because of suppression of mechanical effects that occur *in vivo*, or owing to new conditions imposed by the culture. The curvature that occurs during the elongation of tibias cultured by Wolff and Haffen's method gives an example of the effect of culture conditions on morphogenesis. The elongation of the mandible under the influence of Meckel's cartilage (Jacobson and Fell, 1941) and the segmentation of mammalian sternum under the influence of the ribs (Chen, 1953) are examples of normal morphogenetic processes that may be suppressed by explantation *in vitro*.

4

Culture *in vitro* has often shown that the development of certain anatomical structures is not due to extrinsic factors as generally accepted. Thus, the first stages of formation of the pulmonary interlobar fissures occur *in vitro* despite the absence of any vascularization (Alescio, 1960).

In some cases of culture *in vitro*, certain anatomical and histological differentiations occur as in normal organogenesis, but then regress when culture is prolonged. When a 4-day chick embryo limb bud was explanted at the phase of mesenchymal condensation and cultured for 17 days using Fell and Robinson's method, it was observed that the cartilaginous rudiments of the femur, tibia, and fibula appeared in the first stage of the culture process (Fell and Canti, 1934). These rudiments became very obvious and there was an intermediate space that corresponded to the knee joint. However, after 6 days of culture the articular cartilage had disappeared, the cartilaginous rods had fused, and no articular region was formed. Fell and Canti thought that the regression of the joint was due to the absence of muscular activity *in vitro*.

Finally, some embryonic organs survive well *in vitro* and achieve advanced histological differentiation without true organogenesis. This was observed in the case of the otocyst and the eye when they were cultured using Fell and Robinson's method. In the same way, chick embryo heart when cultured *in vitro* showed continued differentiation of the muscle fibers. These lengthened and the myofibrils developed almost complete striations (Loffredo-Sampaolo and Sampaolo, 1956). Le Douarin (1963) cultured 3-day chick embryo heart using Wolff and Haffen's method. The sinoatrial, ventricular, and bulbotruncal chambers are recognizable at this stage. In the region of the ventricle and the bulb, the epimyocardium and the endocardium are separated by a syncitial layer, the cardiac jelly (Fig. 13a). Structural modifications *in vitro* caused a rapid disappearance of the cardiac jelly, and it became difficult to distinguish the endocardium. Around the central cavity the explant was composed of a fairly compact tissue consisting of anastomosing threads, which tended to subdivide the cavity during the first few days of culture and then to obliterate it almost completely. The explant acquired a progressively more spongy appearance, with the threads surrounding small lacunae (Fig. 13b). The heart remained pulsatile for several days. Transmembrane action potentials characteristic of the different anatomical regions could be recorded during the first 4 days of culture (Le Douarin *et al.*, 1964). Physiological differentiation of the different regions of the heart is retained when the whole organ is explanted, while organogenesis does not occur owing to the absence of blood flow.

Other aspects of embryonic development can also be studied *in vitro;* for instance, the regression of temporary organs such as the Mullerian ducts in the male duck, the phenomenon of the regulation of deficiencies, the histogenetic potentialities of the embryonic rudiments of some mutants, and so on.

The capacity for regulating rudimentary organs in culture is generally limited, determination being irreversible at the time of explantation. Cicatrization of wounds incurred during dissection of the rudiment is usually complete and rapid, and does not interfere with final organogenesis. Long

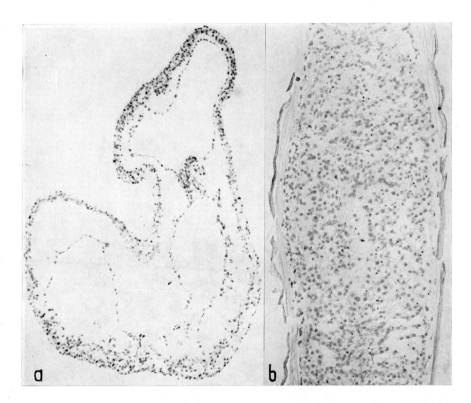

Fig. 13.   Development of chick embryo heart in organ culture on Wolff and Haffen's standard medium (Le Douarin, 1963). a, Three-day embryo heart at the time of explantation; b, heart cultured for 4 days.

bones transplanted at a relatively late stage of development can show partial healing of fractures with the formation of a callus of connective tissue (Weil, 1951; Bucher, 1952). Kieny (1958) showed that in the tibia of 8-day chick embryos a considerable injury could affect the development. If the cartilaginous rudiment was deprived of the articular area of the epiphysis, cicatrization occurred in the region of the cut, but the corresponding morphological differentiations did not take place. Glasstone (1952) studied an unusual case of regulation in the culture of an organ. The first (or second) temporary molar of the rabbit embryo was taken on the 20th day of gestation and was divided into halves which were cultured separately. Each of the halves produced complete morphological development of the crests, although the latter were smaller than when the teeth were cultured intact.

Many recent experiments have been devoted to the analysis of the morphogenetic capacity of the rudiments from mutants, using the methods of organ culture. Thus, Gluecksohn-Waelsch and Rota (1963) have cultured the kidneys of embryonic mice of the mutant strain Sd (short tail). The explants did not differentiate as well as those from normal embryos. In particular, the branching of the ureter was irregular and the branches remained short. Kieny and Abbott (1961, 1962) studied the grown *in vitro* of the tibiotarsus and fibula of the diplopode chick embryo and they compared it with the growth of the same rudiments from normal and creeper embryos. The cartilaginous rudiments were taken after $6\frac{1}{2}$–7 days of incubation and were cultured for 7–8 days using Wolff and Haffen's standard medium and an enriched medium containing chicken plasma. On the standard medium the fibula of the diplopode embryo grew 3 times as long as the tibiotarsus and sometimes formed a distal epiphysis. The tibiotarsus of both creeper and normal embryos grew more rapidly than the fibula. On the enriched medium the growth of the fibula was increased in both mutant and in normal individuals. Kieny and Abbott concluded that in the diplopode embryo the great length of the fibula in relation to the tibiotarsus is due to an accelerated growth of the primary rudiment and not to a simple reduction of the tibia. By contrast, in the creeper embryo it is the slowing down of growth of the tibiotarsus that leads to the relative increase in the length of the fibula.

3. THE RATE OF DIFFERENTIATION DURING CULTURE *in Vitro*

In general, the development of embryonic organs occurs more slowly *in vitro* than under normal conditions. Moreover, growth resulting from cell division must be distinguished from histological differentiation. The former is more often the slower, while the latter may continue at a normal rate in some organs.

In some cases differentiation is accelerated during culture *in vitro*. This was observed by Zaaijer (1953) in the culture of bone rudiments from 6-week human fetus, by Maximov (1925) in the intestine of the rabbit embryo, and by Miszurski (1937) in chick embryo skin.

The physiological activity of organs explanted *in vitro* develops in a variable fashion, according to the organ. Chick embryo thyroid can accumulate iodine in culture at the same rate as it does *in vivo* (Gaillard, 1953; Carpenter et al., 1954). Using a chromatographic method, Gonzales (1954) studied the substances present in the 7-day chick embryo thyroid, when it was cultured in the presence of [131]I. After 1 day of culture monoiodothyronine and inorganic iodine were recovered and after 2 days of culture, diiodothyronine and thyroxine. Up to this stage the thyroid behaves *in vitro* as it does *in ovo*. Physiological and functional differentiation is sometimes faster *in vitro* than it is under normal conditions. In the same way, fragments of 4-day chick embryo liver formed glycogen in increasing quantities between 24 hours and 3 days after the beginning of culture (Dieterlien, 1960). However, chick embryo liver did not contain glycogen after 6 days of incubation. The synthesis of glycogen has thus been accelerated by the conditions encountered during organ culture on Wolff and Haffen's standard medium.

4. Limitations of Differentiation and Survival *in Vitro*

Embryonic organs can be cultured *in vitro* for times varying from several days to many weeks according to conditions. After a certain length of time, an embryonic rudiment explanted *in vitro* will reach a level of differentiation beyond which it cannot progress in culture. Usually the explant can continue to survive *in vitro* after this stage.

Exhaustion of the nutrients in the medium can be avoided by transplanting the tissues onto a fresh medium at regular intervals. Fell and Robinson's method of culture usually requires transplantation every 48 hours when the growth is rapid as in the case of the long bones, or after several days when the growth is slow. Et. Wolff and Haffen (1952) recommended that explants cultured by their method should be washed every 2 days. The explants are washed *in situ* in gently flowing tepid Tyrode's solution, and are then moved and fixed at another point on the surface of the medium. Five to seven day cultures must be transplanted onto fresh medium. Transplantation and washing of the explants ensures good nutritional conditions and removes metabolites and any cell cultures that may surround the organ.

Few experiments have been devoted to the investigation of the intrinsic factors that limit the differentiation and survival of explants in organ culture. Some studies have shown that explants have a diminished ability to utilize atmospheric oxygen (Berman, 1964). The oxygen consumption of explants in relation to their nitrogen retention falls progressively during culture. This decrease in respiration has been demonstrated using chick embryo intestine cultured for 2 days on Wolff and Haffen's medium (Kirrmann and Le Douarin, 1963). The explants showed no signs of degeneration, exhibited peristaltic contraction, and continued to differentiate. The decrease in oxygen consumption was not halted by transferring the organ to a fresh medium (Berman, 1964).

B. Influence of Variations in the Composition of the Culture Medium and of Certain Organic Extracts

Growth and differentiation of embryonic rudiments *in vitro* is strongly influenced by the culture conditions, such as the concentration of saline solutions, pH of the medium, and atmospheric composition. The composition of the culture medium is particularly important.

The influence of these different factors has already been discussed in a previous volume in this series (Et. Wolff, 1956). Some aspects of this problem will be discussed here.

The first question to be answered is whether normal differentiation *in vitro* does or does not depend on the presence of embryonic substances in the culture medium. Most of the culture media used do contain embryo extracts, but the culture medium does not necessarily contain organic material from the same species as the explant. In some cases survival and differentiation of organs is better on a homologous medium (Gaillard, 1950) but as a general rule chick embryo extract can be used as the sole source of nutrient materials for the culture of organs from many species.

Sobel and Moscona (1954) demonstrated that chick embryo rudiments showed the capacity for autodifferentiation when cultured on medium containing only organic material from adult individuals. Fell and Robinson's method was used but the medium was composed of 2 parts of fowl plasma to 1 part adult fowl heart extract. A 4-day chick embryo limb bud was cultured on this medium for 5 days and the same results were obtained as with a medium containing embryo extract.

Under the same conditions the rudiment of the anterior pituitary from a 6-day chick embryo was cultured for 8 days. The cell cords, surrounded by connective tissue, differentiated and contained many acidophile and basophile cells. Differentiation was identical to that seen when the culture medium contained embryo extract. Thus, these embryonic rudiments are capable of developing *in vitro* in the absence of embryonic material in the culture medium.

Wolff and Haffen's method for organ culture has been used by several workers to study the influence of the composition of the medium on the growth and differentiation of several embryonic organs such as the syrinx, tibia, and skin.

Em. Wolff (1957) investigated whether chick embryo extract was the most favorable nutrient for the *in vitro* differentiation of the chick and duck syrinx. Toward the 6th day of incubation the chick embryo syrinx shows a slight enlargement of the junction between the trachea and the bronchi. Subsequently, 4 pairs of cartilaginous arches developed on either side of the midline. In contrast to the chicken syrinx, that of the duck shows sexual dimorphism at a very early stage (10 days of incubation) when the sex hormones begin to circulate in the embryo. The male type is asymmetric and differs markedly from the female type, which is symmetrical and has small cartilaginous arches. The syrinx was taken between $6\frac{1}{2}$ and $8\frac{1}{2}$ days of incubation and was cultured on various natural media as follows: standard medium of Wolff and Haffen, a medium based on a mixture of embryo extract and serum, a medium based on blood serum alone, and a medium based on embryonic extract and serum ultrafiltrate.

The embryonic syrinx did not develop equally well on all of these media. The extract of 7–9 day embryos was not adequate for the development of chick syrinx, nor for that of male duck syrinx, which is the usual form on a hormone-lacking medium (neutral form). The addition of serum improved the nutrient medium (Fig. 14), and in fact the syrinx could grow and differentiate on a medium that contained only blood serum with no embryo extract added. These results, like those of Sobel and Moscona, demonstrate that the cells can multiply in the absence of embryo extract. The "trephones" postulated by Carrel were thus not indispensable. Em. Wolff proved further that the ultrafiltrate did not contain the favorable factors found in horse or bovine serum.

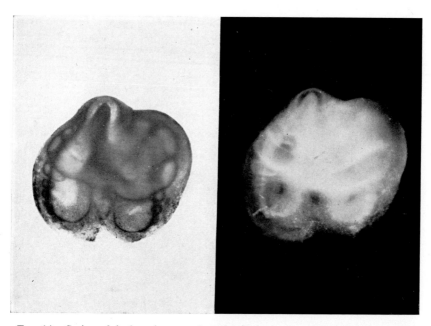

FIG. 14. Syrinx of duck embryo, explanted at 8 days on a medium based on embryo extract and adult horse serum, cultured for 12 days (Em. Wolff, 1957). Male type. *Left :* seen by reflected light; *right :* seen by transmitted light.

Wolff and Kieny (1956) and Kieny (1958) cultured chick embryo tibia on different media. The age of the embryos from which the extracts were prepared had an effect on the growth rate of the explanted tibia. The nutrient value of extracts prepared from embryos younger than 7 days and older than 16 days was less that that of extracts from embryos between these ages. When the embryo extract was replaced by an organic fluid from an adult (such as horse serum or fowl plasma), survival of the tibia was not as good. However, morphogenesis began earlier than on the standard medium and the epiphyses showed more precise modeling. According to Kieny, culture of embryonic tibia *in vitro* is divided into two stages. Cartilaginous maturation (5–6 day tibias) requires both embryo extract and fowl plasma, whilst during true growth embryo extract alone can supply all the necessary nutrients.

Sengel (1958) carried out a similar experiment to check differentiation in chick embryo skin. Fowl plasma alone produced a more advanced differentiation of the feather germs than did embryo extract.

It was also possible to analyze the inductor influence of embryo extracts *in vitro*. The differentiation of cartilage and feather germs was studied in this context by Strudel, by Benoit, and by Sengel.

Strudel (1959, 1962, 1963) showed that the time at which differentiation of chick embryo vertebral cartilage from somite mesenchyme took place in culture depended on two main factors. In the first place, the stage of differentiation that had been reached by the donor embryo was critical. On Wolff and Haffen's standard medium, the mesenchyme would only differentiate into cartilage if the donor embryo had already developed at least 27 pairs of somites. Chondrogenesis also depended on both the composition of the nutrient medium and the method of culture. Thus, cartilaginous differentiation could be obtained at the 17-somite stage when the explant was cultured on a medium containing undiluted embryo extract ("enriched medium") and when it was surrounded by a fragment of vitelline membrane (Et. Wolff, 1960). Lash *et al.* (1957) have shown autodifferentiation of cartilage in somites taken from the 18–20 somite stage. Strudel (1959, 1962) showed that by adding extracts of neural tube and notochord from 3–5 day chick embryos to the medium, differentiation of cartilage from mesenchyme could be induced at a much earlier stage. Thus, on the standard medium, chondrogenesis was obtained from the 17-somite stage. On the enriched medium with vitelline membrane, chondrogenesis was obtained at the 8-somite stage. Consequently, the extract of notochord and neural tube induced cartilage formation in explants incapable of forming it by autodifferentiation. Thus, this extract contained a diffusible inductor material.

Benoit (1960) obtained similar results on the differentiation of the cartilaginous otic capsule in the chicken. Otic mesenchyme taken from 5-day chick embryos never developed typical cartilage when cultured on the standard medium. The precartilage stage was difficult to obtain. By adding extracts of embryonic chick otocyst to the medium it was, however, possible to obtain differentiation of cartilage from the otic mesenchyme. Here again, the induction of cartilaginous differentiation is due to the effect of a diffusible substance. The differentiation of skin *in vitro* can also be influenced by diffusible materials. Sengel (1962) showed that an aqueous extract of chick embryo or adult fowl brain modified the development of skin *in vitro* when it was taken at an undifferentiated stage. No feather germs were developed on the standard medium. If brain extract was added to the medium, the skin developed feather rudiments that progressively differentiated. This action was not entirely specific. In fact, extract of 16-day chick embryo heart also induced the formation of numerous feather germs in explants of undifferentiated skin. However, in this case, the feather germs remained short and round.

C. Influence of Physical Factors

1. TEMPERATURE

Carpenter (1945) subjected 8-day chick embryo thyroid to cold conditions (5°–10°C). When the explants were treated in this way for the first 24 hours of culture and were then warmed up to 38°C, they were able to differentiate at the same rate—or even faster—as control cultures. Longer periods at 5°–10°C affected the survival of the explants. When the explants were subjected to cold conditions after several days of culture their sensitivity to cold increased, according to the degree of differentiation reached at the time of treatment.

Dameron (1960, 1961) studied the effect of various temperatures on the growth of the tibia and on the organization of the intestine in chick embryos. A temperature of 4°C completely stopped growth and differentiation of the tibia in the culture. If the cold treatment was continued for less than 10 days, the increase in length would resume when the culture was returned to normal conditions (38.5°C). Slightly higher temperatures had a less marked effect. Thus, at 10°C the tibia could grow slightly for 2 days. A temporary period (2–5 days) at temperatures between 10°C and 16°C was favorable for growth. When the tibias were returned to 38.5°C, they grew larger than control tibias. The behavior of 10-day embryonic intestine was different. This organ survived and retained its structure when exposed to a temperature of 4°C for 5 days. Temperatures of 30°, 35°, and 40°C were unfavorable to the explants, which lost their normal structure. Dameron concluded that a temperature of 38.5°C was most favorable for the survival, growth, and differentiation of organs cultured *in vitro*, but that periods at other temperatures gave varying results, according to the organs that were used.

2. The Nature of the Substrate

The different methods of culture *in vitro* vary in the nutrient content of the medium and the amount of support that they give to the explant. Some methods that allow differentiation of organ rudiments induce migration of cells from the explant. Wolff and Haffen's method, which is especially favorable for the culture of embryonic organs, is characterized by the relative poverty of the nutrient material in the medium, and by the physical state of the medium. Thus in the latter case the explant is placed on the surface of a gel.

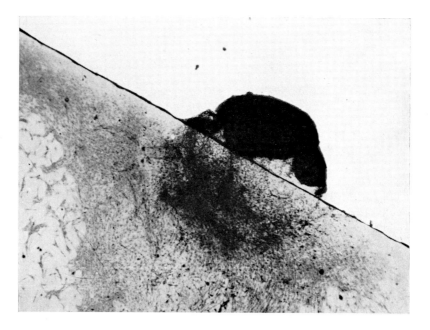

Fig. 15. Development of a piece of embryonic liver cultured in contact with a glass coverslip on Wolff and Haffen's standard medium (Et. Wolff, 1962).

Et. Wolff and Marin (1960) tried to determine whether the physical nature of the substrate plays an important part in the conservation of the organized structure of the explant. Pieces of 6–8 day chick embryo liver were grown on the standard medium. Various small plates and thin lamellae (such as gelatine or glass mica) were placed in contact with the explants. From the day following their establishment in culture the liver fragments placed in contact with glass became spread out, and on the following days gave rise to many migratory cells, especially on the lower surface of the glass (Fig. 15).

The whole explant spread out progressively toward the glass coverslip, and surrounded it with a thin mass with diffuse margins. In this way tissue culture was induced under the conditions of organ culture. The degree of spreading varied with the lamella that was used. Similar results were obtained with other embryonic organs. Thus, under the same nutritional conditions, explants may develop on tissue culture or on organ culture, depending on the surfaces with which they are in contact.

Et. Wolff (1960) has also shown that it is possible to avoid the structural modifications occurring in the first phase of culture which are sometimes a nuisance. A modification of Wolff and Haffen's method of organ culture was carried out by placing the explants not directly on the medium but wrapped in a thin acellular membrane, for example, the vitelline membrane (or chorion) of the hen's egg (Fig. 16). Thus, the vitelline membrane serves both

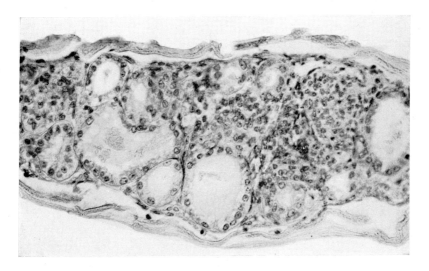

Fig. 16. Explant of 8-day chick embryo mesonephros cultured for 7 days in a sac of vitelline membrane (Et. Wolff, 1961).

as a substrate and as an exchange membrane between the explant and the culture medium. This technique is especially applicable to fragments of organs that do not possess their own limiting membrane. The vitelline membrane acts as the limiting membrane and also allows the explant to spread out into a thin layer, thus improving both nutrition and respiratory exchange. The vitelline membrane is also useful in the culture of some early embryonic rudiments, such as the lung and the metanephros. This new method has also been used to study problems which will be described elsewhere.

BIBLIOGRAPHY

1. Abbott U. K. and Kieny M.   Sur la croissance *in vitro* du tibio-tarse et du péroné de l'embryon de Poulet diplopode. *C. R. Acad. Sc.*, 1961, **252**, 1863–1865.
2. Alescio T.   La culture du poumon embryonnaire de Souris. *1er Congrès Européen d'Anatomie*, Strasbourg, 1960, 143–149.
3. Balinsky B. I.   Histological studies on the development of the mammary gland. *Trans. Roy. Soc. Edinb. B.*, 1949, **62**, 1–31.
4. Benoit J. A. A.   Induction de cartilage *in vitro* par l'extrait d'otocystes d'embryons de Poulet. *J. Embryol. exp. Morph.*, 1960, **8**, 33–38.
5. Bisceglie V.   Studi sui tessuti espiantati. II: L'attivita peristaltica degli espianti di intestino embrionale. *Arch. exp. Zellforsch.*, 1932, **12**, 86–101.
6. Black L. and Comolli R.   La différenciation *in vitro* de l'ébauche du pancréas de l'embryon de Poulet. *Arch. Anat. micr. Morph. exp.*, 1954, **43**, 276–281.
7. Borghese E.   The development *in vitro* of the submandibular and sublingual glands of *Mus musculus. J. Anat.*, 1950, **84**, 287–302.
8. Borghese E.   Lo sviluppo di organi embrionali isolati. *Atti Soc. Ital. Anat.* XVI Convegno sociale, 1955, 92 p.
9. Borghese E.   Lo sviluppo *in vitro* delle gonadi embrionali dei topi anemici w/w. *Sympos. genet.* Pavia, 1956, **5**, 84–130.
10. Borghese E.   Organ differentiation in culture. *A Symposium on Chemical Basis of Development*, W. D. McElroy and B. Glass eds., Johns Hopkins Press, 1958, 704–773.
11. Born G.   Ueber Verwachsungsversuche mit Amphibienlarven (II). *Arch. f. Entwickl.*, 1897, **4**, 517–623.
12. Bucher O.   Untersuchungen über die Regenerationsvorgänge in experimentell gesetzten Knochenbrüchen in der Kultur *in vitro*. *Acta Anat.*, 1952, **14**, 98–107.
13. Bucher O. and Weil J. Th.   L'influence d'un extrait osseux (Ossopan) sur la consolidation de fractures *in vitro*. *Experientia*, 1951, **7**, 38–40.
14. Calame S.   Le rôle des composants épithélial et mésenchymateux du métanéphros, d'après les résultats de la culture *in vitro*. *Arch. Anat. micr. Morph. exp.*, 1961, **50**, 299–308.
15. Carpenter E.   Differentiation of chick embryo thyroids in tissue culture. *J. exp. Zool.*, 1942, **89**, 407–431.
16. Carpenter E.   The effect of exposure to temperatures of 5° to 10°C on the survival and differentiation of embryonic thyroid tissue cultures. *J. exp. Zool.*, 1945, **98**, 79–86.
17. Carpenter E., Beattie J. and Chambers R. D.   The uptake of I[131] by embryonic chick thyroid glands *in vivo* and *in vitro*. *J. exp. Zool.*, 1954, **127**, 249–269.
18. Champy C.   Culture de bulbes plumaires *in vitro*. *C. R. Soc. Biol.*, 1933, **113**, 1450–1452.
19. Chen J. M.   Studies on the morphogenesis of the mouse sternum. II: Experiments on the origin of the sternum and its capacity for self-differentiation *in vitro*. *J. Anat. Lond.*, 1952, **86**, 387–401.
20. Chen J. M.   Studies on the morphogenesis of the mouse sternum. III: Experiments on the closure and segmentation of the sternal bands. *J. Anat. Lond.*, 1953, **87**, 130–149.
21. Chen J. M.   The cultivation in fluid medium of organized liver, pancreas and other tissues of foetal rats. *Exp. Cell Res.*, 1954, **7**, 518–529.

22. Chlopin N. Ueber *in vitro* Kulturen der embryonalem Gewebe der Säugetiere. *Arch. mikr. Anat.*, 1922, **96**, 435–493.

23. Dameron Fl. Influence de la température sur les organes cultivés *in vitro*. I: La croissance des tibias. *Acta Embryol. Moph. exper.*, 1960, **3**, 86–117.

24. Dameron Fl. Influence de la température sur les organes cultivés *in vitro*. III: L'organisation de l'intestin. *Arch. Anat. Hist. Embryol.*, 1961, **44**, 353–366.

25. Dameron Fl. Rôle du mésenchyme dans la différenciation de l'ébauche épithéliale du poumon embryonnaire de Poulet en culture *in vitro*. *Path. Biol.*, 1962, **10**, 811–816.

26. Davidson P. and Hardy M. H. The development of mouse vibrissae *in vivo* and *in vitro*. *J. Anat. London*, 1952, **86**, 342–356.

27. De Jong B. J. and De Haan J. Organ and tissue differentiation in perfused cultures of explants of the oesophagus-stomach-trachea complex of young chicken embryos. *Acta Neerl. Morph.*, 1943, **5**, 26–51.

28. Dieterlen-Lièvre F. Influence du pancréas embryonnaire sur la formation du glyco-gène hépatique chez le Poulet étudiée par la méthode des parabioses *in vitro*. *C. R. Acad. Sc.*, 1960, **250**, 1349–1351.

29. Dorris F. Differentiation of pigment cells in tissue cultures of chick neural crest. *Proc. Soc. exp. Biol. Med.*, 1936, **34**, 448–449.

30. Dorris F. The production of pigment *in vitro* by chick neural crest. *Roux' Arch. Entwickl.*, 1938, **138**, 323–334.

31. Dorris F. Differentiation of the chick eye *in vitro*. *J. exp. Zool.*, 1938, **78**, 385–415.

32. Drukker J. The cultivation of embryonic chick pancreas. Morphological and physiological aspects. *Acta Morph. Neerl. Scand.*, 1964, **5**, 316–328.

33. Fell H. B. Experiments on the differentiation *in vitro* of cartilage and bone. *Arch. exp. Zellforsch.*, 1928, **7**, 390–412.

34. Fell H. B. The development *in vitro* of the isolated otocyst of the embryonic fowl. *Arch. exp. Zellforsch.*, 1928, **7**, 69–81.

35. Fell H. B. Osteogenesis *in vitro*. *Arch. exp. Zellforsch.*, 1931, **11**, 245–252.

36. Fell H. B. The origin and developmental mechanics of the avian sternum. *Philos. Trans. B.*, 1939, **229**, 407–463.

37. Fell H. B. Recent advances in organ culture. *Sc. Progress*, 1953, **162**, 212–231.

38. Fell H. B. and Canti R. G. Experiments on the development *in vitro* of the avian knee-joint. *Proc. Roy. Soc.*, 1934, **116**, 316–351.

39. Fell H. B. and Mellanby E. Metaplasia produced in cultures of chick ectoderm by high vitamin A. *J. Physiol.*, 1953, **119**, 470–488.

40. Fell H. B. and Robinson R. The growth, development and phosphatase activity of embryonic avian femora and limb buds cultivated *in vitro*. *Biol. J.*, 1929, **23**, 767–785.

41. Fell H. B. and Robinson R. The development and phosphatase activity *in vivo* and *in vitro* of the mandibular skeletal tissue of the embryonic fowl. *Bioch. J.*, 1930, **24**, 1905–1921.

42. Fischer A. Cultures of organized tissues. *J. exp. Med.*, 1922, **36**, 393–397.

43. Gaillard P. J. Germinal or covering epithelium. *3ᵉ J. cyto-embryol. belgo-néerl.*, 1949, 4–9.

44. Gaillard P. J. Organ culture technique using embryologic watch glasses. *Methods in Medical Research*, 1951, **4**, 241–246.

45. Gaillard P. J. Growth and differentiation of explanted tissues. *Intern. Rev. Cytol.*, 1953, **2**, 331–401.

46. Gaillard P. J.   Bone primordia and parathyroid secretions *in vitro. Coll. Intern. C.R.N.S., Nogent/Marne*, 1961, 15–32.
47. Glasstone S.   A comparative study of the development *in vivo* and *in vitro* of rat and rabbit molars. *Proc. Roy. Soc. B.*, 1938, **126**, 315–330.
48. Glasstone S.   The development of halved tooth germs. A study in experimental embryology. *J. Anat.*, 1952, **86**, 12–15.
49. Gluecksohn-Waelsch S. and Rota T. R.   Development in organ tissue culture of kidney rudiments from mutant mouse embryos. *Developm. Biol.*, 1963, **7**, 432–444.
50. Gomot L.   Développement et activité phosphatasique alcaline de la glande uropygienne d'embryon de Canard *in vivo* et cultivée *in vitro. C. R. Soc. Biol.*, 1956, **150**, 910–913.
51. Gomot L.   Contribution à l'étude du développement embryonnaire de la glande uropygienne chez le Canard. *Arch. Anat. micr. Morph. exp.*, 1959, **48**, 63–141.
52. Gonzales F.   Evidence of the functional differentiation of the embryonic chick thyroid in tissue culture. *Tex. Rep. Biol. Med.*, 1954, **12**, 828–832.
53. Gozzi R.   Differenziazione e proprieta biologiche del tessuto muscolare liscio embrionale coltivato *in vitro. Arch. ital. Anat. Embriol.*, 1940, **43**, 229–254.
54. Grobstein C.   Analysis *in vitro* of the early organization of the rudiments of the mouse submandibular gland. *J. Morph.*, 1953, **93**, 19–43.
55. Gropp A. and Hilwig I.   Ueber die Entwicklung der Dunenfederanlage des Hühnchenembryos *in vitro. Exp. Cell Res.*, 1954, **7**, 291–302.
56. Hamilton H. L.   A study of the physiological properties of melanophores with special reference to their role in feather coloration. *Anat. Rec.*, 1940, **78**, 525–547.
57. Hardy M. H.   The development of mouse hair *in vitro* with some observations on pigmentation. *J. Anat.*, 1949, **83**, 364–384.
58. Hardy M. H.   The development *in vitro* of the mammary glands of the mouse. *J. Anat.*, 1950, **84**, 388–393.
59. Hardy M. H.   The development of pelage hairs and vibrissae from skin in tissue culture. *Ann. N. Y. Acad. Sc.*, 1951, **53**, 546–561.
60. Harrison J. R.   *In vitro* analysis of differentiation of retinal pigment in the developing chick embryo. *J. exp. Zool.*, 1951, **118**, 209–241.
61. Harrison J. R.   Growth and differentiation of the embryonic chick eye *in vitro*. I: On yolk-albumen fractions obtained with centrifugation and heat. *J. exp. Zool.*, 1954, **127**, 493–510.
62. Holtfreter H.   Ueber die Aufzucht isolierter Teile des Amphibienkeimes. II: Züchtung von Keimen in Salzlösung. *Arch. f. Entwicklungsmech.*, 1931, **124**, 404–467.
63. Jacobson W. and Fell H. B.   The developmental mechanics and potencies of the undifferentiated mesenchyme of the mandible. *Quart. J. micr. Sc.*, 1941, **82**, 563–586.
64. Jolly J. and Lieure C.   La culture du bourgeon caudal des Batraciens et la formation des vaisseaux de l'embryon. *C. R. Soc. Biol.*, 1941, **135**, 702–705.
65. Kapel O.   Einige Untersuchungen über das Verhalten des Epithels *in vitro. Arch. exp. Zellforsch.*, 1929, **8**, 35–129.
66. Kieny M.   Sur l'explantation et la croissance du tibia cartilagineux de l'embryon de Poulet en milieux de culture naturels et synthétiques. *C. R. Soc. Biol.*, 1953, **147**, 868–872.
67. Kieny M.   Contribution à l'étude des besoins nutritifs des tibias embryonnaires d'Oiseau cultivés en milieux naturels et synthétiques. *Arch. Anat. micr. Morph. exp.*, 1958, **47**, 85–169.

68. Kieny M. and Abbott U. K. Contribution à l'étude de la diplopodie liée au sexe et de l'achondroplasie Creeper chez l'embryon de Poulet: culture *in vitro* des ébauches cartilagineuses du tibia et du péroné. *Developm. Biol.*, 1962, **4**, 473–488.

69. Kirrmann J. M. Étude de quelques phénomènes de radioprotection sur un organe embryonnaire de Poulet cultivé *in vitro*. *J. Embryol. exp. Morph.*, 1962, **10**, 27–37.

70. Kirrmann J. M. and Le Douarin G. Effets d'une irradiation aux rayons X sur la consommation d'oxygène et la glycolyse en aérobiose d'organes embryonnaires de Poulet en culture organotypique. *C. R. Acad. Sc.*, 1963, **257**, 3235–3238.

71. Lash J., Holtzer H. and Holtzer S. An experimental analysis of the development of the spinal column. VI: Aspects of cartilage induction. *Exp. Cell Res.*, 1957, **13**, 292–303.

72. Le Douarin G. Étude de l'action des rayons X sur la physiologie et l'organogenèse du cœur embryonnaire chez le Poulet. *Bull. biol. Fr. Belg.*, 1963, **97**, 643–759.

73. Le Douarin G., Obrecht G. and Corabœuf E. Activité électrique transmembranaire du cœur embryonnaire de Poulet explanté en culture organotypique. *C. R. Acad. Sc.*, 1964, **258**, 3911–3914.

74. Lepori N. G. Recherches sur la différenciation *in vitro* de la peau et du pigment chez l'embryon d'Oiseaux. *Arch. Anat. micr. Morph. exp.*, 1953, **42**, 194–208.

75. Loffredo-Sampaolo C. and Sampaolo G. Culture organotipiche di polmone embrionale di pollo, alcuni aspetti istologici e histochimici. *Boll. Soc. ital. biol. sper.*, 1956, **32**, 797–801.

76. Loffredo-Sampaolo C. and Sampaolo G. Indagini sulla differenziazione in coltura organotopica della trachea di embrioni di pollo. *Boll. Soc. ital. biol. sper.*, 1957, **33**, 173–176.

77. Martinovitch P. N. A modification of the watch glass technique for the cultivation of endocrine glands of infantile rats. *Exp. Cell Res.*, 1953, **4**, 490–493.

78. Maximov A. Tissue cultures of young mammalian embryos. *Contribs. Embryol. Carneg. Inst. Wash.*, 1925, **16**, 49–113.

79. Miszurski B. Researches on keratinization of epithelium in tissue-cultures. *Arch. exp. Zellforsch.*, 1937, **20**, 122–139.

80. Monesi V. La differenziazione delle cellule enterocromaffini nell'intestino di embrione di pollo coltivato *in vitro*. *Monit. Zool. ital.*, 1960, **68**, 393–402.

81. Moscona H. and Moscona A. The development *in vitro* of the anterior lobe of the embryonic chick pituitary. *J. Anat.*, 1952, **86**, 278–286.

82. Moszkowska A. L'antagonisme épiphyso-hypophysaire. Étude *in vivo* et *in vitro* chez l'embryon de Poulet Sussex. *Ann. Endocr.*, 1958, **19**, 69–79.

83. Niven J. S. F. The repair *in vitro* of embryonic skeletal rudiments after experimental injury. *J. Pathol. Bacteriol.*, 1931, **34**, 307–324.

84. Niven J. S. F. The development *in vivo* and *in vitro* of the avian patella. *Roux' Arch. f. Entwickl.*, 1933, **128**, 480–501.

85. Reinbold R. Différenciation organotypique *in vitro* de l'œil chez l'embryon de Poulet. *C. R. Sol. Biol.*, 1954, **148**, 1493–1495.

86. Rossi F. and Borghese E. Recherches sur les cultures *in vitro* du duvet des embryons de Poulet. *C. R. Assoc. Anat.*, 1935a, **30**, 440–443.

87. Rossi F. and Borghese E. Sur le comportement des plumes embryonnaires cultivées *in vitro*. *Arch. Anat. micr. Morph. exp.*, 1935b, **31**, 459–478.

88. Sampaolo G. and Loffredo-Sampaolo C. Observations histologiques sur le poumon de fœtus de Cobaye cultivé *in vitro*. *C. R. Assoc. Anat.*, 1959, **46**, 707–714.

89. Sengel Ph. Différenciation *in vitro* des germes plumaires de l'embryon de Poulet. *C. R. Soc. Biol.*, 1956, **150**, 2057–2059.

90. Sengel Ph. Analyse expérimentale du développement *in vitro* des germes plumaires de l'embryon de Poulet. *Experientia*, 1957, **13**, 177–182.

91. Sengel Ph. Recherches expérimentales sur la différenciation des germes plumaires et du pigment de la peau de l'embryon de Poulet en culture *in vitro*. *Ann. Sc. Nat., Zool.*, 1958, **20**, 431–514.

92. Sengel Ph. La différenciation de la peau et des germes plumaires de l'embryon de Poulet en culture *in vitro*. *Ann. Biol.*, 1958, **34**, 29–52.

93. Sengel Ph. Action morphogène de divers extraits de cerveau sur la peau d'embryon de Poulet cultivée *in vitro*. *Arch. Anat. Hist. Embryol.*, 1962, *44 suppl.*, 217–239.

94. Sigot M. Sur le développement du proventricule de l'embryon de Poulet en culture sur des milieux naturels. *C. R. Soc. Biol.*, 1961, **155**, 1210–1212.

95. Sobel H. and Moscona A. Cultivation of embryonic organ rudiments on a medium derived entirely from adult tissues. *Experientia*, 1954, **10**, 502–506.

96. Sorokin S. A study of development in organ culture of mammalian lungs. *Developm. Biol.*, 1961, **3**, 60–83.

97. Strangeways T. S. P. The growth of hair *in vitro*. *Arch. exp. Zellforsch.*, 1931, **11**, 344–345.

98. Strangeways T. S. P. and Fell H. B. Experimental studies on the differentiation of embryonic tissues growing *in vivo* and *in vitro*. I: The development of the undifferentiated limb bud. *Proc. Roy. Soc. London, B*, 1926, **99**, 340–364.

99. Strangeways T. S. P. and Fell H. B. Experimental studies on the differentiation of embryonic tissues growing *in vivo* and *in vitro*. II: The development of the isolated eye of the fowl when cultivated *in vitro*. *Proc. Roy. Soc. London, B*, 1927, **100**, 273–283.

100. Strudel G. Action inductrice de l'extrait de tube nerveux et de la chorde sur la formation du cartilage vertébral. *C. R. Acad. Sc.*, 1959, **249**, 470–471.

101. Strudel G. Induction du cartillage *in vitro* par l'extrait de tube nerveux et de chorde de l'embryon de Poulet. *Developm. Biol.*, 1962, **4**, 67–86.

102. Strudel G. Autodifférenciation de cartilage à partir de mésenchyme somitique cultivé *in vitro*. *C. R. Acad. Sc.*, 1963a, **257**, 2894–2896.

103. Strudel G. Autodifférenciation et induction de cartilage à partir de mésenchyme somitique de Poulet cultivé *in vitro*. *J. Embryol. exp. Morph.*, 1963b, **11**, 399–412.

104. Szabo G. Studies on the cultivation of teeth *in vitro*. *J. Anat.*, 1954, **88**, 31–44.

105. Thomson D., Ebin C. E. and Cantab D. P. Some further researches on the cultivation of tissues *in vitro*. *Proc. Roy. Soc. Med.*, 1914, **7**, 21–46.

106. Tixier-Vidal A. Étude du développement *in vitro* de la thyroïde embryonnaire du Poulet par la méthode de culture d'organes de Wolff. *C. R. Soc. Biol.*, 1955, **149**, 1377–1380.

107. Trowel O. A. A modified technique for organ culture *in vitro*. *Exp. Cell Res.*, 1954, **6**, 246–248.

108. Vidmar B. The development *in vitro* of the embryonic pineal body of the fowl. *J. Embryol. exp. Morph.*, 1953, **1**, 417–423.

109. Vulpian M. A. Note sur les phénomènes de développement qui se manifestent dans la queue de très jeunes embryons de Grenouille après qu'on l'a séparée du corps par une section transversale. *C. R. Acad. Sc.*, 1859, **48**, 807–811.

110. Weil J. T. La consolidation de fractures *in vitro* et l'influence de l'Ossopan. *Rev. Suisse Path. Bact.*, 1951, **14**, 205–224.

111. Wilde C. E. Studies on the organogenesis *in vitro* of the urodele limb bud. *J. Morph.*, 1950, **86**, 73–103.

112. Wolff Em. Nouvelles recherches sur la culture organotypique de la syrinx d'Oiseau.

Culture sur différents milieux naturels et amélioration de ces milieux par des acides aminés. *Arch. Anat. micr. Morph. exp.*, 1957, **46**, 1–38.

113. Wolff Et.   La culture d'organes embryonnaires *in vitro*. *Rev. Scient.*, 1952, **90**, 189–198.

114. Wolff Et.   Les facteurs de la croissance et de la différenciation des organes embryonnaires en culture *in vitro*. Exposés actuels de biologie cellulaire: les facteurs de la croissance cellulaire. J. A. Thomas, éd. Masson, Paris, 1956, 157–188.

115. Wolff Et.   Les propriétés générales des organes embryonnaires en culture *in vitro*. *Acta Anat.*, 1957, **30**, 952–969.

116. Wolff Et.   Sur une nouvelle modalité de la culture organotypique. *C. R. Acad. Sc.*, 1960, **250**, 3881–3882.

117. Wolff Et.   Les principes de la culture d'organes et ses possibilités. 1er Congrès européen d'Anatomie, Strasbourg. *Anat. Anz.*, 1960–1961, suppl. 109, 82–91.

118. Wolff Et.   Utilisation de la membrane vitelline de l'œuf de Poule en culture organotypique. I: Techniques et possibilités. *Developm. Biol.*, 1961, **3**, 767–786.

119. Wolff Et. and Haffen K.   Sur une méthode de culture d'organes embryonnaires *in vitro*. *Texas Rep. Biol. Med.*, 1952, **10**, 463–472.

120. Wolff Et., Haffen K. and Dieterlen F.   Influence des états nutritionnels sur la différenciation et le fonctionnement des glandes endocrines embryonnaires. *Ann. Nutr. Alim.*, 1960, **14**, 11–29.

121. Wolff Et. and Kieny M.   Comparaison des valeurs nutritives de l'extrait embryonnaire et de liquides organiques adultes dans la culture *in vitro* de tibias cartilagineux d'embryon de Poulet. *C. R. Acad. Sc.*, 1956, **243**, 2152–2154.

122. Wolff Et. and Marin L.   Sur les mouvements des explants de foie embryonnaire cultivé *in vitro*. *C. R. Acad. Sc.*, 1957, **244**, 2745–2747.

123. Wolff Et. and Marin L.   Sur les facteurs qui déterminent la transformation d'une culture d'organes en culture de tissus. *C. R. Acad. Sc.*, 1960, **250**, 609–611.

124. Zaaijer J. J. P.   Embryonale pipbenties van de mens *in vitro*. Proefschrift, Leiden, 1953.

125. Zymbal W. E.   Ueber die Verwandlungen des Epithels der Ohrspeicheldrüse im Explantat. *Arch. exp. Zellforsch.*, 1932, **12**, 177–232.

ADDENDUM

I. EXAMPLES OF DIFFERENTIATION IN EMBRYONIC ORGANS

A. Skeletal Rudiments

Skeletal rudiments have been cultured in recent years by various methods: rotating tubes (Endo *et al.*, 1965; White, 1967a), plasma clots (Shaw and Bassett, 1967; Hall, 1967). Shaw and Bassett (1967) studied the influence of oxygen pressure on osteogenesis, and observed that the optimum pressure was 35%; collagen formation and osteogenesis were suppressed if the pO_2 was lower than 5%, while a pO_2 value above 35% led to osteoclasia and chondroclasia. Using a liquid medium and cultured tibias from 10-day chick embryos, White observed that the addition of methyl or propyl *p*-hydroxybenzoate (methyl or propyl paraben) to the medium produced an increase in dry weight when compared to rudiments cultured on standard media. A concentration of $10^{-6}M$ of these substances was sufficient to stimulate growth; the effects of the two substances were not additive and the author suggested that they might act by stabilizing the lysosomes.

Experiments carried out by Abbot and Holtzer (1966), using chick embryo vertebrae, showed particularly the metabolic differences between cells cultured in whole-organ culture and those cultured in tissue culture. When cultured in its entirety, a vertebra incorporated both ^{35}S-sulfate and ^{3}H-proline, which became homogeneously distributed in the cartilaginous matrix. These cells, therefore, actively synthesized the matrix, rather than DNA. Trypsin treatment of the cultured vertebra freed the cells from the matrix. After centrifugation and renewed culture of the sediment, the cells reconstituted a new matrix within 5 hours. After culturing for 5 days, only 3% of cells had synthesized DNA, as in the intact vertebra. If, however, the cells were cultured in a monolayer, they lost their rounded appearance, became stellate, and spread out on the substrate, and rather than synthesizing the matrix chondrin, they synthesized DNA and multiplied actively, resulting in the formation of cell aggregates. These cells required the capacity to synthesize chondroitin sulfate and, in general, stopped the synthesis of DNA. The interaction between associated chondrocytes thus appears to determine the induction and maintenance of chondroitin sulfate synthesis by these cells. The absence of any interaction between the cells leads to DNA synthesis and cell multiplication. The authors proposed the following explanation for this behavior: chondroitin sulfate is secreted by the Golgi apparatus, which is

53

well developed in the rounded chondrocytes. In a monolayer culture, the area of the plasma membrane of the cell is greatly increased and this increase may occur at the expense of the Golgi membranes, which lose their capacity to synthesize chondrin.

One method of organ culture in liquid media (Petrovic and Heusner, 1961; Heusner and Petrovic, 1964) which enables the partial pressure of oxygen to be accurately maintained, has been used for culturing skeletal rudiments (Charlier and Petrovic, 1967; Petrovic and Charlier, 1967). These authors found that cartilage of the mandibular condyle taken from rats aged 5, 10, and 15 days, showed no increase in length when cultured. The spheno-occipital synchondrosis, on the other hand, showed an independent growth potential *in vitro*.

B. Skin

Chang and Maibach (1967) examined the differentiation of skin taken from a pig fetus (10–14 cm) cultured using Trowel's technique (see Ch. II, Trowel, 1954). Medium 199 was used with the addition of varying amounts of horse serum. The organ was placed in a plasma clot containing 0.5 cc of chick plasma and 0.5 cc of embryonic extract. The proportion of horse serum found to be most favorable for differentiation (thickening and keratinization of the epidermis and formation of hair follicles in the dermis) was 20%. Higher levels of horse serum (40%) lead to encystment of the dermis within the epidermis. The latter increased in size and completely surrounded the explant and this process of epiboly was also generally observed in mammalian skin cultures (Sarkany *et al.*, 1965). Many attempts have been made to culture the skin of an adult human; Sarkany *et al.* (1965) used a method based on those of Fell and Robinson (see Ch. II, Fell and Robinson, 1929) and Chen (see Ch. II, Chen, 1954), and obtained good explant growth for 10–11 days. Increased mitotic activity occurred, organ structure was maintained, and keratinization of epidermal cells continued. Using the same material, Reaven and Cox (1965) observed the production of granules of keratohyalin and keratinization *in vitro*. The production of keratohyalin can be affected by modifying the pH of the medium, or by adding glucosamine hydrochloride (Hambrick *et al.*, 1967).

Dodson (1963) made an interesting observation on the factors determining epidermal differentiation *in vitro*. Metatarsal epidermis from a 12-day-old chick embryo did not keratinize and rapidly degenerated when cultured *in vitro*, deprived of dermis. However, when explanted onto a substrate composed of collagen gel, it did differentiate, with abundant keratinization and sometimes forming a basement membrane. This result suggests that the presence of a substrate which permits normal polarization of the basal cells is an important factor in epidermal differentiation. Vanable and Mortensen (1966) cultured the skin from *Xenopus laevis* larvae using a liquid medium and observed the differentiation of cutaneous glands after 6–7 days of culture. The glandular development depended on the degree of maturation which the organ had reached at the time of the explantation.

The epidermal growth factor (EGF) isolated by Cohen (1962) from the submaxillary gland of male mice has been shown to stimulate the growth of chick embryo epidermis in organ culture. The growth factor stimulated cell proliferation and keratinization both in explants of isolated epidermis and in complete skin.

C. Lungs

The stage of development reached by the organ at the time of the explantation greatly influences its subsequent behavior in culture. In a recent paper, Dameron (1968) reported that the pulmonary rudiment from 3- and $3\frac{1}{2}$-day-old chick embryos did not develop in culture. The bronchial epithelium became thinner and necrosis was frequent, even when several rudiments were associated to increase the size of the explant. However, a rudiment taken from a 4-day embryo did show some degree of differentiation, characterized by condensation of the mesenchyme around the bronchi. Ramification of the bronchi starts only if the lung rudiment is explanted when the embryo is at least 114 hours old. The maximum degree of development attained in culture was shown by lungs that had been taken from 7-day embryos. Culture of adult mammalian lung was carried out by Davis (1967) using a continuous gas flow system. The normal lung structure was maintained for 6–7 days, but subsequently the alveolar walls collapsed and the lung tissue became compact. The vascular endothelium degenerated after 3 days in culture.

D. Liver

Organ culture of embryonic liver has made it possible to study the development of certain enzyme activities during the course of differentiation. Unlike the liver of the mammalian fetus, that of the chick embryo is able to synthesize *o*-aminophenyl glucuronide at a very early stage of development. This ability is lost shortly before hatching (19 days) but is regained rapidly and reaches a high level after hatching. The activity of UDP-glucuronyl transferase (UDPGT) shows the same variations (Dutton, 1963; Dutton and Ko, 1966). Ko and Nemeth (1966a,b) cultured fragments of liver from 19-day chick embryos on a medium composed of Tyrode's solution and horse serum, and found that UDPGT activity increased rapidly from zero to the level reached in chick liver after hatching. If the horse serum was replaced by fetal bovine serum, the enzyme activity remained at zero. If the liver was cultured in fetal serum and then transferred to a medium containing horse serum, UDPGT activity reappeared and increased rapidly. The level of enzyme activity reached after 1–2 days of culture in horse serum was maintained if the explant was transferred to fetal bovine serum, and continued to increase if the culture had been in adult serum for at least 3 days. The liver of 11-day-old embryos possesses a level of UDPGT activity, when cultured in horse serum, equal to the level observed in the hatched chick, and this level persisted and increased when fetal bovine serum was used. This phenomenon can be explained by the fact that there is a difference between the enzyme of the young embryo and that of the hatched chick. The loss of UDPGT just before hatching could correspond to the change from the embryonic to the adult form of the enzyme.

E. Nervous System

Bunge *et al.* (1965) cultured the spinal medulla from 17- to 18-day-old rat embryos. After 23, 25, and 76 days of culture the explants were examined under the electron microscope. Nervous tissue differentiates *in vitro* in the same way as *in vivo* and the neurons showed well-developed Nissl and Golgi bodies; the axosomatic and axodendritic synapses were established in the normal way. Certain glial cells remained in a nondifferentiated state. Glycogen stores were also observed in some glial cells and in the terminal ramifications of the neurons.

Lyser (1966) used Wolff and Haffen's method (see Ch. II, Wolff and Haffen, 1952) involving the vitelline membrane (see Ch. II, Wolff, 1961) to study the differentiation of the neural tube *in vitro*. The spinal medulla was removed from chick embryos at differing stages of incubation ranging from 8 somites to 4 days. Association of the neural tube with 8-day-old embryonic mesonephros favored the differentiation of neuroblasts and the formation of histological structures in the medulla. Loffredo Sampaolo (1966) used the same culture method to study the relationships that are established *in vitro* between the chick embryonic spinal ganglia and fragments of skeletal muscle (thigh quadriceps) in culture.

F. Hematopoietic Organs

Salvatorelli (1966, 1967), and Salvatorelli and Gulinati (1967a,b) were able to maintain hematopoiesis for 2 weeks in bone marrow from 18- to 19-day chick embryos by associating it with embryonic liver on Wolff and Haffen's medium (see Ch. II, Wolff and Haffen, 1952). The action of the liver on the bone marrow appeared to be specific. Myeloid cells survived for only limited periods if the marrow cultured alone or associated with another organ such as the mesonephros. Addition to the medium of dialyzed extracts of embryonic liver acted on the bone marrow in the same way as liver explants. Extracts of yeast, mesonephros, or metanephros were incapable of maintaining erythropoiesis in culture for more than 1–2 days. The nature of the erythropoietic factor thus demonstrated is still unknown, but from the way in which the extracts were prepared, the authors deduced its molecular weight to be less than 15,000. Salvatorelli *et al.* (1968) compared hematopoiesis in culture with that normally occurring *in vivo* and found that the amounts of globin, heme, and RNA in the erythrocytes of the explants were less than that in the same cells in the peripheral blood and bone marrow of *in vivo* controls. The hemoglobin synthesized *in vitro* showed the same electrophoretic behavior as *in vivo* controls. A method of organ culture in a continuously oxygenated media has made possible the prolonged culture of spleen, entire thymus, and lymphatic ganglia. In entire culture, the spleens of young mice preserved their fundamental morphological characteristics for up to 42 hours. The megakaryocytes developed to the stage of platelet formation and retained all their ultrastructural characteristics (Petrovic *et al.*, 1964). Pinkel (1964) cultured the thymus of young (2-week-old) mice, using Trowel's method (see Ch. II, Trowel, 1954) and found that the structure of the organ was maintained *in vitro*. Certain cellular elements degenerated rapidly, but the lymphoid tissue survived for 12 weeks.

G. Amphibians

Foote and Foote (1965) developed a culture medium suitable for various organs of axolotl larvae (*Siredon mexicanum*) that was based on Wolff and Haffen's medium (see Ch. II, Wolff and Haffen, 1952). The testes, mesonephros, pancreas, brain, spleen, heart, ovaries, and liver were cultured for 21 days, and, apart from the liver, all the organs survived well. In the spleen, the number of reticulocytes was reduced but the leukocytes survived and multiplied. Heart explants continued to beat for more than 10 days *in vitro*.

Tata (1966) used a method developed by Shaffer (1963) to culture isolated tails from tadpoles of *Rana temporaria*. The culture was carried out in a petri dish, using a liquid medium composed of 150 ml of Gey's solution buffered to pH 7.6, 10 ml of chick embryo extract diluted with Gey's solution, and 10 ml of calf serum. The tails survived *in vitro* for 8 days. Regression could be induced by adding triiodothyronine to the medium. Incorporation of tritiated uridine and ^{14}C-labeled amino acids showed that the regression induced by the thyroid hormone was accompanied by an increase in RNA and protein synthesis. Actinomycin D, puromycin, and cycloheximide all inhibited the regression and the increase in hydrolase activity in tails that had been

subjected to the action of triiodothyronine. Actinomycin D and cycloheximide inhibited the incorporation of ^{3}H-uridine, and puromycin inhibited
the uptake of amino acids. It thus seems that regression of the tadpole tail,
induced by the action of hormones, is accompanied by the continuous
formation of RNA and protein.

The remodeling of connective tissue which occurs during amphibian
metamorphosis, involves degradation of both collagen fibers and the basic
interfibrillar substance. The formation of a collagenolytic enzyme by the
epithelial cells and the production of hyaluronidase by the mesenchyme has
been demonstrated by *in vitro* culture of the two individual tissue components
(Eisen and Gross, 1965).

H. *In Vitro* Differentiation of Chick Embryo Precardiac Mesoderm

The precardiac mesoderm can differentiate in culture without the necessity
of explanting the three embryonic layers that form the presumptive cardiac
region of the blastoderm.

On an agar medium according to Wolff and Haffen's method (see Ch. II,
Wolff and Haffen, 1952) the mesoderm can differentiate into spontaneously
beating myocardial tissue when it is cultured in the presence of either the
ectoderm or the endoderm, the other layer having been removed by trypsin
treatment (Le Douarin *et al.*, 1965a).

This result shows that the differentiation of the precardiac mesoderm into
myocardial tissue can take place at an early stage of development and that it is
not necessary for the mesoderm to be induced by one of the other layers from
the cardiac region. Mesoderm was also cultured alone (after trypsin treatment) on an enriched medium, derived from Wolff and Haffen's standard
medium by substituting foal serum for Tyrode's solution. Mesoderm from the
presomitic stage did differentiate into myocardial tissue (Le Douarin *et al.*,
1966a), but beating persisted for only a few days and the survival period of
the explant was also limited.

Using a technique with a liquid medium, G. Le Douarin and D. Renaud
cultured precardiac mesoderm from chick embryos and obtained the *in vitro*
differentiation of myocardial tissue that survived for a prolonged period. The
medium used was that of Rinaldini (1959), with the following composition:
70% Tyrode's solution, 20% filtered foal serum, and 10% embryonic extract.
In this medium, the layer of explanted precardiac mesoderm soon developed a
rounded outline, became more or less spherical, and grew considerably. This
growth stopped within 24 hours after explantation. Histological examination
showed the cells to be arranged in irregularly concentric rings (Fig. A–1A). At
the periphery the explant was bordered by a layer of flattened cells with an
epithelial appearance, comparable to what is seen in embryonic organs

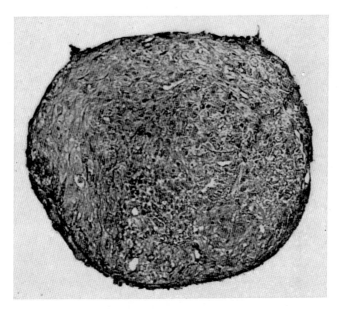

FIG. A-1. A. Histological appearance of myocardial tissue differentiated *in vitro* from precardiac mesoderm, cultured alone. Liquid medium, 2 days of culture. Hematoxylin–eosin stain.

cultured on Wolff and Haffen's agar medium. Spontaneous beating appeared 12–20 hours after explantation. If the culture medium was renewed daily, the cultures could be maintained for 3–4 weeks with persistent spontaneous beating. Analogous results have been obtained with precardiac mesoderm from mouse embryos. The mesoderm was isolated at the time of the formation of the first somites and was cultured using Rinaldini's medium (Le Douarin and Nanot, 1967).

Whichever culture technique was used, either an agar or a liquid medium, the myocardial tissue that differentiated *in vitro* from precardiac mesoderm did not undergo normal organogenesis and histogenesis. Using chick embryo precardiac mesoderm, D. Renaud and G. Le Douarin (1968) studied the influence of adjacent tissues on development when explanted *in vitro*. When the three embryonic layers of the presumptive cardiac region were explanted together onto a liquid medium, the development of the precardiac mesoderm was very different from that observed when the tissue was explanted alone. Very rapidly, within 3–4 hours of culture, the explant tended to form a vesicle within which the precardiac mesodermal cells condensed. This vesicle formed in the anterior region of the cardiac area, i.e., in the zone to which the cells migrate during normal development. A cardiac tube that pulsated spontaneously thus became progressively organized and underwent the beginning of organogenesis, as seen by a double curvature and constrictions (Fig. A–1B). Histological examination showed histogenesis very similar

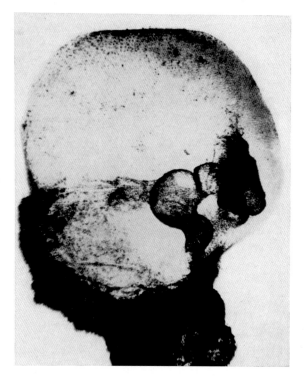

FIG. A-1. B. Cardiac tube formed during culture *in vitro* with all three layers of the presumptive cardiac region explanted. Liquid medium, 2 days of culture.

to that observed in a normal heart in the early stages of development. The epimyocardium was composed of 3–4 cell layers and was separated by an anhistic space from a thin endocardial layer of flattened cells (Fig. A–1C), The different parts of the cardiac tube, as defined by the constrictions. communicated with each other, as do the sinoatrial, ventricular, and bulbar chambers of the normal heart. If either the ectodermal or the endodermal layer of the cardiac region was removed by trypsin action prior to explantation in a liquid medium, then morphogenesis proceeded differently from normal, but the precardiac mesoderm still developed into a thin-walled vesicular or tubular structure. The same result was obtained when precardiac mesoderm was cultured in association with fragments of ectoderm or of endoderm taken from the posterior region of 3-day-old embryos.

Thus, the precardiac mesoderm becomes organized into a thin-walled

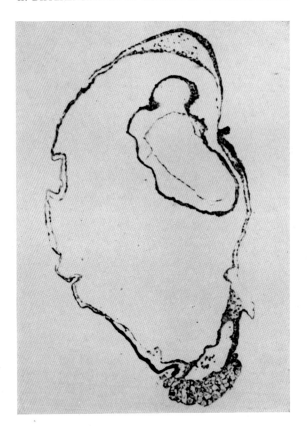

FIG. A-1. C. Histological appearance of the cardiac tube formed in culture. The epimyocardium is thin and the endocardium has differentiated (Renaud and Le Douarin, 1968).

vesicular or tubular structure when cultured in the presence of an epithelial support, whereas it forms a compact tissue when explanted alone.

I. Transmembrane Electrical Activity in Chick Embryo Heart after Explantation and Culture

The cardiac rudiment of 3-day chick embryos is differentiated into three regions: the sinoatrial chamber, the ventricle, and the bulbus. Organ culture of this rudiment using Wolff and Haffen's method (see Ch. II, Wolff and Haffen, 1952) makes it possible to study under good experimental conditions the transmembrane electrical activity of the various cell types in the embryonic myocardium (Le Douarin *et al.*, 1965b). The action potentials, recorded by transmembrane microelectrodes according to Corabœuf and Weidmann's method (1949), are characteristic for each anatomical region of the cardiac rudiment (Fig. A–2A). In the region of the sinus the membrane potential

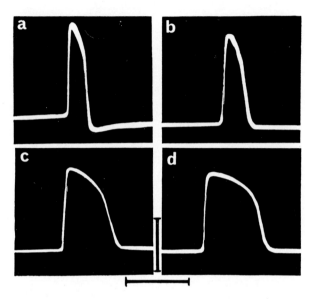

FIG. A-2. Characteristic action potentials from the different heart regions of 3-day chick embryo. (a) atrium, near the sinus; (b) another region of the atrium; (c) ventricle; (d) bulbus. Calibration: vertically, 50 mV; horizontally, 400 msec (Le Douarin *et al.*, 1966b).

showed a slow diastolic depolarization that was not observed in the atrial regions at some distance from the sinus. This indicated that the automatism remained localized in the sinus under organ culture conditions. The ventricular and bulbar cells had longer-lasting action potentials of the "rectangular" type, with the slow phase of repolarization constituting the plateau being of longer duration for bulbar than for ventricular cells. Despite the progressive morphological rearrangements which the cardiac rudiment undergoes when explanted *in vitro*, the atrial, ventricular, and bulbar action potentials remained remarkably constant during the first 4 days of culture. Thus, the electrophysiological characteristics of embryonic myocardial cells are maintained in organ culture on an agar medium.

When isolated heart fragments from 3- to 4-day-old embryos were cultured, the development of electrical activity varied, depending on whether the tissue fragments were of atrial or ventricular origin. When of atrial origin, the characteristic (prepotential and diastolic depolarization) extended progressively to the whole explant. On the contrary, the center of automatism which appeared in isolated ventricular explants remained confined to a well-defined region of the explant, which itself retained action potentials of characteristic ventricular type (Fig. A–3).

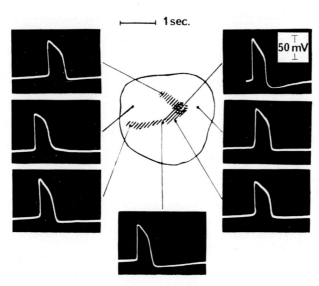

1 sec.

50 mV

FIG. A-3. Examples of transmembrane potentials recorded in a ventricular fragment from a 4-day-old heart, cultured for 3 days. Hatched area indicates the approximate localization of the center of automatism (Coraboeuf *et al.*, 1965).

The automatic activity of ventricular explants could be inhibited by association with a fragment of atrial tissue beating at a more rapid rate. When an atrial and a ventricular fragment were placed in contact with each other on the culture medium, the two explants beat at their own individual rates for a certain length of time; recordings of transmembrane electrical activity showed that each of them possessed a localized automatism. After about 12 hours of culture, the two explants united and from then on the beats of the whole tissue complex were coordinated; the pulsation rate of the ventricular fragment was then controlled by the atrial portion and all the ventricular action potentials were indicative of this regulation, with no loss of diastolic depolarization. A single atrial fragment, associated as a mosaic with several ventricular fragments all beating at different rates, could regulate the whole preparation once explant fusion had taken place.

Organ culture has been used in the electrophysiological study of the appearance and development of automatism in the embryonic heart (Le Douarin *et al.*, 1965b, 1966b; Obrecht-Coutris *et al.*, 1968b). When the cardiac rudiment was removed shortly before the appearance of spontaneous beating, i.e., from embryos with 8 to 9 somites and then cultured *in vitro*, beating appeared a few hours after explantation. Two types of ventricular action potential were recorded (Fig. A–4). One had an isopotential

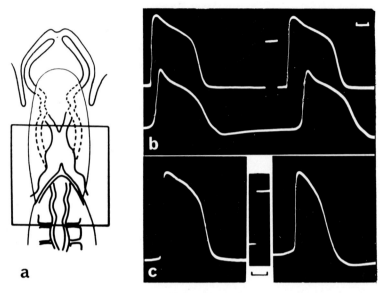

FIG. A-4.   a. Diagram to indicate removal of the cardiac rudiment (9-somite embryo). b. Action potentials of the ventricular type recorded after a few hours in culture. The lower tracing shows characteristics of automatism. c. Recording taken on Day 7 of culture. Left, ventricular potential; right, atrial potential. Calibration: horizontally, 100 msec; vertically, 50 mV (Obrecht-Coutris *et al.*, 1968b).

diastole while the other, corresponding to the region of the cardiac tube where the excitomotor impulse originated, possessed the characteristics of automatism. After a few days of culture, recordings indicated cellular activity of the sinoatrial type with the characteristics of automatism while the ventricular action potentials were now all of the "regulated" type. After the early phase of cardiac automatism, which was of the ventricular type, the sinoatrial material was incorporated into the cardiac tube where it subsequently differentiated and imposed its rhythm on the whole cardiac complex.

De Haan (1963) showed that fragments at the cardiac region from chicks at stages 4 to 8 (Hamburger and Hamilton, 1951) differentiated *in vitro* into spontaneously beating vesicles. The cardiac tissue formed by fragments from the posterior region of the cardiac area was found to beat at a more rapid rate than the tissue which had differentiated from fragments from the middle region, and the anterior fragments gave rise to cardiac tissue that was found to beat at a very slow rate. It, therefore, seems that, at an early stage, the histogenetic potentialities of the cardiac area are not uniformly distributed. As the cellular types in the myocardium can be distinguished by their electrophysiological characteristics, it can be demonstrated that the anterior part of the cardiac area contains the future bulbar cells, the mid-portion—the future ventricular cells—and the posterior portion—the future sinoatrial cells. The action potentials characteristic of these cellular types (Fig. A–5)

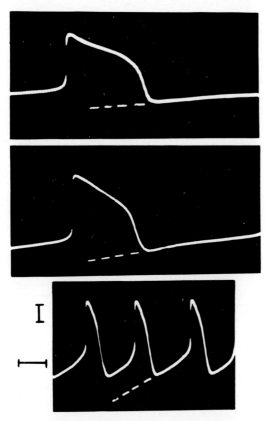

FIG. A-5. Action potentials recorded in myocardial tissue differentiated *in vitro* from three fragments of the presumptive cardiac region (from top to bottom: anterior, intermediate, and posterior fragments). These three types of action potential show a slow depolarization phase (extended on this figure by the discontinuous line) characteristic of automatism. Calibration: horizontally, 200 msec; vertically, 10 mV (Le Douarin *et al.*, 1966)b.

are recorded in the pulsating vesicles that differentiate respectively from the anterior, intermediate, and posterior portions of the cardiac area (Le Douarin, *et al.*, 1966b). Since the phase of slow diastolic depolarization is observed for all three types of electrical activity, it is deduced that spontaneous beating does not result from the activity of specific pacemaker cells but is a property common to all myoblasts at the particular developmental stage reached by the culture. Certain characteristics of automatic activity in noninnervated myocardium have been studied in fragments of chick embryo heart cultured *in vitro* using Wolff and Haffen's method. G. Obrecht, E. Corabœuf, and G. Le Douarin (1966) studied the aftereffects of electrical stimulation on atrial and ventricular fragments taken from chick embryo hearts at different stages of incubation, ranging from 2 to 11 days. When the explants were stimulated electrically for a certain period, in such a way that they beat more rapidly than their spontaneous rate, the cessation of stimulation was followed by a temporary suppression of beating. This poststimulatory inhibition was observed in both atrial and ventricular preparations, whatever the developmental stage of the embryo from which the heart fragment had been removed. In the early stages of development cardiac tissue is not innervated, and the poststimulatory inhibition cannot be attributed to the liberation of acetylcholine by intracardiac nerve endings. Poststimulatory inhibition is suppressed by atropine at concentrations of 10^{-6} gm/ml which suggests the presence in the embryonic heart of endogenous substances of acetylcholine type prior to the establishment of cardiac innervation. G. Obrecht-Coutris, E. Corabœuf, and G. Le Douarin (1968a) have demonstrated the liberation of acetylcholine or a related substance by the noninnervated heart of young chick embryos and it is possible that this substance may play a part in regulating the cardiac rhythm prior to the establishment of cardiac innervation. It has also been found (Crepin and Le Douarin, 1966) that in organ culture using Wolff and Haffen's method differentiation of mesenchyme from the cardiac region of the chick embryo gives rise to a myocardial tissue in which acetylcholinesterase activity can be detected.

J. The Respiratory Metabolism of Embryonic Organs Cultured *in Vitro* Using Wolff and Haffen's Method (see Ch. II, Wolff and Haffen, 1952)

The development of respiratory metabolism in cell and tissue cultures has been extensively studied. Generally speaking, the metabolism of chick embryo cells cultured *in vitro* has been shown to be glycolytic in nature with the glycolysis/respiration ratio varying according to the density of cells in the medium. The optimal oxygen tension has been shown to vary according to the culture technique used. The use of air as the gas phase is generally suitable for cells cultured in suspension or in monolayer culture.

Air is also used as the gas phase in Wolff and Haffen's culture method, with one of the explant surfaces being in direct contact with air.

Various types of respirometers have been used to study metabolism *in vitro*. Lucas (1965) developed an apparatus adapted for Trowel's culture method.

Bermann (1964) adapted Warburg's manometric technique for use with Wolff and Haffen's culture method on an agar medium, the medium used being based on Wolff and Haffen's standard medium. It is a "maintenance medium" slightly deficient in protein, with the Tyrode solution replaced by saline. The pH can be maintained at an appropriate value for several days, despite aerobic glycolysis of the embryonic explants. Each measurement made, using the respirometer, is composed of two parts. First, the change in pressure ΔP_1 is measured, which corresponds to the absorption of oxygen and the production of carbon dioxide during a time interval ΔT_1 (usually about 5 hours). Immediately afterward, the carbon dioxide is rapidly absorbed by connecting the flask to a side-arm containing alkali and the corresponding variation in pressure ΔP_2 is measured over a time interval ΔT_2 (about half an hour). Under these conditions the average hourly respiration rate of the explants in the flask, during the time $\Delta T_1 + \Delta T_2$, is given by the formula: $R\mu l\ O_2/h = K(\Delta P_1 + \Delta P_2)/(a\Delta T_1 + \Delta T_2)$ where K and a are parameters depending on the units chosen and the flask constant. The results are related to an "explant value" based on an evaluation of the total nitrogen level at the end of the culture (N_f) and that of equivalent explants at the beginning of culture (N_i), so assuming a linear variation in nitrogen level during the time of culture T, the "explant value" is given by $(N_i + N_f)/2T$ in μg N/hour.

Determination of the level of lactic acid which has accumulated in the culture medium permits an evaluation of glycolysis to be made. Bermann studied the development of respiration in culture of skin fragments from chick embryos of about 8 days' incubation. The duration of culture was 5 to 6 days. The pO_2 measured during the first 13 hours of culture was around $0.1\ \mu l\ O_2/\mu g$ N/hour. The oxygen consumption subsequently diminished, and the curve obtained by plotting oxygen consumption against time was hyperbolic. The glycolysis/respiration ratio was close to 0.3, showing that in organ culture the metabolism remained predominantly of the oxidative type, in contrast to that occurring in tissue culture. In cultures of 10-day-old embryonic intestine and 4-day-old embryonic heart (Kirrmann and Le Douarin, 1964, 1965) the oxygen consumption decreased linearly with time, but oxidative metabolism was still predominant during the culture period of 6 days. It should be noted that Bermann's manometric method enables the development of respiration to be observed for several days of culture, but each measurement requires about 5 hours. The initial value of oxygen consumption can only be obtained by extrapolation of the curve obtained, but it is in full agreement with the value for embryonic intestine in culture using a simple microspirometric method (Le Douarin and Kirrmann, 1964).

BIBLIOGRAPHY

1. Abbot J. and Holtzer H.   The loss of phenotypic traits by differentiated cells. The reversible behavior of chondrocytes in primary cultures. *J. Cell Biol.*, 1966, **28**, 473–487.
2. Bermann F.   Étude manomètrique du métabolisme respiratoire d'une culture d'organe embryonnaire. *Arch. Sc. Physiol.*, 1964, **28**, 89–113.

3. Bunge R. P., Bunge M. B. and Peterson E. R. An electron microscope study of cultured rat spinal cord. *J. Cell Biol.*, 1965, **24**, 163–191.

4. Chang L. W. and Maibach H. I. Fetal pig skin organ culture in dermatologic investigation. *J. invest. Dermatol.*, 1967, **49**, 486–496.

5. Charlier J. P. and Petrovic A. Recherches sur la mandibule de rat en culture d'organes: le cartilage condylien a-t-il un potentiel de croissance indépendant. *L'Orthodontie Française*, 1967, **38**, 1–11.

6. Cohen S. Isolation of a mouse submaxillary gland protein accelerating incisor eruption and eyelid opening in the newborn animal. *J. biol. Chem.*, 1962, **237**, 1555–1562.

7. Cohen S. The stimulation of epidermal proliferation by a specific protein (EGF). *Developm. Biol.*, 1965, **12**, 394–407.

8. Corabœuf E., Le Douarin G. and Obrecht G. Morphologie de l'activité électrique transmembranaire du cœur embryonnaire de Poulet en culture organotypique. *C. R. Soc. Biol.*, 1965, **159**, 110–114.

9. Corabœuf E. and Weidmann S. Potentiel de repos et potentiel d'action du muscle cardiaque mesurés à l'aide d'électrodes intracellulaires. *C. R. Soc. Biol.*, 1949, **143**, 1329–1331.

10. Crepin M. and Le Douarin G. Activités cholinestérasiques du tissu cardiaque différencié *in vitro* par le mésenchyme de l'aire cardiaque de l'embryon de poulet. *C. R. Acad. Sc.*, 1966, **263**, 1479–1481.

11. Dameron Fl. Étude expérimentale de l'organogenèse du poumon chez l'embryon de poulet. Mise en évidence et chronologie des interactions épithélio-mésenchymateuses. *Ann. Embryol. Morph.*, 1968, **1**, 373–393.

12. Davis J. M. G. The structure of guinea-pigs lung maintained in organ culture. *Brit. J. exp. Pathol.*, 1967, **48**, 371–378.

13. De Haan R. Regional organization of pre-pacemaker cells in the cardiac primordia of the early chick embryo. *J. Embryol. exp. Morph.*, 1963, **11**, 65–76.

14. Dodson J. W. On the nature of tissue interactions in embryonic skin. *Exp. Cell Res.*, 1963, **31**, 233–235.

15. Dutton G. F. *Ann. N. Y. Acad. Sc.*, 1963, **111**, 259. Also see Ko and Nemeth (1966a,b).

16. Dutton G. J. and Ko V. *Biochem. J.*, 1966, **99**, 550. Also see Ko and Nemeth (1966a,b).

17. Eisen A. Z. and Gross J. The role of epithelium and mesenchyme in the production of a collagenolytic enzyme and a hyaluronidase in the anuran tadpole. *Developm. Biol.*, 1965, **12**, 408–418.

18. Endo H., Enomoto H. and Warkabayashi K. Ossification of chick embryo femur growing in natural liquid media. *Tissue Cult., Proc. Seminar*, Baroda, India, 1965, **24**, 27–30.

19. Fell H. B. The technique of organ culture. *Tissue Cult., Proc. Seminar*, Baroda, India, 1965a, **24**, 9–16.

20. Fell H. B. The application of organ culture to medical and biological research. *Tissue Cult., Proc. Seminar*, Baroda, India, 1965b, **24**, 17–26.

21. Foote F. M. and Foote C. L. Organs of the larval axolote (Siredon mexicanum) grow singly or in combination *in vitro*. *Trans. Illinois State Acad. Sc.*, 1965, **58**, 164–175.

22. Hall B. K. The formation of adventitious cartilage by membrane bones under the influence of mechanical stimulation applied *in vitro*. *Life Sc.*, 1967, **6**, 663–667.

23. Hambrick G. W., Lamberg S. I. and Bloomberg R. Observations on keratinization of human skin *in vitro*. *J. invest. Dermatol.*, 1967, **47**, 541–550.

24. Heusner A. and Petrovic A. *Med. Electron. Biol. Eng.*, 1964, **2**, 381. Also see Petrovic and Charlier (1967).
25. Kirrmann J. M. and Le Douarin G. Consommation d'oxygène et glycolyse en aérobiose d'organes embryonnaires en culture organotypique; effets d'une irradiation aux rayons X. *Arch. Sc. Physiol.*, 1964, **28**, 383–402.
26. Kirrmann J. M. and Le Douarin G. Le métabolisme respiratoire d'organes embryonnaires cultivés *in vitro*. *C. R. Soc. Biol.*, 1965, **159**, 114–117.
27. Ko V. and Nemeth A. M. Synthesis of glucuronide by organ cultures of liver. *Biochem. J.*, 1966a, **100**, 27.
28. Ko V. and Nemeth A. M. Factors affecting induction and development of UDP-glucuronyltransferase in cultured liver from chick embryos of different ages. *Bioch. J.*, 1966b, **100**, 27–28.
29. Le Douarin G. and Kirrmann J. M. Inhibition précoce de la consommation d'oxygène de l'intestin embryonnaire de Poulet en culture organotypique provoquée par une irradiation aux rayons X. *C. R. Acad. Sc.*, 1964, **258**, 2917–2920.
30. Le Douarin G., Le Douarin N. and Cuminge D. Étude ultrastructurale des capacités d'autodifférenciation du mésoderme de l'aire cardiaque chez l'embryon de Poulet. *C. R. Acad. Sc.*, 1965a, **260**, 6998–7001.
31. Le Douarin G. and Nanot J. Différenciation *in vitro* de tissu myocardique à partir du mésoderme de l'embryon de Souris. *C. R. Soc. Biol.*, 1967, **161**, 1811–1813.
32. Le Douarin G., Nanot J. and Renaud D. Sur la différenciation *in vitro* du mésenchyme précardiaque. *C. R. Soc. Biol.*, 1966a, **160**, 1733–1735.
33. Le Douarin G., Obrecht G. and Corabœuf E. Activité électrique transmembranaire de vésicules pulsatiles différenciées en culture organotypique par des fragments de l'aire précardiaque de l'embryon de Poulet. *C. R. Acad. Sc.*, 1965b, **260**, 287–290.
34. Le Douarin G., Obrecht G. and Corabœuf E. Déterminations régionales dans l'aire cardiaque présomptive mises en évidence chez l'embryon de poulet par la méthode microélectrophysiologique. *J. Embryol. exp. Morph.*, 1966b, **15**, 153–167.
35. Le Douarin G. and Renaud D. Différenciation en milieu liquide et culture de longue durée du tissu myocardique embryonnaire. *C. R. Soc. Biol.*, 1967, **161**, 436–440.
36. Loffredo Sampaolo C. Indagini sulle correlazioni strutturali tra gangli nervosi spinali e frammenti di muscolo scheletrico associati in coltura organotipica. *Quaderni di Anatomia Pratica*, 1966, serie XXII, 1–4.
37. Lucas D. R. A respirometer for organ cultures. *Bioch. J.*, 1965, **97**, 769–775.
38. Lyser K. M. Différenciation du tube neural de l'embryon de Poulet en culture organotypique. *Arch. Anat. micr. Morph. exp.*, 1966, **55**, 37–53.
39. Obrecht G., Corabœuf E. and Le Douarin G. Inhibition poststimulative de l'automatisme de fragments de cœur embryonnaire de Poulet cultivés *in vitro*. *J. Physiol.*, Paris, 1966, **58**, 577.
40. Obrecht-Coutris G., Corabœuf E. and Le Douarin G. Libération d'acétylcholine par le cœur embryonnaire de Poulet avant le stade de l'innervation. *C. R. Acad. Sc.*, 1968a, **267**, 1102–1104.
41. Obrecht-Coutris G., Le Douarin G. and Corabœuf E. Aspects électrophysiologiques de l'automatisme du myocarde ventriculaire chez l'embryon de poulet. *C. R. Acad. Sc.*, 1968b, **267**, 765–768.
42. Petrovic A. and Charlier J. P. La synchondrose sphéno-occipitale de jeune rat en culture d'organes: mise en évidence d'un potentiel de croissance indépendant. *C. R. Acad. Sc.*, 1967, **265**, 1511–1513.
43. Petrovic A. and Heusner A. *C. R. Acad. Sc.*, 1961, **253**, 3066. Also see Petrovic and Charlier (1967).

44. Pinkel D.   Cultivation of mouse thymus in organ culture. *Proc. Soc. exp. Biol. Med.*, 1964, **116**, 54–56.
45. Reaven E. P. and Cox A. J.   Organ culture of human skin. *J. invest. Dermatol.*, 1965, **44**, 151–156.
46. Renaud D. and Le Douarin G.   Influence de l'environnement tissulaire et des conditions de culture sur l'évolution du mésoderme précardiaque de l'embryon de Poulet. *C. R. Acad. Sc.*, 1968, **267**, 431–434.
47. Rinaldini L. M.   An improved method for the isolation and quantitative cultivation of embryonic cells. *Exp. Cell Res.*, 1959, **16**, 477–505.
48. Salvatorelli G.   Observations sur l'hématopoïèse *in vitro* dans la moelle osseuse embryonnaire de Poulet. *C. R. Acad. Sc.*, 1966, **262**, 666–668.
49. Salvatorelli G.   Réactivation de l'érythropoïèse de la moelle osseuse de Poulet *in vitro* par l'apport de foie embryonnaire. *C. R. Acad. Sc.*, 1967, **265**, 1219–1222.
50. Salvatorelli G., Callegarini C., Gulinati A. M. and Gardenghi G.   Observations sur la différenciation *in vitro* des cellules myéloïdes d'embryons de Poulet. *J. Embryol. exp. Morph.*, 1968, **19**, 145–155.
51. Salvatorelli G. and Gulinati A. M.   L'effetto eritropoietico del fegato di diversa età su culture organotipiche di midollo osseo embrionale di pollo. *Atti Accad. Nazl. Lincei, Rend. Classe Sc. Fis. Mat. Nat.*, 1967a, **43**, 1–4.
52. Salvatorelli G. and Gulinati A. M.   Alcuni dati sperimental sulla eritropoiesi nel pollo. *Atti Accad. Sc. Ferrara*, 1967b, **44**, 1–6.
53. Sarkany I., Grice K. and Caron G. A.   Organ culture of adult human skin. *Brit. J. Dermatol.*, 1965, **77**, 65–76.
54. Shaffer B. M.   The isolated *Xenopus laevis* tail: a preparation for studying the central nervous system and metamorphosis in culture. *J. Embryol. exp. Morph.*, 1963, **11**, 77–90.
55. Shaw J. L. and Bassett C. A.   The effects of varying oxygen concentrations on osteogenesis and embryonic cartilage *in vitro*. *J. Bone Joint. Surg.*, 1967, **49**, 73–80.
56. Tata J. R.   Requirement for RNA and protein synthesis for induced regression of the tadpole tail in organ culture. *Developm. Biol.*, 1966, **13**, 77–94.
57. Teaford M. E. and White A. A.   *Proc. Soc. exp. Biol. Med.*, 1964, **117**, 536. Also see White (1967b).
58. Vanable J. W. Jr. and Mortensen R. D.   Development of *Xenopus laevis* skin glands in organ culture. *Exp. Cell Res.*, 1966, **44**, 436–442.
59. White A. A.   Stimulation of the growth of organ cultures by methyl and propyl parabens. *Proc. Soc. exp. Biol. Med.*, 1967a, **126**, 588–591.
60. White A. A.   *Proc. Soc. exp. Biol. Med.*, 1967b, **126**, 436–442.

CHAPTER III

CULTURE OF EMBRYO ORGANS
IN SYNTHETIC MEDIA

Madeleine Kieny

INSTITUT D'EMBRYOLOGIE EXPÉRIMENTALE DU COLLÈGE DE FRANCE ET DU C.N.R.S.
PARIS, FRANCE

I. INTRODUCTION

Many experiments on the nutrition and differentiation of embryonic organs require the ideal conditions that are provided by the use of synthetic media. Owing to their simplicity and constant composition, these media provide an ideal means of studying the assimilation of foodstuffs, and the role of growth factors and morphogenic substances. Several examples will be considered.

To be effective a synthetic medium must provide good conditions for the survival of the explanted organs. The integrity of the structure of the explanted organ must be preserved, and neither its subsequent differentiation nor its functional activity must be affected. The effects of the addition or subtraction of a certain ingredient can then be examined.

The objectives of culture in synthetic media differ according to whether embryonic or adult organs are studied. With the latter, the aim is to preserve the histological structure of the explant and to maintain *in vitro* one or other of its normal functions. All growth is avoided since this involves the risk of dedifferentiation of a part of the organ.

An example of such a culture is that of the lymphatic glands of the mouse (18), in which lymphocyte production can be maintained *in vitro*.

On the contrary, in the case of embryonic organs, the aim is to obtain some development of the explants *in vitro*. The media employed often favor growth, either by an increase in the number and size of the cells, or by an increase in the amount of intercellular material. In addition, the media often encourage histogenetic and morphogenetic differentiation of the organs. Such organs are often explanted as undifferentiated rudiments.

This chapter will be limited to reporting the main results obtained in the culture of embryonic organs. Various synthetic mixtures are effective in allowing the survival of embryonic organs *in vitro*. These media mainly contain amino acids, vitamins, sugars, and sometimes hormones and other metabolites. The explants use these materials either for growth or for differentiation, but rarely for both at the same time.

The research considered at present has been concerned more with the aspects of differentiation than with growth. The embryonic organs involved are the gonads, the syrinx, the skin and its derivatives, the thyroid gland, and the tibiotarsus. The reason is that simple synthetic media have not yet been perfected to the point where, like natural media, they can maintain a normal growth rate.

II. METHODS FOR THE CULTURE OF ORGANS IN SYNTHETIC MEDIA

The culture media used in the investigation of the nutritional requirements for growth and differentiation of embryonic organs vary widely in complexity, ranging from the very simple media for organ culture described by Et. Wolff and his school (30) to the very complex media for cell culture that have been described by various workers.

The simple synthetic solutions in the method of Et. Wolff are incorporated into an agar base, while the other mixtures are used as liquids.

A. Gel Media

The culture method using synthetic media was only a variant of that described by Et. Wolff and Haffen (26). The embryo extract was replaced by a solution of nitrogenous substances in Tyrode's physiological solution (30).

Solutions B and C, the compositions of which are given in Tables I and II, represent the more complex mixtures of amino acids.

TABLE I

Solution B of Wolff et al.

Amino acid	Concentration (mg/100 ml)
L-Lysine-2HCl	60.4
L-Arginine	30.8
DL-Methionine	10.4
DL-Histidine HCl	12.4
L-Glutamic acid	56.4
DL-Aspartic acid	23.6
L-Proline	20.4
L-Cysteine-HCl	6.0
L-Tryptophan	20.0

Solution C contained amino acids found in blood fibrin (2) in addition to those amino acids that were essential to growth (14).

Using media B and C, it was possible for the first time to culture organs on synthetic media containing only specific chemical compounds.

TABLE II

SOLUTION C OF WOLFF *et al.*

Amino acid	Concentration (mg/100 ml)	Amino acid	Concentration (mg/100 ml)
L-Lysine-2HCl	60.4	DL-Isoleucine	40.0
L-Arginine	30.8	DL-Threonine	48.0
DL-Methionine	10.4	DL-Valine	56.0
DL-Histidine-HCl	12.4	Glycine	10.0
L-Glutamic acid	56.4	L-Tyrosine	4.0
DL-Aspartic acid	23.6	L-Hydroxyproline	10.0
L-Proline	20.4	Taurine	20.0
L-Cysteine-HCl	6.0	Ornithine-2HCl	20.0
L-Tryptophan	20.0	DL-Serine	50.0
DL-Phenylalanine	28.0	L-Asparagine	20.0
L-Leucine	36.0		

To culture the thyroid (29), solution C was used as described; to culture the syrinx (23), the gonads (16), and the uropygial gland (8), solutions B and C were diluted by half; and to culture the tibiotarsus (12), and the dorsal skin (15), solutions B and C were diluted tenfold. All of the organs for culturing were derived from bird embryos.

The minimum concentration of amino acids in the nutrient medium was generally that given in solution C, adapted to the organ in question.

B. Liquid Media

Two organs have been cultured on liquid media. They are the tibiotarsus (14) and the tarsometatarsal skin of the chick embryo (20, 21).

An organ explanted in a liquid medium requires some support. The tibiotarsus was explanted on floating lens paper using Chen's technique (5). Skin cultured by Trowell's method (17) was placed on a perforated metal grid.

Synthetic solutions that had been perfected for the prolonged survival and multiplication of mouse fibroblasts (strain L) in tissue culture contained many ingredients such as amino acids, vitamins, coenzymes, purines, and pyrimidines.

The tibiotarsus was explanted in Healy, Fisher, and Parker's solution 828 (9), the composition of which is given in Table III, and in their solution 929, which differs from solution 828 in that the concentration of the amino acids is doubled.

TABLE III

MEDIUM 858 OF HEALY, FISHER, AND PARKER

Ingredients	Concentration (mg/100 ml)	Ingredients	Concentration (mg/100 ml)
L-Arginine	7.0	p-Aminobenzoic acid	0.005
L-Histidine	2.0	Vitamin A	0.01
L-Lysine	7.0	Calciferol	0.01
L-Tyrosine	4.0	α-Tocopherol phosphate	0.01
L-Tryptophan	1.0	Menadione	0.001
L-Phenylalanine	2.5	Ascorbic acid	5.0
L-Cystine	2.0	Diphosphopyridine nucleotide	0.7
L-Methionine	1.5	(NAD)	
L-Serine	2.5	Triphosphopyridine nucleotide	0.1
L-Threonine	3.0	(NADP)	
L-Leucine	6.0	Coenzyme A	0.25
L-Isoleucine	2.0	Cocarboxylase	0.1
L-Valine	2.5	Flavine adenine nucleotide	0.1
L-Glutamic acid	7.5	Uridine triphosphate	0.1
L-Aspartic acid	3.0	Glutathione	1.0
L-Alanine	2.5	Adenine deoxyriboside	1.0
L-Proline	4.0	Guanine deoxyriboside	1.0
L-Hydroxyproline	1.0	Cytosine deoxyriboside	1.0
L-Cysteine	26.0	5-Methyldeoxycytidine	0.01
Glycine	5.0	Thymidine	1.0
Pyridoxine	0.0025	Sodium acetate	5.0
Pyridoxal	0.0025	Sodium glucuronate	0.42
Biotin	0.001	L-Glutamine	10.0
Folic acid	0.001	Tween 80 (oleic acid)	0.5
Inositol	0.005	Cholesterol	0.02
Choline	0.05		

Skin was cultured in Waymouth's solution MB 752/1, the composition of which is given in Table IV (19).

III. CULTURE OF THE GONADS

These experiments were carried out by Stenger-Haffen (16).

The gonads of chicken and duck embryos were taken before sexual differentiation had occurred. Tissue was taken from chick embryos after 8 days of incubation, and from duck embryos after 9 days of incubation (Plate I, Fig. 1).

When explanted onto relatively complex media (B and C), the gonads developed in the same way as controls on the natural medium based on embryo extract (Plate I, Figs. 2 and 3).

TABLE IV

WAYMOUTH'S MEDIUM MB 752/1

Ingredients	Concentration (mg/100 ml)	Ingredients	Concentration (mg/100 ml)
Glucose	500.0	L-Lysine-HCl	24.0
Ascorbic acid	1.75	L-Histidine-HCl	15.0
Cysteine-HCl	9.0	L-Glutamic acid	15.0
Glutathione	1.5	L-Threonine	7.5
Choline-HCl	25.0	L-Arginine-HCl	7.5
Hypoxanthine	2.5	L-Valine	6.5
Glutamine	35.0	L-Aspartic acid	6.0
Thiamine-HCl	1.0	Glycine	5.0
Calcium pantothenate	0.1	L-Proline	5.0
Riboflavine	0.1	L-Leucine	5.0
Pyridoxine-HCl	0.1	L-Methionine	5.0
Folic acid	0.04	L-Tyrosine	4.0
Biotin	0.002	L-Phenylalanine	5.0
m-Inositol-2H$_2$O	0.1	L-Tryptophan	4.0
Nicotinamide	0.1	L-Isoleucine	2.5
Vitamin B$_{12}$	0.02	L-Cystine	1.5

Genetically male gonads developed into testes. The development of the genetically female gonads depended on whether they were taken from the right or the left side. Usually gonads from the left side continued to differentiate, while those from the right regressed. In the duck embryo, the left gonad differentiated into a typical ovary and the right gonad remained undifferentiated (27). In the chicken, the development of the female gonads was atypical; the left gonad developed into an ovotestis, while the right gonad flattened and assumed a testicular form (28).

A. Minimum Requirements of Amino Acids

When they were cultured on a medium that contained only mineral salts and glucose but no nitrogenous material, male and female gonads taken at the undifferentiated stage survived for 3–4 days but never became differentiated. To obtain sexual differentiation of the female gonad, it was necessary to add only a single amino acid, cysteine, to the medium (Plate I, Fig. 4).

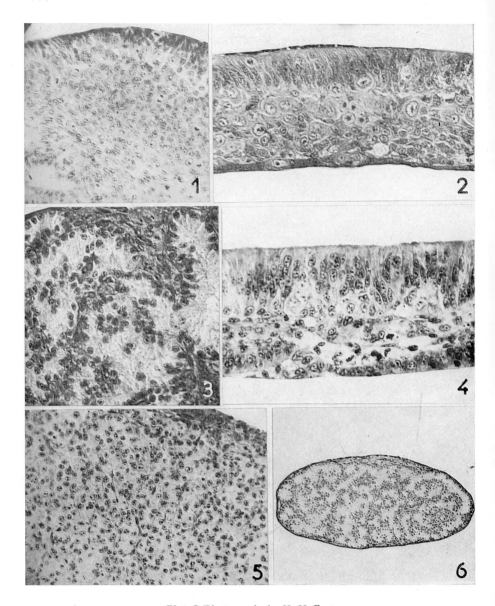

Plate I (Photographs by K. Haffen)

FIG. 1.   Detail of the left gonad from an 8-day duck embryo (undifferentiated stage).
The thick germinal epithelium contains germinal cells. The medulla is composed of thick,
diffuse cords that are also fertile.

FIG. 2.   Structure of an 8-day duck embryo ovary, showing differentiation after 5

In contrast, this medium did not allow the differentiation of male gonads (Plate I, Fig. 5). These required the presence of four additional amino acids: methionine, arginine, histidine, and glutamic acid (or lysine) (Plate I, Fig. 6).

A certain number of other amino acids, without being essential, favored differentiation and growth. These were hydroxyproline, ornithine, glycine, glutamine, tryptophan, phenylalanine, and threonine.

B. Vitamin Requirements

Vitamins added to the minimum medium, as will be defined, and to media B and C, favored the growth of male chick embryo gonads as long as the vitamins were added as a mixture and not singly. The useful vitamins were ascorbic acid, folic acid, p-aminobenzoic acid, nicotinamide, pyridoxine, biotin, aneurin, m-inositol, calcium pantothenate, riboflavine, and vitamin B_{12}.

None of the vitamins, whether added to the culture medium singly or in combination, had any effect on sexual differentiation in male or female duck embryo gonads.

C. Sugar Requirements

Glucose was indispensable for the differentiation and survival of the gonads, whatever the composition of the synthetic medium. Necrosis occurred rapidly in its absence. However, glucose could always be replaced by mannose, and, with less advantage, by galactose, fructose, or xylose (Plate II Fig. 2).

D. Anomalies of Sexual Differentiation in Relation to the Nutrient Medium

The differentiation of male duck embryo gonads on certain synthetic culture media was sometimes accompanied by anomalies similar to those seen

---

days of culture on medium C. Deep in the cortex are oogonia, both resting and in mitosis, which have formed groups.

FIG. 3.   Structure of a testicular explant from an 8-day duck embryo, showing differentiation after 6 days of culture on medium C. The spaces are seminiferous tubules.

FIG. 4.   Detail of a duck ovary differentiated in part from an undifferentiated 7-day rudiment cultured on a synthetic medium containing only cysteine (medium 27). Characteristic ovarian structure is seen, although the cortex is partly sterile.

FIG. 5.   Detail of an 8-day male gonad after 5 days of culture on medium 27. The medullary cords are undifferentiated.

FIG. 6.   Low power view of a testis from a late 8-day embryo, showing differentiation after 13 days of culture on the minimum synthetic medium (containing arginine, cysteine, methionine, glutamic acid, and histidine). Seminiferous tubules with wide lumens are separated from the coelomic epithelium by the connective tissue of the tunica albuginea.

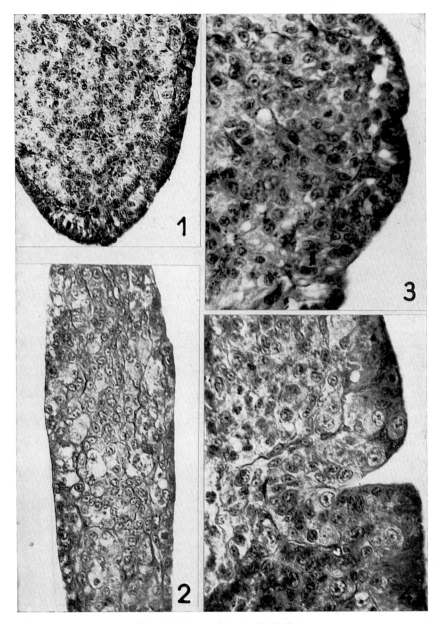

Plate II (Photographs by K. Haffen)

FIG. 1. Detail of left gonad from an 8-day duck embryo grown on medium 27 (compare with Plate I, Fig. 5) and acted on by crystalline female hormone (estradiol dipropionate). A thick cortex with one germinal cell is developed in mitosis. The medulla is undifferentiated.

when testes were grown on a natural organic medium with added female hormone.

Thus, some media brought about an apparent type of intersexuality indicated by persistence of the germinal epithelium and poor differentiation of the medullary cords. These were medium B containing 9 poorly balanced amino acids, the minimum medium without histidine (see Section A), and the favorable media in which glucose had been replaced by fructose or galactose.

E. The Effect of Sex Hormones on Male Gonads

When male gonads were cultured on the inadequate media that have been described above they often developed an intermediate structure that resembled a type of intersexuality. Does the addition of male hormone to the medium allow the reestablishment of normal male differentiation, or does the addition of female hormone to the deficient synthetic medium induce complete transformation from male to female gonad?

1. INFLUENCE OF MALE HORMONE

Male hormone had no effect on the development of female gonads whatever the composition of the synthetic medium. Even on a deficient medium, male hormones did not favor testicular differentiation in the male. These results clearly showed that the atypical development was due to a nutritional defect.

2. INFLUENCE OF FEMALE HORMONE

Female hormones could induce sexual inversion of a male gonad *in vitro* so long as it was grown on an adequate synthetic medium, such as the minimum medium or medium C (Plate II, Fig. 4).

Female hormone would not feminize a male gonad that had been explanted

---

FIG. 2. Detail of female gonad from an 8-day duck embryo, grown on the minimum medium with glucose replaced by xylose. Note the absence of differentiation in the cortex. The gonad is reduced to a medulla formed by undifferentiated cords and surrounded by a thin epithelium.

FIG. 3. Gonad from genetically male duck embryo grown on medium B for 5 days. The medulla is composed of poorly differentiated cell cords. It is covered by a thick germinal epithelium which is reminescent of a cortex. Note the germinal cells inserted between the cortical cells. Taken after 8 days of incubation.

FIG. 4. Detail of male gonad from a $7\frac{1}{2}$-day duck embryo. Feminization has occurred after addition of crystalline female hormone to medium B. A thick fertile cortex is invaginating into the medulla, where lacunas analogous to those seen in the ovary begin to appear. (Compare with Plate I, Fig. 2).

onto a medium inadequate for male differentiation. The male germinal epithelium persisted, and the medulla retained its usual structure (Plate II, Fig. 1). However, when the male gonads were kept under conditions where the nutrients were favorable for normal development, they reacted to the presence of female hormone. In this case they developed into characteristic ovotestes (Plate II, Fig. 3).

These experiments by Stenger-Haffen (16) showed that the nutrient medium had an important effect on the differentiation of the gonads. The conditions required for normal development of the male gonads were more stringent than those for the female gonad. Female sexual differentiation required only a single sulfhydryl-containing amino acid (cysteine) in addition to glucose. Male differentiation required the presence of at least four other amino acids.

It is interesting to note that female sexual differentiation occurred on a very simple medium in which the only nitrogenous component was cysteine, but that on the same medium, the male gonad could not respond to the effect of the female hormone. The female hormone could only induce feminization of the male gonad under conditions that allowed normal testicular differentiation.

This demonstrates the close relationship between the nutritional and hormonal factors necessary for the sexual differentiation of avian gonads.

F. Secretory Activity of the Gonads

Em. Wolff and Lutz-Ostertag (25) used the syrinx as a means of showing that the explanted female gonads continued to secrete female hormones. Undifferentiated duck syringes were grown on medium C with fragments of differentiated ovary from 12–16 day duck embryos. Under these conditions, the syringes differentiated into the symmetrical female type, whilst the controls grown without ovarian fragments acquired the asymmetric male shape. This proved that the synthetic medium C could support the functional activity of the female gonad for at least 12 days.

IV. CULTURE OF THE SYRINX

These experiments were carried out by Em. Wolff (23, 24).

The syrinx is the vocal organ in birds. It is situated at the junction of the trachea and the bronchi and is composed of 5 pairs of cartilaginous arches which form its skeleton.

The object of culturing the syrinx on synthetic media was twofold.

1. Investigation of the materials necessary for, and favorable to, the differentiation of the cartilaginous arches (23).

2. Study of the role of nutrition in the sexual differentiation of the syrinx (24).

The first was studied on the syrinx of chick embryos, the second on the syrinx of duck embryos.

A. Nutritional Requirements of the Syrinx

In the chick embryo the syrinx is a symmetrical organ, with the same structure in both sexes (Plate III, Fig. 1).

At the time of explantation, after $7\frac{1}{2}$ days of incubation, the syrinx was composed of an endodermal canal surrounded by homogeneous connective tissue in the middle of which the cartilaginous arches would develop. Two faint mesenchymal condensations were already visible at this stage. They were the rudiments of the first bronchial arches (Plate III, Fig. 3).

Syringes from $7\frac{1}{2}$ day embryos (but not those taken from younger embryos) could differentiate on medium B. On medium C syringes from 7-day embryos taken at the beginning of their differentiation could form their cartilaginous skeletons. Moreover, medium C prolonged the survival of the $7\frac{1}{2}$ day syrinx, and the differentiation was more elaborate than that seen when a medium based on embryo extract was used (Plate III, Fig. 2). For totally undifferentiated syringes of less than 7 days' incubation, neither medium B nor medium C was adequate. The explants became necrotic within 5 days.

1. SPECIFIC REQUIREMENTS FOR AMINO ACIDS AND VITAMINS

The syrinx survived for 3–4 days, on a medium that contained no nitrogenous material but contained glucose, but it neither grew nor differentiated.

Five amino acids were necessary for the culture of the syrinx. These constituted the minimum medium, allowing the explants to live long enough to complete histological differentiation of the bronchial arches (Plate III, Fig. 4). They were cysteine, methionine, arginine, histidine, and lysine (or glutamic acid). The absence of cysteine induced necrosis of the explants in less than 24 hours. When cysteine was used alone explants of $7\frac{1}{2}$–8 days incubation survived for more than 5 days, and two pairs of arches differentiated.

The minimum medium could be modified in several ways. The cysteine content could be increased fourfold or cysteine could be replaced by glutathione. Other amino acids (phenylalanine, asparagine, ornithine, tryptophan, glycine, aspartic acid, serine) or vitamins (ascorbic acid, m-inostitol, calcium pantothenate, folic acid, riboflavine, pyridoxine, p-aminobenzoic acid) could be added.

All these modified media assured survival, growth, and differentiation equal to or close to those obtained with medium C.

2. SUGAR REQUIREMENTS

Glucose was essential to the survival of the syrinx. Whatever else the medium contained, an absence of glucose produced rapid death of the explants. Of all the sugars tested, only mannose could replace glucose.

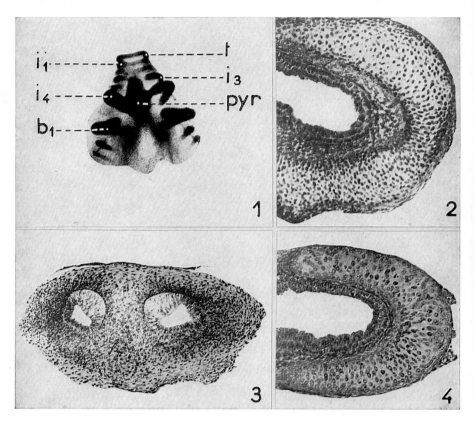

Plate III (Photographs by Em. Wolff)

FIG. 1. Syrinx of 12-day chick embryo. b_1, First bronchial arch, which is the arch below the syrinx; pyr, anterior pyramid; i_1–i_4, intermediate arches; t, first tracheal ring. The organ is divided into two chambers by a partial partition which ends anteriorly in a pyramid to which the cartilaginous arches become attached.

FIG. 2. Transverse section across the cartilaginous arch b_1 of a syrinx grown on medium C for 12 days. The epithelium lining the cavity of the syrinx is stratified and villous.

FIG. 3. Histological section of the syrinx of an 8-day chick embryo. Section taken across the middle. The rudiments of the arches b_1 are beginning to condense.

FIG. 4. Cartilaginous arc i_3 of a syrinx explanted at 8 days onto the minimum medium, containing arginine, glutathione, methionine, lysine, and histidine. Culture discontinued after 14 days.

B. Nutrition and Sexual Differentiation of the Syrinx

In ducks the syrinx shows marked sexual dimorphism (Plate IV, Fig. 1). In the female, the syrinx is small and bilaterally symmetric. In the male it is large and asymmetric, the left half being much larger than the right.

Previous experiments (22, 31) had clearly established that the male type of syrinx corresponded to the neutral type with deficient hormones. This type developed in castrated embryos and in undifferentiated syringes explanted on a natural medium.

How does sexual differentiation occur in the duck syrinx on chemically defined media ?

On a synthetic medium containing cysteine as the only nitrogenous material, all syringes taken at the undifferentiated stage developed into the symmetric female type regardless of the sexual genetics of the embryo from which they were taken (Plate IV, Fig. 2). On the minimum medium containing five amino acids the syrinx developed better, tending toward the asymmetric form, again regardless of the sex of the donor (Plate IV, Fig. 3). The same mixture of amino acids with the cysteine content increased fourfold allowed morphogenesis that tended more toward the typical male form, although this was never completely attained. On these media of intermediate quality the syrinx developed into a form recalling certain types of intersexuality (Plate IV, Fig. 4).

Medium C, with an increased cysteine content, was most appropriate for inducing typical male differentiation of the syrinx whatever its genetic origin (Plate IV, Fig. 5).

Finally the male form developed on a medium that was quantitatively and qualitatively rich in the nutrients required for the development of the syrinx. On a poor medium, although the same pieces of cartilage formed, the smaller and bilaterally symmetric female syrinx was developed.

The asymmetric development of the cartilaginous arches on the left-hand side could be inhibited by poor nutrition. Crystalline female hormone and hormones secreted by embryonic ovaries had the same effect. The normal mode of differentiation of the syrinx has been described by Em. Wolff. At first the differentiation was equal on both sides and then, when the medium was rich enough when the female hormone was lacking, the hypertrophic growth of the cartilaginous arches occurred. However, this hypertrophy did not occur until the arches on both right and left sides had reached a certain stage of development.

It is tempting to think that female hormone acts *in vivo* by controlling and restraining the utilization of nutrients by the syrinx.

When cultured on synthetic media, the two types of sexual organs, gonads and syringes, react in the same way to the nitrogenous content of the medium.

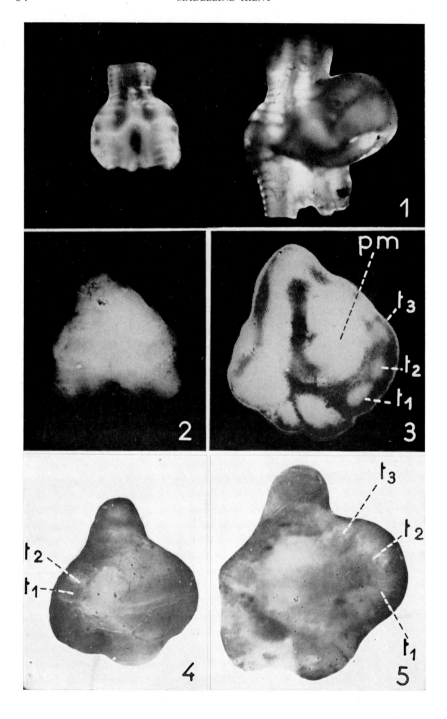

Female morphogenesis requires little while male morphogenesis is more demanding. The sexual morphogenesis of the syrinx of either the male or the female can be completely inverted by altering the available nutrients. With the gonads, only the development of the male gland can be modified. Moreover, this modification never goes beyond the stage of intersexuality.

V. CULTURE OF THE SKIN

Various aspects of the development of the skin have been investigated using synthetic media. These are skin pigmentation (15), the differentiation of the uropygial gland (8), and keratinization of the epidermis (20, 21).

A. Pigmentation of the Dorsal Skin of Chick Embryos *in Vitro*

The feather germs of skin taken from 8-day embryos continued to grow *in vitro* even if the explants were cultured in an amino acid-deficient medium. The addition of different amino acids scarcely altered the results of culture. However, cysteine encouraged survival of the explants.

In contrast to the growth of the feather germs, pigment formation was sensitive to the composition of the culture medium. This was shown when embryonic skin was explanted from either a black or a white strain.

Natural media based on embryo extract were favorable to pigment deposition in the skin of both strains of chickens. Explants from the black strain showed intense pigmentation, those from the white strain showed little pigmentation; the latter formed more pigment if the extract was prepared from older embryos.

Plate IV (Photographs by Em. Wolff)

Fig. 1. Syrinx from an 18-day duck embryo. Female syrinx on the left, male syrinx on the right.

Fig. 2. Genetically male syrinx explanted at $8\frac{1}{2}$ days onto a medium containing only cysteine as the source of nitrogenous material. Culture discontinued after 9 days. The explant is symmetrical.

Fig. 3. Genetically female syrinx explanted at $8\frac{1}{2}$ days onto a minimum medium containing 5 amino acids (arginine, cysteine, methionine, glutamic acid, and histidine). Asymmetry is noticeable with the mamillary protuberance (p.m.) prominent. Culture discontinued after 11 days.

Fig. 4. Genetically female syrinx explanted at $8\frac{1}{2}$ days onto a minimum medium with the amount of cysteine quadrupled. Asymmetry is marked. 12 days culture.

Fig. 5. Genetically female syrinx explanted at $8\frac{1}{2}$ days onto medium C with a raised cysteine content. The asymmetry is typically male. 12 days culture. t_1, t_2, t_3, Cartilaginous arches of the syrinx.

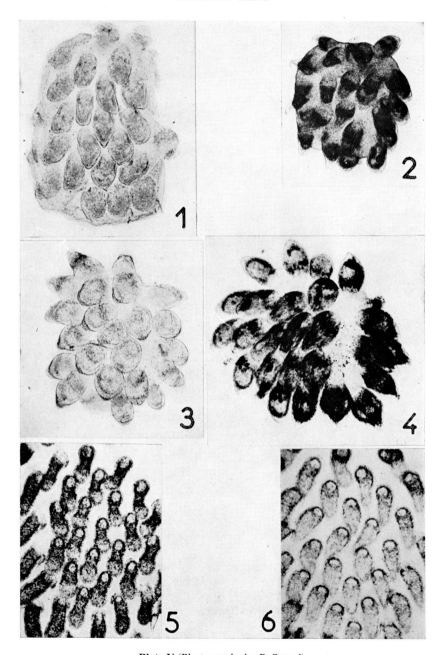

Plate V (Photographs by P. Sengel)

FIG. 1.   Fragment of skin from the Alsace black strain grown for 5 days on synthetic medium B. There is an inhibition of pigment formation (compare with Fig. 2).

1. BLACK STRAIN

The role of the amino acids in solution B (30) in pigment production was studied in the black strain (Alsace black). This solution contained arginine, cysteine, methionine, glutamic acid, lysine, histidine, aspartic acid, proline, and tryptophan. Most of these amino acids inhibited pigmentation. Solution B, and in particular cysteine and methionine, suppressed synthesis of the pigment in skin from the black strain (Plate V, Figs. 1–4). Only arginine was slightly favorable to pigmentation (Plate V, Figs. 5 and 6).

In the absence of all other amino acids, tyrosine could increase the amount of pigment produced in skin from the black strain. In the presence of the amino acids in solution B this action was much less pronounced. When added to a solution of amino acids containing arginine, cysteine, methionine, glutamic acid, histidine, and lysine, tyrosine could overcome the inhibition induced by the sulfhydryl-containing amino acids. An intense pigmentation was induced. This may have been due to the favorable presence of arginine.

2. WHITE STRAIN

Tyrosine also induced pigment production in a white strain of chickens (White Leghorn). When tyrosine was present, 10 times as many melanocytes were seen in the feather germs as in controls grown on medium B without tyrosine (Plate VI, Figs. 1 and 2). The melanocytes that differentiated in the presence of added tyrosine were identical to those seen in the pigmented strain (Plate VI, Fig. 3). After 5 days of culture, pigment was deposited in the epidermal cells, just as it was in the pigmented strain. In this way pieces of skin from the white strain, when grown on medium B plus tyrosine, developed the appearance of skin from the black strain. The degree of pigmentation (115 melanocytes per feather germ) was of the same order as that seen in skin from the black strain when it was grown on a medium containing glucose and inorganic salts but no nitrogenous material.

FIG. 2.   Control to Fig. 1. Skin from the Alsace black strain grown for 5 days on a glucose medium with no nitrogenous material. Normal pigment formation.

FIG. 3.   Fragment of skin from the Alsace black strain grown for 5 days in the presence of cysteine (medium 27). There is inhibition of pigment formation (compare with Fig. 4).

FIG. 4.   Control to Fig. 3. Skin from the Alsace black strain grown for 5 days on a glucose medium with no nitrogenous material. Normal pigment formation.

FIG. 5.   Fragment of skin from the Alsace black strain grown for 5 days in the presence of arginine. Increased pigmentation. (Compare with Fig. 6.)

FIG. 6.   Control to Fig. 5. Skin from the Alsace black strain grown for 5 days on a glucose medium with no nitrogenous material. Pigmentation less marked than in the presence of arginine.

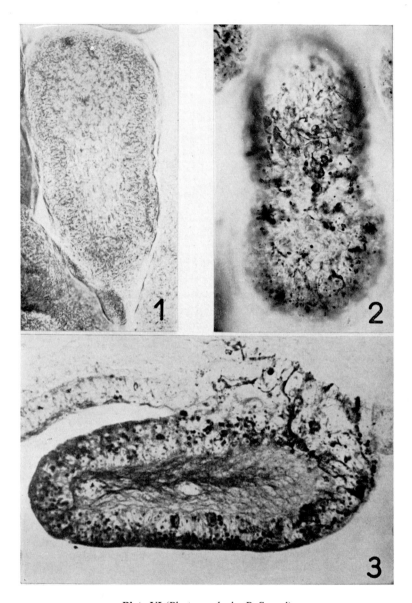

Plate VI (Photographs by P. Sengel)

FIG. 1.   Control to Fig. 2. Feather germ from the White Leghorn strain grown for 5 days on medium B. No pigment is present.

FIG. 2.   Feather germ from the White Leghorn strain grown for 5 days on medium B with added tyrosine. Tyrosine induces the differentiation of many melanocytes (see histological section Fig. 3).

FIG. 3.   Detailed view of a feather germ from the White Leghorn strain grown for 5 days on medium B with added tyrosine. Note the numerous melanocytes transferring their pigment to the epidermal cells.

These facts indicate that of the three factors necessary for the synthesis of melanin, that is, propigment, enzyme, and oxygen, only the propigment is lacking in the white strain. In fact, the white strain certainly contains tyrosinase, since the tyrosine provided in culture was oxidized. As oxygen was also utilized, it seems that the only reason that melanoblasts do not differentiate in this white strain is the absence of free tyrosine in the skin or pigment cells.

By simple modification of a chemically defined medium this mode of culture results in true pigment phenocopies of skin. The presence of tyrosine transforms skin from the white strain into skin having the appearance of that from the black strain. In contrast, cysteine causes skin from the black strain to assume the appearance of skin from the white strain.

B. Differentiation of the Uropygial Gland of the Duck Embryo

The uropygial gland is the only skin gland to be found in birds. The undifferentiated dorsal skin of the tail bud of a 9–10 day duck embryo, cultured on a natural medium containing embryo extract, underwent autodifferentiation to produce, within 8–10 days, the typical glandular invaginations (7).

When no nitrogenous material was available, and the culture medium contained only inorganic salts and glucose, only the rudimentary invaginations continued to deepen and the survival of the explants was limited to a few days. When skin from $9\frac{1}{2}$–10 day embryos was used together with medium C (30) the resulting morphogenesis was comparable to that obtained if a medium based on embryo extract had been used (Plate VII, Fig. 1). Skin taken from 9-day embryos did not differentiate on medium C, containing 21 amino acids, and survived for a shorter time than on the natural medium.

Gomot and Pascal (8) tried to define the role of certain amino acids on the differentiation of the uropygial gland. This work followed that of Em. Wolff on the syrinx, of Stenger-Haffen on the gonads, of Kieny on the tibiotarsus, and of Sengel on the feather germs.

The simplest medium that permitted glandular differentiation, similar to that obtained with a natural medium, contained arginine, methionine, cysteine, glutamic acid, lysine, and histidine (Plate VII, Figs. 2 and 4).

If one of these 6 amino acids was omitted, developmental deficiencies occurred in the explants. These deficiencies varied according to which amino acid was omitted from the solution.

Glutamic acid and arginine were essential for autodifferentiation of the uropygial gland (Plate VII, Figs. 3 and 5). Cysteine and methionine prolonged the survival of the explants permitting better morphogenesis with deeper invaginations.

Lastly, lysine and histidine acted in different ways. The withdrawal of

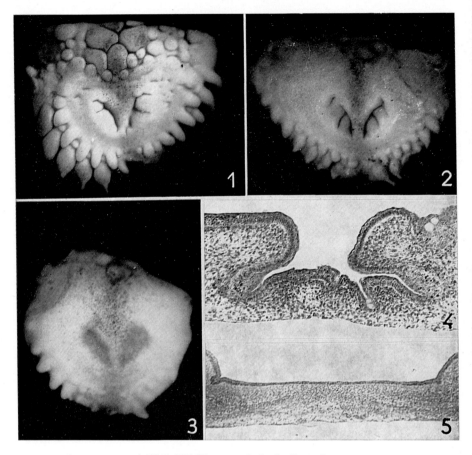

Plate VII (Photographs by L. Gomot)

FIG. 1.   Explant of tail skin from a 10-day duck embryo grown for 5 days on medium C. The invaginations are almost completely closed again. Transverse epidermal folds can be seen at the origin of the gland buds.

FIG. 2.   Dorsal tail skin of a 10-day duck embryo after 5 days of culture on a medium with six amino acids (arginine, cysteine, methionine, glutamic acid, lysine, and histidine). The invaginations are closed as on medium C (compare Fig. 3).

FIG. 3.   Explant of uropygial skin grown for 5 days on the same medium as the explant in Fig. 2 but in the absence of glutamic acid. Development stopped on the second day of culture; many necrotic regions can be seen and the invaginations are blurred.

FIG. 4.   Transverse section of an explant grown under the same conditions as that in Fig. 2. The floor of the invaginations shows areas of epidermal proliferation at the base of the glandular tubules.

FIG. 5.   Transverse section of an explant grown under the same conditions as that in Fig. 3. No folds have appeared on the floor of the invaginations and only the lateral borders are slightly raised. Glutamic acid is essential to the autodifferentiation of the uropygial invaginations (compare Fig. 4).

either from the synthetic solution produced a reduction in the percentage of invaginations.

Used as the sole source of nitrogen, glutamic acid permitted only a short survival, although it was essential for glandular differentiation. Meanwhile, cysteine, which was not indispensable to morphogenesis, prolonged the survival of the explants.

As in the cases of the syrinx, the gonads, the tibiotarsus, and the dorsal skin, the ability to utilize the amino acids depended on the presence of glucose. If glucose was absent from a synthetic medium, no matter what else it contained, the explants of the tail bud did not survive, and became necrotic in less than 24 hours.

C. Keratinization of the Epidermis of the Tarsometatarsal Skin in Chick Embryos

Keratinization of the tarsometatarsal skin of 8–10 day chick embryos has been studied by Wessells (20, 21), who used Trowell's method (17) with Waymouth's synthetic medium MB 752/1 (19). This medium contains 19 amino acids and 11 vitamins, besides hypoxanthine, minerals, salts, and glucose.

The main stages of normal differentiation of tarsometatarsal skin *in vivo* are as follows. After 9–10 days of incubation the epidermis is composed of three layers of cells. At 11 days birefringent material appears in the superficial layer, the peridermis. After 14 days keratohyalin particles appear in the peridermis, whilst tonofibrils differentiate in the underlying layer of subperidermis. Finally, after 16 to 17 days the true cornified layer forms by the flattening and keratinization of the outer layers of the epidermis.

1. Development of Skin Taken at 11–12 Days

Tarsometatarsal skin taken before 10 days of incubation did not differentiate in the synthetic medium used. However, 11–12 day skin differentiated *in vitro* and reached a stage corresponding to 15–16 days of normal incubation. Thus the tonofibrils differentiated but the cornified layer did not develop. Complete keratinization was obtained by trebling the amount of methionine in the medium. In contrast, if, methionine was omitted from medium MN 752/1, the explants did not survive longer than 3–4 days. The other sulfur-containing compounds in this medium were cysteine, cystine, glutathione, and magnesium sulfate. Thus methionine is an essential amino acid for the survival of the skin and for the completion of keratinization.

Neither cysteine nor cystine was necessary for the development of the tonofibrils but their presence encouraged differentiation of the cornified layer.

The basal layers and superficial layers of the epidermis did not have the same requirements for sulfur-containing amino acids. The cytoplasm of the basal layers where keratin fibrils are synthesized required methionine. The superficial layers, where the transition was from the fibrous state to the cornified state, required the presence of cystine and cysteine.

2. EXPERIMENTAL INDUCTION OF KERATINIZATION IN 8–10 DAY SKIN

As with other organs, it is difficult to obtain differentiation of the skin *in vitro*. However, once it has differentiated it is easy to maintain in culture. One of the aims of organ culture is to discover the factors that will induce differentiation *in vitro*.

It has been shown that 8–10 day skin would not differentiate normally in medium MB 752/1. Neither keratohyalin particles nor tonofibrils were formed but the skin showed atypical swellings that resulted from disorganized growth of the basal layer. Bartels (1) showed that thyroxine injected into the embryo hastened epidermal differentiation, and Wessells (21) suggested that keratinization was induced by the onset of thyroid activity at 10–11 days of incubation.

To prove the hypothesis, Wessells added 200 μg/100 ml of thyroxine to his basic culture medium. Under these conditions, instead of proliferating into a disorganized mass of cells, the epidermis progressively acquired all its characteristics. Keratohyalin particles appeared in the peridermis and tonofibrils appeared in the subperidermis. Finally, complete keratinization of the outer layers took place.

Short contact with a high concentration of thyroxine (1 hour at 2,000 μg/100 ml) induced partial differentiation, but never resulted in the formation of cornified layers.

Thus thyroxine could induce the onset of differentiation of tarsometatarsal skin of 8–10 days of incubation. Its activity was not limited to the initiation of keratinization. The continued presence of thyroxine in the medium was necessary for complete keratinization. Wessell's experiments also showed that 8-day skin was already capable of differentiation. That keratinization *in vivo* does not begin until 11 days is probably due to the lack of thyroxine in the embryonic circulation.

VI. THYROID CULTURE

Undifferentiated chick embryo thyroid gland retained a typically inactive structure of cell cords when it was cultured on Parker's medium (6) 199 or Earle's medium (6) 1098 (29) (Plate VIII, Figs. 2 and 3). Only medium C (30) containing 21 amino acids in high concentration (see methods) allowed differentiation of the gland with abundant formation of the thyroid

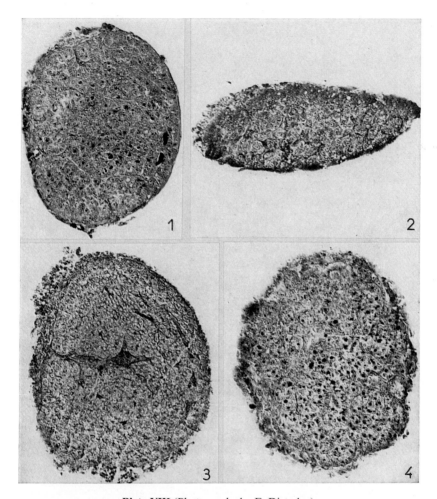

Plate VIII (Photographs by F. Dieterlen)

FIG. 1.   Thyroid gland from a 7-day chick embryo grown for 3 days on the "standard" natural medium of Wolff and Haffen. Droplets of intracellular colloid are present. After this period of culture, the explant has not yet developed the typical follicular structure.

FIG. 2.   Thyroid gland from a 7-day chick embryo grown for 3 days on the synthetic medium B (diluted by half). The thyroid has not differentiated. The cells are small and closely packed and are arranged in compact cords.

FIG. 3.   Thyroid gland of a 7-day chick embryo grown for 3 days on the synthetic medium 199 of Parker *et al.* This has the same appearance as the thyroid in Fig. 2.

FIG. 4.   Thyroid gland of a 7-day chick embryo grown for 3 days on synthetic medium C (undiluted). Quite large intracellular droplets of thyroid colloid have formed throughout the explant.

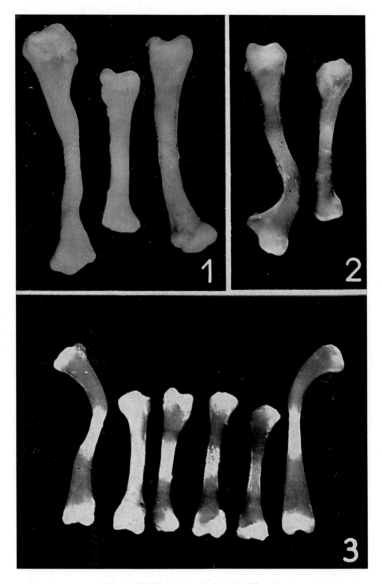

Plate IX (Photographs by M. Kieny)

FIG. 1.   Comparison of the development of 7-day chick embryo tibiotarsus grown on (from left to right) standard natural medium, glucose medium with no added nitrogenous material, and medium B with added p-aminobenzoic acid. Growth is significant on the synthetic medium, but never equals that obtained on the standard natural medium.

FIG. 2.   Tibiotarsus from a 7-day chick embryo grown for 7 days on the minimum medium with added p-aminobenzoic acid (left) and on the same medium without p-

colloid, even when no iodine was present in the medium (Plate VIII, Fig. 4). This indicated that the iodine concentrated by the embryonic organ before it was explanted was sufficient for the gland for several days.

These results demonstrated that the thyroid of the chick embryo will show autodifferentiation on an appropriate synthetic medium. The beginning of hormone synthesis was established in the absence of pituitary control.

VII. CULTURE OF THE TIBIOTARSUS

A 7-day chick embryo tibiotarsus continued to grow in length and weight when explanted onto a natural medium containing chick embryo extract. The morphogenetic processes that accompanied this growth resulted in the final modeling of the bone. The tibiotarsus autodifferentiated and developed as in the normal embryo, but the process occurred more slowly (Plate IX, Fig. 1).

The tibiotarsus is thus of use in the study of the nutritional requirements for growth *in vitro*.

The analysis of the nutritional requirements for nitrogenous materials was carried out in two ways. The first method (11, 12) involved adding selected substances (amino acids and vitamins) that had a favorable effect on the development of the tibiotarsus to media that contained no nitrogenous material, or that contained only a few amino acids. In this way it was possible to define the minimum requirements of the tibiotarsus *in vitro*.

In the second method, amino acids were removed one by one from a complex mixture containing 59 ingredients (amino acids, vitamins, and other organic compounds). In this way, it was possible to find the effect of the deficiency of a single amino acid on the growth of the tibiotarsus (3).

A. Simple Synthetic Media

These experiments were carried out by Kieny (11, 12).

The first synthetic media used were the solutions B and C of Wolff *et al.* (30). When added to the culture mixture, neither medium was adequate for the survival or growth of a tibiotarsus from one 7-day chick embryo. It was necessary to add a growth factor which would enable the tibiotarsus to utilize the amino acids provided. *p*-Aminobenzoic acid (0.002 mg per 100 ml

---

aminobenzoic acid (right). This vitamin encourages the development of the embryonic tibiotarsus *in vitro.*

FIG. 3. Action of different hexose sugars on the development of 7½-day chick embryo tibiotarsus grown on the minimum synthetic medium with added *p*-aminobenzoic acid. The media contained (from left to right) added mannose, added galactose, added fructose, added sorbose, no additional sugar, and added glucose. It is clear that only mannose can replace glucose completely.

of Tyrode's solution) stimulated growth in length and an increase in weight (Plate IX, Figs. 1 and 2).

It could not be shown that p-aminobenzoic acid had the same effect on the embryo under normal conditions. It could be replaced by folic acid, biotin, cocarboxylase, dicarnitine (vitamin B_1), or carnitine. When p-aminobenzoic acid and one of these other compounds were added to the medium together, there was no summation of the effects.

1. Amino Acid Requirements

The specific requirements of the tibiotarsus were defined by testing many combinations of amino acids. Glutamic acid was essential. In its absence, the explant died rapidly, regardless of the other components of the medium. Methionine, lysine, and histidine were active and their effects were additive to that of glutamic acid.

Other amino acids with smaller activity were added singly or together to the basic minimum medium that contained arginine, methionine, glutamic acid, histidine, and p-aminobenzoic acid. These amino acids were serine, valine, threonine, and taurine.

Other amino acids were favorable if they were added singly to a synthetic medium. When they were added together there was a decrease in growth. When added separately, lysine and histidine induced good development, but when they were added together there was a decrease in the growth of the tibiotarsus. Similarly, cysteine could be used alone to increase survival and growth of the explant, but it hindered growth when other amino acids were present.

It should be noted that in these combinations of a few amino acids, the action of one given acid depended very closely on the composition of the medium.

2. Sugar Requirements

Glucose was an essential nutrient in synthetic media; the explants became totally necrotic within 24 hours if glucose was absent. Among the carbohydrates that have been tested, only mannose could replace glucose (Plate IX, Fig. 3).

In conclusion, it seems that the described synthetic media were not as effective as a natural medium based on embryo extract. On a natural medium, the growth was accompanied by a considerable increase in the total nitrogen content of the explant (55–91%). On synthetic media, despite increases in length and weight, the nitrogen content was not increased. The growth in length must exceed 50% after 5 days of culture if there is to be a measurable increase in the total nitrogen. On synthetic media, growth never exceeds this amount.

B. Complex Synthetic Media

The experiments described above show that synthetic minimum media ensure a certain amount of development of cartilaginous rudiments. However, synthetic media are not as effective as natural media based on embryo extract.

In H. B. Fell's laboratory a group of investigators has been attempting to define the nutritional requirements of the tibiotarsus, and to find the point at which a complex synthetic medium becomes equivalent to a natural medium (Biggers *et al.*).

The first tested medium 770 of Healy, Fisher, and Parker (9), developed for culturing mouse cells. This contains 20 amino acids, 17 vitamins (A, B, C, D, E, and K), cholesterol, coenzymes (NAD, NADP, and coenzyme A), and other organic compounds.

When tibiotarsi from $6\frac{1}{2}$–7 day chick embryos were explanted by Chen's technique (5), they increased in length by 20%, there was slight morphological differentiation, and they survived for one week. These results were poor when compared with those obtained using a natural medium.

The first improvement in culture conditions was made by increasing the glucose content from 1 to 2.25%. The second improvement was made by using only L-amino acids (medium 858, see Section II) and by the addition of 7 derivatives of nitrogenous bases (3).

1. SUGAR REQUIREMENTS

When the glucose content was increased in medium 858, and particularly in medium 929 (see Section II), explants of tibiotarsus behaved as on a natural medium. After 10 days' culture there was an increase in length of 120%. Only mannose could replace glucose entirely. Galactose and fructose were ineffective.

2. AMINO ACID REQUIREMENTS

Amino acids were removed singly from medium 929 so that their effect on growth could be determined. Eleven amino acids were found to be essential (arginine, lysine, histidine, methionine, valine, isoleucine, threonine, tyrosine, phenylalanine, leucine, and tryptophan). The absence of certain amino acids (threonine, arginine, and tryptophan) greatly affected growth, and this effect was seen within 48 hours of culture. The absence of other amino acids, such as lysine, showed its effects much later.

Nine amino acids were not essential. These were hydroxyproline, alanine, serine, proline, glycine, cystine, cysteine, glutamic acid, and aspartic acid.

3. SYNTHESIS OF AMINO ACIDS FROM GLUCOSE

Using a medium containing glucose labeled with ^{14}C and many of the compounds from medium 858, Biggers et al. were able to show that glucose could be used as the precursor for six nonessential amino acids. These were alanine, aspartic acid, glutamic acid, serine, glycine, and proline.

Very complex synthetic media are apparently as effective as natural ones. However, when medium 929 was compared with a natural medium based on cockerel serum, there were still differences to be observed in the tibiotarsus. These differences were based on three criteria: an increase in length, an increase in weight, and an increase in the total nitrogen content. While there was no difference between the increases in length on these two media, the increase in weight and the increase in total nitrogen were always smaller on the synthetic medium.

Recently, Biggers et al. (4) have described a relatively simple medium that gave an increase in length, an increase in weight, and an increase in the total DNA content with the embryonic tibiotarsus from chick and turkey embryos, and with the embryonic tibia from rats and mice.

This medium contained 12 amino acids (all the essential amino acids plus cysteine), 11 vitamins, glutamine, and adenosine. Using this medium, Biggers et al. showed the importance of both the combined amino acids and glutamine.

Cartilaginous rudiments could not increase in length or in total weight on a medium lacking amino acids or glutamine.

C. Comparison between the Two Methods

As a result of experiments based on the two methods described above, the amino acids have been classified as essential or nonessential (see Table V).

The results agree for 10 amino acids. Arginine, lysine, histidine, methionine, valine, isoleucine, and threonine are essential; proline, cysteine, and aspartic acid are not.

As regards the results that do not agree, five amino acids are essential in simple media but not in complex ones. Four of these (glutamic acid, alanine, serine, and glycine) can be synthesized from glucose, as shown by Biggers et al. This sugests that in rich media the tibiotarsus does not need these four amino acids since it can synthesize them from the high concentration of glucose that is present. In contrast, the nutritional conditions of simple media are such that these amino acids cannot be synthesized and must be provided in the medium.

Finally, the results obtained from the two methods disagree for five amino acids. These are hydroxyproline, tyrosine, phenylalanine, leucine, and tryptophan.

TABLE V

AMINO ACID REQUIREMENTS OF CHICK EMBRYO TIBIOTARSUS WHEN STUDIED BY TWO DIFFERENT METHODS (4, 12)

Amino acid	Essential amino acids		Nonessential amino acids	
	Simple	Complex	Simple	Complex
Arginine	+	+		
Lysine	+	+		
Histidine	+	+		
Methionine	+	+		
Valine	+	+		
Isoleucine	+	+		
Threonine	+	+		
Proline			+	+
Cysteine			+	+
Aspartic acid			+	+
Glutamic acid	+			+
Hydroxyproline	+			+
Alanine	+			+
Serine	+			+
Glycine	+			+
Tyrosine		+	+	
Phenylalanine		+	+	
Leucine		+	+	
Tryptophan		+	+	

VIII. CONCLUSIONS

Organ culture techniques using synthetic media have made an important contribution to the knowledge of the nutritional requirements of embryonic organs, but this is not their only use. It is possible to study under ideally simple conditions the effects of a single factor on the mechanisms of differentiation. Thus, with skin, it has been possible to show the effects of tyrosine on pigmentation and of thyroxine on keratinization. In the syrinx, simple changes in nutritive conditions have been shown to induce male or female differentiation. In cultures of whole blastoderms, the suppression of some amino acids (by the use of antagonists) causes disturbances in development, as in the case of phenylalanine which affects the nervous system, and leucine which affects the muscles (10).

Only a short period of embryonic development can be investigated using the technique of organ culture on synthetic media. This is usually the period between the determination and the differentiation of an organ rudiment. Usually an undifferentiated organ is cultured up to the stage of morphological, histological, and functional differentiation. The techniques used do not allow embryonic organs to survive and grow indefinitely like cell cultures (6).

One of the main characteristics of organ culture as opposed to cell culture is the amount of reserve nutrient material carried by the explanted organs. This explains the ability of explanted organs to survive on minimum media that contain only a few ingredients. As far as the tibiotarsus is concerned, these resources seem to undergo marked seasonal variations. In the spring the increase in the growth of the tibiotarsus is optimum (37%) on a given medium. In winter, on the same medium, the increase in growth is markedly decreased (18%). This suggests that in the "poor" season, the tibiotarsus possesses fewer reserves of enzymes, vitamins, and other nutrients than it has in the "good" season (12) (Fig. 1).

Until now, the morphological processes studied using culture on synthetic media have been devoted to the investigation of the appearance of certain new tissues from the initial explants rather than to the increase in the mass of the living tissues.

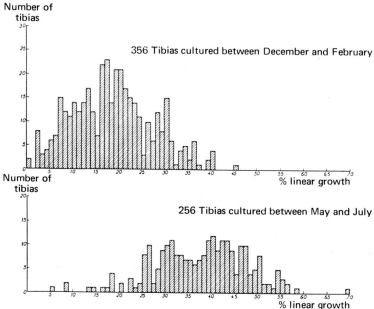

FIG. 1.   Histogram showing the linear growth of 612 tibiotarsi explanted on a synthetic medium containing glucose, 6 amino acids, and *p*-aminobenzoic acid in "good" (top) and "poor" (bottom) seasons.

BIBLIOGRAPHY

1. Bartels E. A. Morphogenetische Wirkungen des Schilddrüsenhormons auf das Integument von Vogelembryonen. *Roux' Arch. Entw.-mech.*, 1943, **142**, 763–816.
2. Bergmann M. and Niemann C. On blood fibrine. A contribution to the problem of protein structure. *J. Biol. chem.*, 1936, **115**, 77–85.
3. Biggers J. D., Webb M., Parker R. C. and Healy G. M. Cultivation of embryonic chick bones on chemically defined media. *Nature, London*, 1957, **180**, 825–828.
4. Biggers J. D., Gwatkin R. B. L. and Heyner S. Growth of embryonic avian and mammalian tibiae on a relatively simple chemically defined medium. *Exp. Cell. Res.*, 1961, **25**, 41–58.
5. Chen J. M. The cultivation in fluid medium of organised liver, pancreas and other tissues of fœtal rats. *Exp. Cell. Res.*, 1954, **7**, 518–529.
6. Evans V. J., Bryant J. C., Mc Quilkin W. T., Fioramonti M. C., Sanford K. K., Westfall B. B. and Earle W. R. Studies of nutrient media for tissue cells *in vitro*. II: On improved protein-free chemically defined medium for long term cultivation of strain L 929 cells. *Canc. Res.*, 1956, **16**, 87–94.
7. Gomot L. Contribution à l'étude du développement embryonnaire de la glande uropygienne chez le Canard. *Arch. Anat. micr. Morph. exp.*, 1959, **48**, 63–141.
8. Gomot L. and Pascal P. Recherches des besoins de la peau dorsale du bourgeon caudal de l'embryon de Canard pendant la différenciation des invaginations uro-pygiennes en culture *in vitro* sur milieux synthétiques. *Ann. Scient. Univ. Besançon*, 1962, **17**, 67–85.
9. Healy G. M., Fisher D. C. and Parker R. C. Nutrition of animal cells in tissue culture. Synthetic medium No. 858. *Proc. Soc. exp. Biol. Med.*, 1954, **89**, 71–77.
10. Herrmann H. Interference of amino acid analogues with normal embryonic development. *J. Embryol. exp. Morph.*, 1953, **1**, 291–295.
11. Kieny M. Les besoins nutritifs spécifiques des tibias d'embryon de Poulet en culture *in vitro* sur milieux synthétiques. *C. R. Soc. Biol.*, 1955, **149**, 418–421.
12. Kieny M. Contribution à l'étude des besoins nutritifs des tibias embryonnaires d'Oiseau cultivés en milieux naturels et synthétiques. *Arch. Anat. micr. Morph. exp.*, 1958, **47**, 86–169.
13. Morton J. H., Morgan J. F. and Parker R. C. Nutrition of animal cells in tissue culture. Initial studies on a synthetic medium. *Proc. Soc. exp. Biol. Med.*, 1950, **73**, 1–8.
14. Rose W. C. The nutritive significance of the amino acids. *Physiol. Rev.*, 1938, **18**, 109–136.
15. Sengel P. Recherches expérimentales sur la différenciation des germes plumaires et du pigment de la peau de l'embryon de Poulet en culture *in vitro*. *Ann. Sc. nat. Zool.*, 1958, 11ᵉ série, **20**, 431–514.
16. Stenger-Haffen K. Étude des besoins nutritifs des gonades embryonnaires d'Oiseau cultivées en milieux synthétiques. *Arch. Anat. micr. Morph. exp.*, 1957, **46**, 521–607.
17. Trowell O. A. A modified technique for organ culture *in vitro*. *Exp. Cell. Res.*, 1954, **6**, 246–248.
18. Trowell O. A. The culture of lymph nodes in synthetic media. *Exp. Cell. Res.*, 1955, **9**, 258–276.
19. Waymouth C. Rapid proliferation of sublines of NCTC clone 929 (strain L) mouse cell in a simple chemically defined medium. (MB 752/1). *J. Nation. Canc. Inst.*, 1959, **22**, 1003–1015.

20. Wessells N. K. An analysis of chick epidermal differentiation *in situ* and *in vitro* in chemically defined media. *Dev. Biol.*, 1961, **3**, 355–389.

21. Wessells N. K. Thyroxine initiation of epidermal differentiation as studied *in vitro* in chemically defined medium. *Exp. Cell. Res.*, 1961, **24**, 131–142.

22. Wolff Em. La différenciation sexuelle normale et le conditionnement hormonal des caractères sexuels somatiques précoces, tubercule génital et syrinx, chez l'embryon de Canard. *Bull. Biol.*, 1950, **84**, 121–193.

23. Wolff Em. Analyse des besoins nutritifs d'un organe embryonnaire, la syrinx d'Oiseau, cultivée en milieu synthétique. *Arch. Anat. micr. Morph. exp.*, 1957, **46**, 407–468.

24. Wolff Em. La différenciation sexuelle de la syrinx de l'embryon de Canard, explantée *in vitro* sur des milieux chimiquement définis. *Bull. Biol.*, 1957, **91**, 271–283.

25. Wolff Em. and Lutz-Ostertag Y. Free-martinisme spontané et expérimental chez l'embryon de Canard. *Arch. Anat. micr. Morph. exp.*, 1961, **50**, 439–468.

26. Wolff Et. and Haffen K. Sur une méthode de cultures d'organes embryonnaires *in vitro*. *Tex. Rep. Biol. Med.*, 1952, **10**, 463–472.

27. Wolff Et. and Haffen K. Sur le développement et la différenciation sexuelle des gonades embryonnaires d'Oiseau en culture *in vitro*. *J. exp. Zool.*, 1952, **119**, 381–404.

28. Wolff Et. and Haffen K. Sur la différenciation sexuelle des gonades embryonnaires de l'embryon de Poulet en culture *in vitro*. *Ann. Endocrinol.*, 1952, **13**, 724–731.

29. Wolff Et., Haffen K. and Dieterlen F.—Influence des états nutritionnels sur la différenciation et le fonctionnement des glandes endocrines embryonnaires. *Ann. Nutr. Alim.*, 1960, **14**, 11–29.

30. Wolff Et., Haffen K., Kieny M. and Wolff Em. Essais de culture *in vitro* d'organes embryonnaires en milieux synthétiques. *J. Embr. exp. Morph.*, 1953, **1**, 55–84.

31. Wolff Et. and Wolff Em. Le déterminisme de la différenciation sexuelle de la syrinx de Canard en culture *in vitro*. *Bull. Biol.*, 1952, **86**, 325–350.

ADDENDUM

Since the publication of the first part of this chapter, numerous new data have been obtained on the behavior of many organs cultivated in synthetic media. Among them, those concerning the skin, the bone, and the teeth are of particular interest. The addendum which follows will deal with the effect of various environmental factors on the survival and differentiation of these organs.

I. SKIN

A. The Effect of Excess Vitamin A on Keratinization

The addition to the natural medium of excess vitamin A has a profound effect on the explants of 13-day shank and foot skin (19): keratinization is inhibited, epidermis undergoes a mucous metaplasia. The biochemical investigation on keratinization and vitamin A action on the epidermis was attempted in a chemically defined system [modified BGJ medium (7); Table A–I] by Rothberg. In contrast to natural medium, defined medium supplemented with vitamin A dissolved in ethanol does not produce epidermal changes. To obtain the hypervitaminosis A effects, it was necessary to introduce a small quantity of purified serum albumin (0.5 mg/ml) into the medium, according to Lasnitzki (49), who investigated the effect of excess vitamin A on mouse postnatal vaginal epithelium grown in a chemically defined medium and found that a serum carrier was needed. Thus stabilized and carried by a protein solution, the vitamin A produces the same effect on 13-day metatarsal skin in defined medium as in natural media: arrest of keratinization and formation of mucous material. Compared to the effect on chick embryonic skin, vitamin A has only a reduced antikeratinizing action on fetal mouse skin grown in defined media (57).

With this synthetic system on hand, the study of the interrelationship between epidermal protein synthesis and keratinization should yield precise data on the mode of action of the vitamin A.

II. BONES

A. Generalities on the Behavior of Long Bones in Liquid Media

Schryver (69) compared the increase in length, wet weight, dry weight, DNA content, and chondroitin sulfate content of 8-day tibiotarsi grown in medium BGJ (Table A-I) with that of older tibiotarsi *in ovo*. The data showed

103

TABLE A-I

Composition of Medium BL_1 and BGJ (mg/100 ml)

	BL_1	BGJ		BL_1	BGJ
I. Amino acids and related compounds					
L-Lysine HCl	7	24	L-Valine	2.5	6.5
L-Histidine HCl	2	15	L-Aspartic acid	3.0	—
L-Arginine HCl	7	7.5	L-Alanine	2.5	—
L-Glutamic acid	7.5	—	L-Proline	4.0	—
L-Tryptophan	1.0	4.0	L-Hydroxyproline	1.0	—
L-Phenylalanine	2.5	5.0	L-Tyrosine	4.0	4.0
L-Methionine	1.5	5.0	L-Cystine	2.0	
L-Serine	2.5	—	L-Cysteine HCl	26.0	9.0
L-Threonine	3.0	7.5	Glycine	5.0	—
L-Leucine	6.0	5.0	L-Glutamine	10.0	20.0
L-Isoleucine	2.0	3.0	Glutathione	1.0	—
II. Vitamins					
Pyridoxine HCl	0.0025	—	Riboflavin	—	0.02
Pyridoxal	0.0025	0.02	Calcium pantothenate	—	0.02
Biotine	0.001	0.02	Vitamin B_{12}	—	0.004
Folic acid	0.001	0.02	Vitamin A acetate	0.01	—
Choline chloride	0.05	5.0	Calciferol	0.01	—
meso-Inositol	0.005	0.02	Tocopherol		
Nicotinamide	—	2.0	phosphate	0.001	0.1
Thiamine HCl	—	0.4	Vitamin K	0.001	—
p-Aminobenzoic acid	0.005	—	L-Ascorbic acid	5.0	—
III. Nucleosides					
Deoxyadenosine	1.0	—	Deoxycytidine HCl	1.0	—
Deoxyguanosine	1.0	—	Thymidine	1.0	—
IV. Coenzymes					
Diphosphopyridine			Flavin adenine		
nucleotide	0.7	—	dinucleotide	0.1	—
Triphosphopyridine			Cocarboxylase	0.1	—
nucleotide	0.1	—	Uridine triphosphate	0.1	—
Coenzyme A	0.25	—			
V. Salts					
Sodium chloride	800.0	800.0	Potassium chloride	40.0	53.0
Magnesium sulfate			Calcium chloride	14.0	—
(7 H_2O)	20.0	20.0	Calcium lactate	—	55.5
Disodium dihydrogen			Ferric nitrate	0.072	—
phosphate	6.0	—	Sodium bicarbonate	140.0	350.0
Potassium dihydrogen					
phosphate	6.0	16.0			
VI. Miscellaneous					
Glucose	225–400	500	Streptomycin	10.0	5.0
Phenol red	2.0	2.0	Penicillin	—	10,000 units

that, despite an important gain, the rate and magnitude of growth are slower *in vitro* than *in vivo*. Furthermore, the organs reveal a progressive decline in their dry weight/wet weight ratio. This phenomenon, at first described by Biggers (2, 3) on medium BL_1 (Table A-I), seems to be related to an abnormal water uptake after a 5-day cultivation period, leading to a deficient matrix; this deficiency is also visualized by the chondroitin sulfate/dry weight ratio which increases when bone is grown *in vitro*, while it remains approximately stationary *in ovo*. We shall see below that ascorbic acid may prevent these deficiencies.

It has been shown, however, that the medium BGJ, which is quite adequate for 7- to 8-day embryonic chick tibiotarsi, is not sufficient for larger 11- to 12-day bones. The medium must be supplemented with some nonessential amino acids, folinic acid, orthophosphate, and specially with a high dose of ascorbic acid (200 μg/ml) (28, 30). Thus, the growth set up in a 6-day period *in vitro* is equivalent to the growth in a 2-day period *in ovo*. Similar results have been obtained by cultivating somewhat younger 10-day tibiotarsi on a slightly modified medium 858 (see Table III, main part) (13). After a 12-day cultivation period, the chemical composition of the rudiments is about the same as that of a 12-day tibiotarsus *in ovo* (Table A-II).

TABLE A-II

GROWTH AND CHEMICAL COMPOSITION OF 10-DAY EMBRYONIC TIBIAE AFTER 12 DAYS
in Vitro COMPARED TO THAT AFTER 2 MORE DAYS *in Ovo*
(Prepared from the data of Chokshi and Ramakrishnan, 13)

	Age of the tibiae		
	10 Days *(in ovo)*	10 Days + 12 days *in vitro*	12 Days *(in ovo)*
Length (mm)	7.6	13.0	10.9
Wet weight (mg)	3.6	10.8	12.2
Dry weight (mg)	0.38	0.96	1.47
Calcium (μg)	9.8	35.4	57.4
Phosphorus (μg)	7.7	18.7	34.8
Nitrogen (μg)	11.7	32.1	88.0
Ca/P	1.28	1.89	1.65
Ca/N	0.85	1.10	0.65
Citric acid (μg)	1.06	0.00	3.23
Hexosamine (μg)	12.0	26.8	Unknown (197 at 14 days)

As concerns the nutritional requirements of long bones grown *in vitro* on synthetic media, a comparison between the results obtained in semisolid media and the ones derived from the use of liquid media has already been done and various discrepancies have been explained (46, 47). The comparison between both methods indicates furthermore that the choice of a reference medium remains arbitrary. This is particularly cogent with the findings concerning glutamic acid to which a role as precursor of collagen proline and hydroxyproline has been recently ascribed (40). In a mixture of a small number of ingredients, glutamic acid is required for survival and growth (44, 45). However, its omission from complex medium 858 does not affect growth (10). But, when the number of ingredients is lowered from 60 to 37 (medium BGJ), then its improving action on growth can again be demonstrated (4, 5). All these results show that amino acid requirements depend on the qualitative composition of the medium.

Besides, the concentration of a given substance within the medium has its importance, too. Let us take glutamine, for example. Biggers (5, 6) showed that the responses in length, wet weight, and dry weight are highly dependent on the concentration of glutamine, within a range from 1 to 25 mg/ml medium. In her experiments, the author (45) reported that glutamine, which was employed at a very low concentration (0.16 mg/ml), had no beneficial effect on growth. It may well be that the latter concentration was too low to produce any measurable increase of growth.

B. Environmental Factors on Intercellular Material

This part will deal with extracellular material of cartilage (long bone) and bone (long bone and skull) which is constituted by protein-polysaccharides and collagen secreted by chondroblasts as well as by osteoblasts. Explants from embryonic chicken and rats have been grown in chemically defined media to which has been added a substance which acts upon one or another component of the matrix. Therefore, the numerous results have been grouped in two sections, those concerning the protein-polysaccharides and those concerning the collagen.

1. PROTEIN-POLYSACCHARIDES

The chondroitin sulfate-protein complex of cartilage, chondromucoid, is made up of sulfated glucosaminoglycans intimately associated with 10 to 20% of noncollagenous protein. The chemical composition of the former is uronic acid, sulfate, and hexosamine. Biggers, Lawson, Lucy, and Webb (8) showed from studies on extraction with trichloroacetic acid, that chick embryonic limb bones contain at least three glycosaminoglycans: chondroitin sulfate A, a polysaccharide characterized by a high content of glucosamine (similar to orosomucoid), and keratosulfate.

a. Action of Proteolytic Enzymes. The question is whether the cells may replace the glycosaminoglycans after the intercellular matrix of the tissues has been depleted from them. The method chosen is enzymatic depletion, the enzyme being added directly in the synthetic medium (papain or hyaluronidase) or an enzyme release being provoked in the tissues by the presence of vitamin A in excess or by sucrose in the medium. The action of three of these factors had been studied in biological media: Fell and Thomas (27) and Girard (32) for papain; Paff and Seifter (55) for testicular hyaluronidase; Fell and Mellanby (26) and Hebertson (39) for excess of vitamin A. (See Chapter of F. Dieterlen.)

Papain. Vegetable protease papain acts against the linkage region of the protein polysaccharide liberating the glycosaminoglycans from the protein moiety of the ground substance. Its effect has been studied on 11- to 12-day embryonic chick tibiotarsi grown on a modified (by Fitton-Jackson), BGJ medium for older embryonic bones (11). When papain is administered for a 24-hour period, large amounts of glycosaminoglycans are released from the tissues. This release is not accompanied by a loss of collagen, whose status remains practically unchanged. In response to the loss of the glycosaminoglycans from the matrix, increased amounts of precursor hexosamine and polymerized glycosaminoglycans are produced by the explants during its recovery (Fig. A-1).

The variations of the histological structure of the explants agree with the biochemical data. After the 24-hour treatment, the metachromasia disappears completely. After depletion of their chondroitin sulfate and their keratosulfate, the cartilage and the ossified portions of the low-treated rudiments (8 μg/ml), within 48 hours, have completely restored their metachromatic material. The restoration is more difficult during recovery from the highest dose level at 80 μg/ml. Indeed, the newly synthesized macromolecules are not held within the tissues and are released into the medium (Fig. A-1D), because the matrix during the first 2 days of recovery is structurally unable to accommodate these macromolecules. Bosmann assumes that the network of the remaining collagen fibers (about 50% of the cells are lost) is not sufficient to retain the cells in their necessary structural configuration. Subsequently, the treated explants increase in length and weight. New collagen fibers are produced, correct glycosaminoglycans are synthesized and incorporated into the matrix. It must be noted that the explants never lost their normal shape.

This investigation demonstrates that depletion of a macromolecular constituent of the extracellular environment induces an increased rate of synthesis of the lost macromolecules by the tissue.

Hyaluronidase. As papain, hyaluronidase acts against a specific component of the matrix, chondroitin sulfate. Two-thirds of the hexosamine-containing material is removed from 11- to 12-day embryonic chick tibiotarsi grown during a 36- to 48-hour period in the presence of hyaluronidase (28, 29, 31).

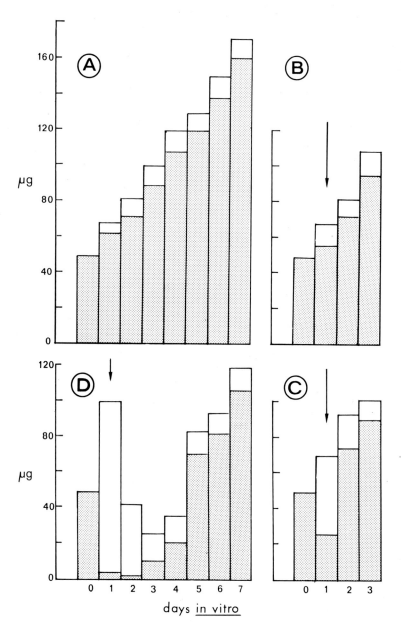

Fig. A-1. Histograms showing the effects of various levels of papain on the hexosamine content per explant. A, control; B, 1.6 μg/ml; C, 8 μg/ml; D, 80 μg/ml. The shaded area represents the amount of hexosamine present in the ossified and the cartilaginous portions of the explant. The unshaded area represents the amount of hexosamine released in the synthetic medium per explant. The arrow indicates that the enzyme was present for the first 24 hours only; control medium thereafter. Prepared from data of Bosmann (11).

When the treated explants are allowed to recover in normal synthetic medium, the cells reestablish their normal environment by replacing the lost macromolecules at an increased rate of synthesis. It takes about 5 days to obtain a similar content of hexosamine to that observed in the controls.

In contrast to the papain-treated rudiments, metachromasia is never completely lost in the hyaluronidase-treated ones, perhaps because keratosulfates are not attacked. Besides, it is interesting to note that the two enzymes, papain and hyaluronidase, each one digesting a different part of the protein polysaccharide complex, induce similar patterns of rapid replacement of the lost intercellular components. When the repair is complete, the rates of synthesis return to normal.

Hypervitaminosis A. The work on the action of excess vitamin A provides an example in which organ culture method has proved ideal for the elucidation of a physiological problem. Excess vitamin A causes the disappearance of metachromatic material from cartilage and bone matrix in defined as in biological media (Dingle *et al.* and Fell *et al.*). These changes are accompanied by a decrease in wet and dry weight, and a decrease of total hexosamine. These results resemble strongly those obtained after a temporary treatment of the rudiment by the proteolytic enzymes, papain or hyaluronidase. Indeed, Fell and Dingle (21) showed that the alterations in the case of hypervitaminosis A are due to the release of acid hydrolases from lysosomal particles of the cartilaginous and osseous cells. Vitamin A in an excessive dose alters the structure of lipoprotein plasma membranes and of the intracellular particles such as the lysosomal bags. Those alterations are followed by a change in enzyme distribution that provokes the extracellular alterations and ground substance depletion (14, 16). Dingle, Fell, and Lucy (15) have shown that $6-6\frac{1}{2}$-day embryonic chick limb bones grown in medium BGJ supplemented with excess vitamin A release hydroxyproline and hexosamine. But the total synthesis of hexosamine and hydroxyproline is not inhibited. On the contrary, it is found to be considerably active. Under hypervitaminosis, synthesis and degradation may occur simultaneously, but when very high doses of vitamin A are employed, a drastic breakdown of cartilage matrix is observed, because not only release of lysosomal enzymes occur, but the synthesis of the connective tissue components is inhibited.

It is possible that under normal conditions, vitamin A not only plays a role in the biosynthesis of polysaccharides but regulates the permeability of the membrane systems and acts upon the stability of the lysosome membrane.

Sucrose. Studying the action of complement-sufficient antisera on cartilage and bone *in vitro*, Fell, Dingle, and Coombs (23) stumbled upon an unexpected phenomenon in osmolarity control experiments. In the presence of 0.08 *M* sucrose, the morphological effect (breakdown of intercellular material by means of lysosomal protease) of the antiserum was much enhanced, the release and total synthesis of lysosomal acid protease was considerably increased. After that, the action of sucrose was investigated in more detail (22).

Chick embryonic limb bones of 13–14 days have been cultured in defined media. The cells of the ossified shafts become distended with vacuoles and the bone matrix undergoes a curious lysis. The total synthesis of lysosomal acid protease and acid phosphatase (activity of explant and activity in the medium) is increased.

In the case of 8-day limb rudiments, the effect of sucrose is less drastic. The matrix surrounding the articular chondrocytes is degraded only there where severe vacuolation at the cell surface occurs.

Electron microscopic studies have shown that the vacuoles in the articular chondrocytes, after 48 hours of culture in the presence of sucrose, contain fibrils identical in appearance to those in the surrounding matrix. It is yet unknown whether these fibrils are newly synthesized or destroyed ones. When the 8-day rudiments, treated with sucrose for 2 days, are transferred to normal medium the number of cytoplasmic vacuoles diminishes. It seems that the vacuoles move toward the surface of the cell and release their contents into the matrix after having fused with the plasma membrane.

These experiments show that accumulation of undigested material in cells stimulates the release as well as the synthesis of lysosomal enzymes. It can be assumed that in normal turnover of the tissues, breakdown products of intercellular material, through endocytosis and subsequent intracellular digestion, regulate the supply of newly synthesized constituents. Such feedback regulation is an essential mechanism in growth control.

b. Action of Hormones. Bone rudiments cultured in BGJ medium for more than 5 days undergo a progressive hydration. This terminal hydration can be arrested by adding small doses of hydrocortisone to the medium (67, 68). The suppression of the excessive waterlogging prevents disruption of the cells and consequent destruction of the surrounding matrix. Reynolds (60), too, shows that hydrocortisone considerably increases the metachromasia and reduces hypertrophy of diaphyseal cells compared to the nontreated bones, where an abnormal "foamy" intercellular matrix is seen throughout the rudiment. No substantial changes in the sulfate/uronic acid ratio occurs; and it remains unknown why the cortisol-treated rudiments are less hydrated than their paired controls (1).

Dingle, Fell, and Lucy (15) expressed the possibility that hydrocortisone could stabilize lysosomal membranes. When combined in a physiological concentration with excess vitamin A, the hormone cannot prevent the characteristic effects of the vitamin, but at relatively high concentrations, it retards the action of excess vitamin A. So it seems possible, but not proved, that hydrocortisone diminishes the rate of degradation of the cartilage matrix by inhibiting or slowing down the release of lysosomal enzymes.

2. COLLAGEN

a. Synthesis of Collagen: Action of Vitamin C. Collagen formation is one of the most thoroughly studied biological function of vitamin C (cf. 37). Studies have led to the assumption that ascorbic acid is involved in hydroxylation reactions and specially in microsomal hydroxylation of proline to hydroxy-proline in collagen precursor.

The question of the role of vitamin C in the building up of extracellular material has been investigated *in vitro* by growing chick limb bone rudiments in synthetic media (199 or BGJ) in the presence of a high dose of ascorbic acid (41–43, 61, 62). In the presence of vitamin C (50 $\mu g/ml$), the long bones undergo higher growth (length and dry weight), they maintain their structure (Figs. A-2–5), the terminal waterlogging usually observed after 5 days in protein-free medium is prevented and collagen synthesis is greatly stimulated as indicated by the hydroxyproline amount in the rudiments. Whether ascorbic acid is present or not in the medium, hexosamine contents and DNA contents are similar. These data show conclusively that the maintenance (12) and the synthesis of collagen are dependent upon the presence of ascorbic acid.

Ascorbic acid analogues have been tested for the synthesis of collagen. Isoascorbic acid is about 50% (42) or 33% (62) as effective as ascorbic acid, whereas dehydroascorbic acid [perhaps because no extra cysteine has been added to the medium (70)], and glucoascorbic acid are inactive and fail to prevent waterlogging and to promote collagen production.

The fact that vitamin C and some of its analogues both increase collagen synthesis and prevent the terminal excessive hydration suggests that the two effects may be interdependent. In this view, it is interesting to mention the existence of hydrophobic interactions as a stabilizing factor in collagen structure in skin (66). These interactions can be weakened experimentally by various aliphatic alcohols.

The following experiments seem to indicate that vitamin C and its analogues are also involved in bone cellular energy metabolism. Eighteen-day chick embryonic diaphyseal bones, freed from the marrow, have been cultured in modified Eagle's minimum medium by adding the following substances: glucine, proline, $CaCl_2$, glucose, vitamin B_{12}, vitamin D_3, para-aminobenzoic acid, biotine, and a daily dose of 50 $\mu g/ml$ of ascorbic acid, D-isoascorbic acid, or dehydroascorbic acid. The cultures are gassed with a mixture of 5% CO_2, 75% N_2, and 20% O_2. In these conditions, Ramp and Thornton (59) observed an enhanced O_2 consumption and depressed lactic

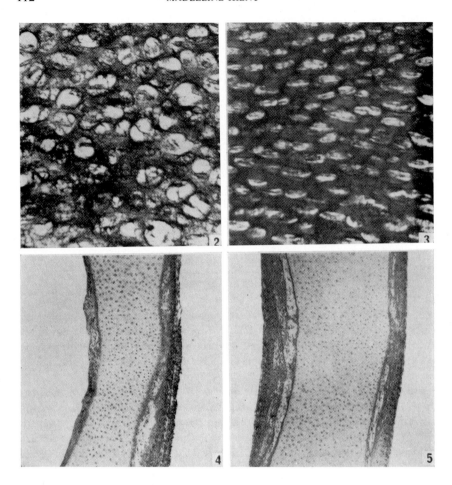

Figs. A-2 to A-5.   Cultures of chick long bones in synthetic medium supplemented with 50 μg/ml ascorbic acid. From Reynolds (61).

Fig. 2.   Zone of flattened cells in the epiphyseal region of a 7-day chick femur grown in synthetic medium for 6 days. Note the bubbly appearance of the matrix. Toluidine blue. × 540.

Fig. 3.   Zone of flattened cells in the epiphyseal region of a 7-day chick femur grown in synthetic medium with 50 μg/ml ascorbic acid for 6 days; the matrix appears normal. Toluidine blue. × 540.

Fig. 4.   Diaphyseal region of a 7-day chick femur grown in synthetic medium for 6 days. Note the thin ossified collar. Celestin blue, Mayer's hemalum, and van Gieson's stain. × 100.

Fig. 5.   Diaphyseal region of a 7-day chick femur grown in synthetic medium with 50 μg/ml ascorbic acid for 6 days. Note ossified collar and hypertrophied cells. Celestin blue, Mayer's hemalum, and van Gieson's stain. × 100.

acid production. This report suggests that ascorbic acid and, to a lesser extent, its analogues influence energy metabolism in connective tissues.

b. Degradation of Collagen. Excess Vitamin A. Bone resorption in rat calvaria is accompanied by collagen degradation, which is enhanced by the presence of parathyroid hormone in the biological medium. The degradation and release of collagen is provoked by enzymes whose action is similar to that of bacterial collagenase (71).

Since vitamin A in excess also causes the release of enzymes, it was tempting to submit skull bone to its destructive action (63). Thus fetal rat calvaria have been grown in modified BGJ medium (61) supplemented with 22 IU of retinol/ml of medium. Bone resorption is induced in the same manner as does parathyroid hormone: there is a concomitant loss of weight and mineral; histologically, many multinucleate osteoclasts form, osteocytes are no more recognizable and osteoblasts take a fibroblastic shape.

The effect of excess vitamin A can be partially counteracted by calcitonin (thyroid polypeptide hormone) (63, 64). Its presence in the medium inhibits bone resorption (release of calcium, perhaps the breakdown of mature collagen) but does not inhibit the release of lysosomal proteolytic enzymes. Furthermore, calcitonin suppresses the multinucleate osteoclasts, but does not prevent the loss of osteocytes and the fibroblastic transformation of osteoblasts.

Collagenase. It has already been shown that the degradation of protein polysaccharides by a proteolytic enzyme has a feedback effect on the synthesis of their components. Does the depletion of collagen have a similar effect on its subsequent synthesis? To answer this question, collagenase has been tested on 11- to 13-day chick embryonic long bones grown in synthetic media (53, 54). In this case, there is a rapid loss of cartilage matrix, chondrocytes get loose and the clumps of cells remain without visible intercellular material. The digestion of collagen leads to a drastic and general loss of intercellular material. The release of collagen peptides is accompanied by that of hexosamine-containing materials, which are not degraded (cf. 31). After withdrawal of the enzyme, the normal rates of synthesis are not restored. However, cartilage, and to a lesser extent bone are regenerated.

Finally, these reports indicate that the removal of the structural protein, collagen, affects the general shape of the rudiment which cannot be maintained because the destruction of the collagen framework leads to a disruption of the whole intercellular materials. The reestablishment of the matrix is difficult and slow. The removal of the ground substance, on the contrary, does not affect the organization of the long bones, and the removed components rapidly resynthesized, can be retained in the unaffected collagenic network. Lucy, Webb, and Biggers showed that the ground substance components—

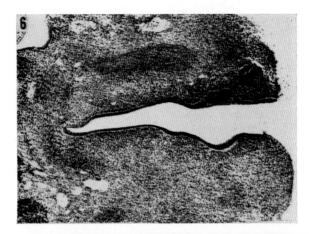

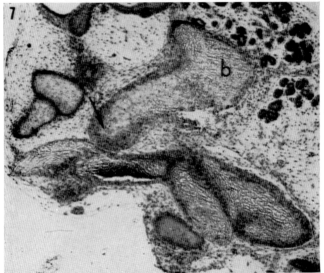

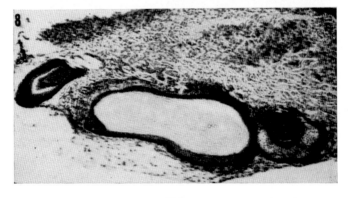

glucosamine and galactosamine—are synthesized by $6\frac{1}{2}$- to 7-day chick tibiae and femora directly from ^{14}C-labeled glucose introduced in chemically defined media 858 and BL_1.

III. TOOTH GERMS AND TOOTH PRIMORDIA

Considerable degree of development is undergone by isolated mammalian tooth germs in biological media (33, 34, 38, 50). Anatomical development is complete, the cusps develop, and, like the epiphysis of long bones (45), their shape is acquired independently of extrinsic factors. However, the histological development is not always complete; tubular dentine develops, but it fails to calcify; enamel is seldom produced.

Grown in medium BL_1 (Table A-I), tooth germs undergo the same degree of development (35) as in biological media. Tooth germs form cusps, histological differentiation progresses but the dentine formed does not calcify. To obtain a complete histological development it is necessary to supplement the defined medium by adding the following: serum (15%), ascorbic acid (15 mg/ml) and to expose the explants to a special gas phase. Indeed, in such conditions, Wigglesworth (72) obtained consistent differentiation of isolated rat tooth germs with deposition of characteristic matrices of dentine and enamel. Tooth development can be obtained even when culturing the presumptive area in biological (56) or in defined (36) media. Similar conditions as those necessary for isolated tooth germs are necessary for growing jaws of 13-day mouse embryos, containing the tooth primordia (Fig. A-6), in synthetic media BL_1 or 199. Next to mandibular bones (Fig. A-7), teeth form (Fig. A-8) in which dentine is present and whose cusps differentiate.

FIGS. A-6 to A-8.   Culture of mouse embryo jaws in supplemented synthetic medium BGJ. (Courtesy of Dr. S. Glasstone. The work supported by a grant under Medical Research Council has been published in *Nature*, 1968, see reference 36.)

Fig. 6.   The upper and lower jaws of a 13-day mouse embryo. The anlage of the incisor tooth can be seen and the mesenchymal condensation of Meckel's cartilage. (Hematoxylin–eosin stain. $\times 51$).

Fig. 7.   Section of a 13-day tissue culture showing ossification of the squamosal bone, formation of the condylar cartilage (arrow), and an articular disc. Mandibular bone (b) is present. Malleus and incus can be seen on the left and the submandibular gland on the right. Meckel's cartilage developed fully but cannot be seen in this section. (van Gieson stain. $\times 56$).

Fig. 8.   Section of a 12-day tissue culture showing the incisor and molar formed during cultivation. There is dentine present in the incisor, and cusps of the molar have developed but cannot be seen in this section. A large epithelial cyst has formed. (van Gieson stain. $\times 57$).

Thus, complete tooth differentiation has not yet been obtained in fully synthetic media. It seems, nevertheless, that the techniques devised can be used for the study of the metabolic changes which accompany morphogenesis, because, as for chondrogenic and osteogenic cells, the terminal differentiated state of the odontogenic cells is their ability to synthesize collagen and mucopolysaccharides to form the organic matrices. It will be of great interest to see whether in this tissue similar breakdown and recovery reactions occur as those described for cartilage and bone. There are some histochemical data indicating that the glycosaminoglycans present in the stellate reticulum of tooth germs are not sulfated but rather carboxylated (58).

BIBLIOGRAPHY

1. Barrett A. J., Sledge C. B. and Dingle J. T.   Effect of cortisol on the synthesis of chondroitin sulphate by embryonic cartilage. *Nature, London*, 1966, **211**, 83–84.
2. Biggers J. D.   The growth of embryonic chick tibiotarsi on a chemically defined medium. *J. exp. Zool.*, 1960, **144**, 233–256.
3. Biggers J. D.   The growth in dry weight and wet weight of embryonic chick tibiotarsi grown *in vivo* and *in vitro*. *J. exp. Zool.*, 1960, **145**, 227–242.
4. Biggers J. D.   The effect of L-glutamic acid on the weight of embryonic tibiotarsi cultivated *in vitro*. *Nature, London*, 1961, **192**, 664–665.
5. Biggers J. D.   Studies on the development of embryonic cartilaginous long-bone rudiments *in vitro*. *In* "Symposium on Organ Culture." *Nation. Canc. Inst. Monogr.*, 1963, **11**, 1–18.
6. Biggers J. D.   Cartilage and bone. *In* "Cells and Tissues in Culture. Methods. Biology, and Physiology" (E. N. Willmer, ed.), Vol. 2, pp. 197–260. Academic Press, New York, 1965.
7. Biggers J. D., Gwatkin R. B. L. and Heyner S.   The growth of embryonic avian and mammalian tibiae on a relatively simple chemically defined media. *Exp. Cell Res.*, 1961, **25**, 41–58.
8. Biggers J. D., Lawson K. A., Lucy J. A. and Webb M.   The chemical composition of long bone rudiments from embryonic chick. *Biochim. biophys. Acta*, 1961, **54**, 236–248.
9. Biggers J. D. and Lucy J. A.   Composition and preparation of small batches of a modification of medium 858 (Denoted BL1). *J. exp. Zool.*, 1960, **144**, 253–256.
10. Biggers J. D., Webb M., Parker R. C. and Healy G.   Cultivation of embryonic chick bones on chemically defined media. *Nature, London*, 1957, **180**, 825–828.
11. Bosmann H. B.   Cellular control of macromolecular synthesis; rates of synthesis of extracellular macromolecules during and after depletion by papain. *Proc. roy. Soc., London, B*, 1968, **169**, 399–425.
12. Candlish J. K. and Tristram G. R.   The resistance to dispersion of collagen fibres formed *in vitro* in the presence of ascorbic acid. *Biochim. biophys. Acta*, 1963, **78**, 289–294.
13. Chokshi H. R. and Ramakrishnan C. V.   Studies on chick embryonic tibiae cultivated in a chemically defined medium. *Indian J. exp. Biol.*, 1967, **5**, 211–215.
14. Dingle J. T.   Studies on the mode of action of excess of vitamin A. 3. Release of a bound protease by the action of vitamin A. *Biochem. J.*, 1961, **79**, 509–512.

15. Dingle J. T., Fell H. B. and Lucy J. A.   Synthesis of connective-tissue components. The effect of retinol and hydrocortisone on cultured limb-bone rudiments. *Biochem. J.*, 1966, **98**, 173–181.

16. Dingle J. T., Glauert A. M., Daniel M. and Lucy J. A.   Vitamin A and membrane systems. 1—The action of the vitamin on the membranes of cells and intracellular particles. *Biochem. J.*, 1962, **84**, 76P.

17. Dingle J. T. and Lucy J. A.   Studies on the mode of action of Vitamin A. 2—The release of a bound protease by the action of vitamin A. *Biochem. J.*, 1961, **78**, 11P.

18. Dingle J. T., Lucy J. A. and Fell H. B.   Studies on the mode of action of excess of vitamin A. 1—Effect of excess of vitamin A on the metabolism and composition of embryonic chick-limb cartilage grown in organ culture. *Biochem. J.*, 1961, **79**, 497–509.

19. Fell H. B.   The effect of excess vitamin A on cultures of embryonic chicken skin explanted at different stages of differentiation. *Proc. roy. Soc. London, B*, 1957, **146**, 242–256.

20. Fell H. B.   The effect of vitamin A on the breakdown and synthesis of intercellular material in skeletal tissue in organ culture. *Proc. Nutr. Soc., Engl. Scot.*, 1965, **24**, 166–170.

21. Fell H. B. and Dingle J. T.   Studies on the mode of action of excess of vitamin A. 6—The release of a lysosomal protease. *Biochem. J.*, 1963, **87**, 403–408.

22. Fell H. B. and Dingle J. T.   Extracellular release of lysosomal enzymes in response to sucrose. *Biochem. J.*, 1966, **98**, 40P.

23. Fell H. B., Dingle J. T. and Coombs R. R. A.   Recent experiments on the degradation and synthesis of bone and cartilage matrix in organ culture. *Proc. 4th European Symp. Calcified Tissues*, Noordwijk aan Zee, 1966, 27–29.

24. Fell H. B., Dingle J. T. and Webb M.   Studies on the mode of action of excess of vitamin A. 4—The specificity of the effect on embryonic chick-limb cartilage in culture and on isolated rat liver lysosomes. *Biochem. J.*, 1962, **83**, 63–69.

25. Fell H. B., Lucy J. A. and Dingle J. T.   Studies on the mode of action of excess vitamin A. 1—The metabolism, composition and degradation of chick-limb cartilage *in vitro*. *Biochem. J.*, 1961, **78**, 11P.

26. Fell H. B. and Mellanby E.   The effect of hypervitaminosis A on embryonic limb bones cultivated *in vitro*. *J. Physiol., London*, 1952, **116**, 320–349.

27. Fell H. B. and Thomas L.   Comparison of the effects of papain and vitamin A on cartilage. II. The effects on organ cultures of embryonic skeletal tissues. *J. exp. Med.*, 1960, **111**, 719–744.

28. Fitton-Jackson S.   Factors concerned in the growth of embryonic limb-bones (chick) cultured in a chemically defined medium. *Strangeways Res. Lab. ann. Rep.*, 1966, 29–30.

29. Fitton-Jackson S.   Factors concerned in the maintenance of the synthetic balance of intercellular macromolecules. *Biochem. J.*, 1967, **104**, 13P.

30. Fitton-Jackson S.   The nutritional requirements of tibiae from $11\frac{1}{2}$–12 day embryonic chicks. *Strangeways Res. Lab. ann. Rep.*, 1967, 32–33.

31. Fitton-Jackson S.   The morphogenesis of collagen. *In* "Treatise on Collagen. Vol. 2, Part B: Biology of Collagen" (B. S. Gould, ed.), pp. 1–67. Academic Press, New York, 1968.

32. Girard H.   Influence de la papaïne sur le tibia embryonnaire de Poulet cultivé *in vitro*. *J. Embryol. exp. Morphol.*, 1962, **10**, 231–247.

33. Glasstone S.   The development of tooth germs *in vitro*. *J. Anat.*, 1936, **70**, 260–266.

34. Glasstone S.   A comparative study of the development *in vivo* and *in vitro* of rat and rabbit molars. *Proc. roy. Soc. London, B*, 1938, **126**, 315–350.

35. Glasstone S. Cultivation of mouse tooth germs in a chemically defined protein-free medium. *Arch. oral Biol.*, 1964, **9**, 27–30.
36. Glasstone S. Tissue culture of the mandible and mandibular joint of mouse embryos. *Nature, London*, 1968, **220**, 705–706.
37. Gould B. S. "Treatise on Collagen. Vol. 2, Parts A and B: Biology of Collagen." Academic Press, New York, 1968.
38. Hay M. F. The development *in vivo* and *in vitro* of the lower incisor and molars of the mouse. *Arch. oral Biol.*, 1961, **3**, 86–109.
39. Hebertson M. A. The reversibility of the effect of hypervitaminosis A on embryonic limb-bones cultivated *in vitro*. *J. Embryol. exp. Morphol.*, 1955, **3**, 355–365.
40. Ishibashi S., Ide T. and Tsurufuji. Role of glutamic acid as a precursor of collagen proline and hydroxyproline. *Biochim. biophys. Acta*, 1968, **165**, 296–299.
41. Jeffrey J. J. and Martin G. R. Ascorbic acid dependent synthesis of collagen by embryonic chick tibia grown in tissue culture. Abstracts of the 6th International Congress of Biochemistry, New York, July 1964. *Collagen Currents*, 1964, **5**, 63.
42. Jeffrey J. J. and Martin G. R. The role of ascorbic acid in the biosynthesis of collagen. I. Ascorbic acid requirement by embryonic chick tibia in tissue culture. *Biochim. biophys. Acta*, 1966, **121**, 269–280.
43. Jeffrey J. J. and Martin G. R. The role of ascorbic acid in the biosynthesis of collagen. II. Site and nature of ascorbic acid participation. *Biochim. biophys. Acta*, 1966, **121**, 281–291.
44. Kieny M. Les besoins nutritifs spécifiques des tibias d'embryon de Poulet en culture *in vitro* sur milieux synthétiques. *C. R. Soc. Biol.*, 1955, **149**, 418–421.
45. Kieny M. Contribution à l'étude des besoins nutritifs des tibias embryonnaires d'Oiseau cultivés en milieux naturels et synthétiques. *Arch. Anat. micr. Morphol. exp.*, 1958, **47**, 86–169.
46. Kieny M. La culture d'organes embryonnaires en milieux synthétiques. "Exposés actuels de Biologie cellulaire. Les cultures organotypiques," pp. 57–89. 1965.
47. Kieny M. The culture of embryonic cartilaginous organs in synthetic media. *Proc. 4th European Symp. Calcified Tissues*, Noordwijk aan Zee, 1966, p. 94.
48. Koch W. *In vitro* development of tooth rudiments of embryonic mice. *Anat. Rec.*, 1965, **152**, 513–524.
49. Lasnitzki J. Effects of excess vitamin A on the normal and oestron-treated mouse vagina grown in a chemically defined medium. *Exp. Cell Res.*, 1961, **24**, 37–46.
50. Lefkowitz W. and Swayne P. *In vitro* cultivation of rat molar tooth germs. *J. dent. Res.*, 1956, **35**, 523–531.
51. Lucy J. A. and Dingle J. T. Vitamin A and membrane systems. 2—Membrane stability and protein-vitamin A—lipid interactions. *Biochem. J.*, 1962, **84**, 76P–77P.
52. Lucy J. A., Dingle J. T. and Fell H. B. Studies on the mode of action of excess of vitamin A. 2—A possible role of intracellular proteases in the degradation of cartilage matrix. *Biochem. J.*, 1961, **79**, 500–508.
53. O'Dell D. S. The use of collagenase in investigating the synthetic balance of the intercellular materials. *Exp. Cell Res.*, 1965, **40**, 432–435.
54. O'Dell D. S. The effect of changes in the microenvironment of the cells on macromolecular synthesis. 2. The effect of collagenase. *Strangeways Res. Lab. ann. Rep.*, 1967, 36–37.
55. Paff G. H. and Seifter J. The effect of hyaluronidase on bone growth *in vitro*. *Anat. Rec.*, 1950, **106**, 525–537.
56. Pourtois M. Comportement en culture *in vitro* des ébauches dentaires de Rongeurs

prélevées aux stades de prédifférenciation. *J. Embryol. exp. Morphol.*, 1964, **12**, 391–405.

57. Pullar P. Keratin formation in tissue culture. *In* "Progress in the Biological Sciences in Relation to Dermatology" (A. Rook and R. H. Champion, eds.), 1964, pp. 213–226.

58. Quintarelli G., Sajdera S. and Dziewiatkowski D. Modifications of connective tissue matrices by an enzyme extracted from cartilage. *Histochemie*, 1968, **15**, 1–20.

59. Ramp W. K. and Thornton P. A. The effect of ascorbic acid on the glycolytic and respiratory metabolism of embryonic chick tibias. *Calcified Tissue Res.*, 1968, **2**, 77–82.

60. Reynolds J. J. The effect of hydrocortisone on the growth of chick bone rudiments in chemically defined medium. *Exp. Cell Res.*, 1966, **41**, 174–189.

61. Reynolds J. J. The effect of ascorbic acid on the growth of chick bone rudiments in chemically defined medium. *Exp. Cell Res.*, 1966, **42**, 178–188.

62. Reynolds J. J. The synthesis of collagen in chick bone rudiments *in vitro*. *Exp. Cell Res.*, 1967, **47**, 42–48.

63. Reynolds J. J. Inhibition by calcitonin of bone resorption induced *in vitro* by vitamin A. *Proc. roy. Soc. London, B.*, 1968, **170**, 61–69.

64. Reynolds J. J. and Dingle J. T. The induction and inhibition of bone resorption *in vitro*. Sixth European Symposium on Calcified Tissues, 1968. *Calcified Tissue Res.*, 1968, **2**, No. 50.

65. Rothberg S. The cultivation of embryonic chicken skin in a chemically defined medium and the response of the epidermis to excess of vitamin A. *J. invest. Dermatol.*, 1967, **49**, 35–38.

66. Schnell J. Evidence for the existence of hydrophobic interactions as a stabilizing factor in collagen structure. *Arch. Biochem. Biophys.*, 1968, **127**, 496–502.

67. Schryver H. F. The influence of hydrocortisone on the water uptake of embryonic chick tibiotarsi in organ culture. *Exp. Cell Res.*, 1965, **37**, 327–337.

68. Schryver H. F. The effect of hydrocortisone on chondroitin sulfate production and loss by embryonic chick tibiotarsi in organ culture. *Exp. Cell Res.*, 1965, **40**, 610–618.

69. Schryver H. F. A quantitative comparison of the growth of the embryonic chick tibiotarsus *in vivo* and *in vitro*. *J. exp. Zool.*, 1966, **161**, 81–88.

70. Shimizu Y., McCann D. S. and Keech M. K. Human dermal fibroblasts in monolayer tissue culture. Effect of ascorbic acid analogues. *J. Lab. clin. Med.*, 1965, **66**, 659–666.

71. Stern B. D., Glimcher M. J., Mechanic G. L. and Goldhaber P. Studies of collagen degradation during bone resorption in tissue culture. *Proc. Soc. exp. Biol. Med.*, 1965, **119**, 96–100.

72. Wigglesworth D. J. Formation and mineralisation of enamel and dentine by rat tooth germs *in vitro*. *Exp. Cell Res.*, 1968, **49**, 211–215.

CHAPTER IV

SEXUAL DIFFERENTIATION
AND INTERSEXUALITY *IN VITRO*

Katy Haffen

INSTITUT D'EMBRYOLOGIE ET DE TÉRATOLOGIE EXPÉRIMENTALE DU
C.N.R.S. ET DU COLLÈGE DE FRANCE
PARIS, FRANCE

I. INTRODUCTION

The *in vitro* culture of sex organs (gonads and secondary sexual structures) has resolved many of the problems of sexual morphogenesis. These problems are concerned with autodifferentiation of the genital glands, sexual inversion, and the role of the embryonic gonads in the differentiation of the genital tract.

The most important experiments have been carried out on birds and mammals. Some work has also been done on amphibians. The culture of the sex organs in invertebrates is now in the course of development and will not be discussed in this chapter.

II. BIRDS

A. Development and Differentiation of the Sex Organs of Avian Embryos When Cultured *in Vitro*

Et. Wolff and Haffen (69, 70) developed a technique for studying the development of avian embryo gonads *in vitro*. This technique is useful for the culture of many embryonic organs. The composition of the culture medium used is as follows:

1% gelatin in Gey's solution	6 parts
7–9 Day chick embryo extract	3 parts
Tyrode's solution	3 parts

1. SPONTANEOUS SEXUAL DIFFERENTIATION OF DUCK EMBRYO GONADS

The sexual differentiation of duck embryo gonads occurs between the end of the 9th and the beginning of the 10th day of incubation. Et. Wolff and

121

Haffen (71) cultured sexually undifferentiated gonads from 7–8 day duck embryos. Testes explanted on the culture medium developed swollen tubules similar to those of the normal embryo. After 5 days of culture, they consisted of a fairly well-developed tunica albuginea with typical seminiferous tubules lying beneath it. These contained spermatogonia undergoing mitosis and in the interphase (Fig. 1).

Genetically female gonads developed differently from male gonads. The left ovary flattened out on the medium and became surrounded by a wide transparent fringe. The center of the organ contained large refringent granules. Histological sections showed that the cortex was composed of several layers of prismatic cells with nuclei oriented perpendicularly to the surface. The reduced medulla was composed of cell cords with no definite structure. These were sometimes closely packed and sometimes formed lacunae (Fig. 2).

The right gonads of the female embryo appeared as small plaques, granular and flat, without a fringe. They showed marked proliferation of the peripheral cells, and regular central atrophy. *In vitro*, these organs underwent regression analogous to the normal regression. In structure, they resembled the ovarian medulla (Fig. 3).

2. CULTURE OF ISOLATED GERMINAL EPITHELIUM FROM DUCK EMBRYO GONADS

Et. Wolff and Haffen (75) took the germinal epithelium from the left gonads of 5–9 day duck embryos. Moscona's technique (37) of digestion with dilute trypsin was used to separate the germinal epithelium from the medulla. Culture of the germinal epithelium was unsuccessful unless the organ was grown with a piece of tissue (mesonephros) for suppport and to prevent disintegration of the epithelium. The right gonads were grown separately to determine the genetic sex of the germinal epithelium taken from the left gonads.

a. Development of the Male Germinal Epithelium. Male germinal epithelium explanted at the time of sexual differentiation ($8\frac{1}{2}$–9 days) or a little earlier ($7\frac{1}{2}$–8 days) gave rise to a medulla. In most of the explants this medulla acquired all the characteristics of a testicular medulla (Fig. 4).

Male germinal epithelium taken at an earlier stage of embryonic development (less than $6\frac{1}{2}$ days) survived but did not differentiate.

b. Development of the Female Germinal Epithelium. Female germinal epithelium from 5–10 day embryos developed and differentiated into an ovarian cortex. It was thick, many-layered and in its deeper parts contained islets of oogonia (Fig. 5). These explants were similar in shape and cellular

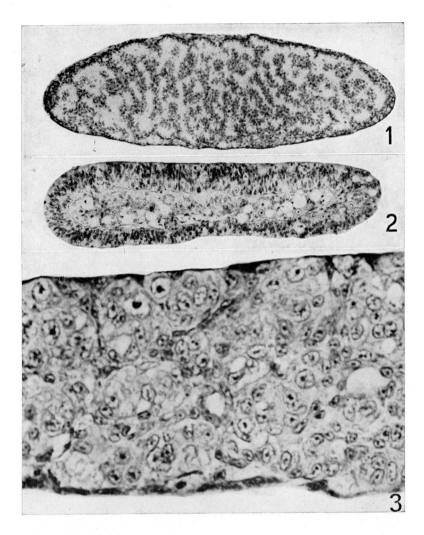

Fig. 1.   Left gonad from an 8-day duck embryo, cultured for 10 days and showing characteristic testicular structure. After Et. Wolff and K. Haffen.

Fig. 2.   General appearance of 8-day duck embryo ovary, cultured for 5 days. A thick cortex completely surrounds the medulla, which is composed of diffuse cords and lacunae. Oogonia occupy almost the entire thickness of the organ. After Et. Wolff and K. Haffen.

Fig. 3.   Detail of the right gonad taken from an 8-day female duck embryo and cultured for 5 days. It is surrounded by a very flattened epithelium, and is formed of diffuse, un-differentiated medullary cell cords, containing numerous germ cells. After Et. Wolff and K. Haffen.

arrangement to duck ovaries cultured *in vitro*, differing from cultured ovaries only in the lack of a regressing, lacunar medulla.

Thus the germinal epithelium can develop alone to form structures analogous to those which develop in the entire ovary, complete with its medulla. This result definitely confirms the often disputed classical theory relating to the formation of the medulla.

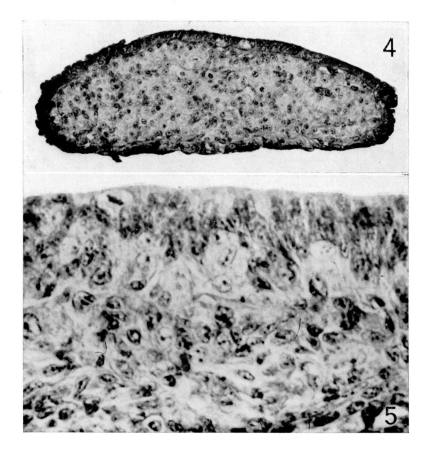

Fig. 4. Differentiation of germinal epithelium from a male duck embryo after 5 days of culture. The tissue was taken after $7\frac{1}{2}$ days of incubation. A single layer of epithelial cells covers extensive medulla where the cell cords already show some tendency to differentiate into seminiferous tubules. After Et. Wolff and K. Haffen.

Fig. 5. Differentiation of the germinal epithelium from a female duck embryo after 5 days of culture. The tissue was taken after $7\frac{1}{2}$ days of incubation. The thick multilayered cortex covers a deeper zone, occupied by oogonia lying singly and in groups. This structure is similar to that of the whole ovary cultured *in vitro*. After Et. Wolff and K. Haffen.

3. Spontaneous Sexual Differentiation of Chick Embryo Gonads

Sexual differentiation of chick embryo gonads occurs on the 9th day of incubation. Et. Wolff and Haffen (72) explanted 7–8 day gonads. Sex can be determined visually by the 8th day using as the criterion the morphological differentiation of the gonads. Male gonads are symmetric and those in the female slightly asymmetric.

The external appearance of the gonads changed soon after explantation. Two types of morphological differentiation were seen. One type appeared as cylindrical, often spindle-shaped tubules resembling testes. When the left gonad developed in this way, the right gonad developed in the same manner. The second type appeared as flattened structures on the medium, and became surrounded by a transparent fringe. These structures resembled ovaries. Meanwhile the corresponding right gonads did not undergo such a clear-cut regression as the right gonad does in the duck. They developed the appearance of small, somewhat flattened testes.

The right and left gonads in the male usually had the typical structure of testes. Histological studies of the female gonads showed an aberrant differentiation. They did not have the structure of ovaries but of ovotestes (Fig. 6). The cortex was usually well developed with a normal structure, and contained oogonia. The medulla was massive, with a male structure. The lacunar zone present in the normal embryo was greatly reduced in these ovotestes. The right female gonads had the structure of testes. They differed from testes taken from male embryos only in their flatness and small size. As will be seen later, this apparent intersexuality of the female gonads did not correspond to a functional intersexuality, for despite its structure the medulla secreted a feminizing hormone.

Weniger (52) succeeded in growing much younger gonads (4–6 days of incubation) from both sexes, and obtained similar results. Chick embryo gonads taken after sexual differentiation had occurred (9–18 days of incubation) continued to develop. The oogonia became oocytes showing the different stages of meiosis (leptotene, pachytene). Ovaries taken toward the end of incubation differentiated as far as the stage of primary follicles (Haffen, unpublished work).

B. Hormonal Intersexuality and Sexual Inversion of Male Gonads under the Influence of Female Hormones

It has been shown (5, 60, 68) that estrogenic hormones injected *in ovo* can feminize the gonads and genital tract of male embryos. E. Wolff (64) showed that grafts of female gonads into male embryos had the same effect. Experiments carried out *in vitro* by Et. Wolff and Haffen (73) confirmed these results.

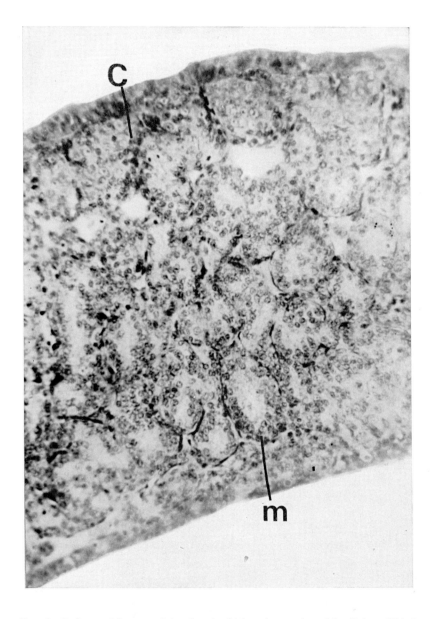

FIG. 6.   Left gonad from an 8-day female chick embryo cultured for 5 days. This has
the structure of an ovotestis. A fertile ovarian cortex and a testicular medulla are present.
After Et. Wolff and K. Haffen.

These authors induced intersexuality of duck embryo gonads by two experimental procedures:

1. By associating two gonads of different sexes in the same culture.

2. By using the direct effect of crystalline female hormone on gonads in the process of differentiation.

1. PARABIOSIS

Pairs of left gonads from different embryos (6, 7, or 8 days old) were cultured parabiotically on the surface of the culture medium. They fused more or less intimately at the surfaces in contact. The corresponding right gonads were cultured separately to determine the genetic sex of the gonads. The pairs of gonads and the right gonads were cultured for 4–6 days, during which period sexual differentiation normally occurs.

In heterosexual pairs of gonads the female gonad was a characteristic ovary, and the male gonad was feminized. Its structure was intermediate between an ovary and an ovotestis. A thick cortex covered the two associated gonads. The medulla of the male partner was much larger, and was composed of nontesticular epithelial cords (Fig. 7). The male partner had no effect on the differentiation of the female partner.

Et. Wolff and Haffen (74) obtained the same results when they cultured an undifferentiated left male gonad with a 7–10 day right female gonad. The female right gonad, although regressing, feminized the left male gonad (Fig. 8).

2. EFFECT OF CRYSTALLINE FEMALE HORMONE

An oily emulsion of the hormone (estradiol benzoate at a concentration of 5 mg/ml) was poured onto the surface of the medium. At the time of explantation a few droplets were brought into direct contact with the gonad. In genetically male gonads female hormone induced a cortical proliferation seen as transparent lacy lobes on the surface of the gonad.

Histologically, the left gonads were seen as intersexual glands covered by an irregular lobed cortex. The medulla was composed of closely packed cords which showed neither ovarian nor testicular structure (Fig. 9).

Thus these experiments indicate again the role of the sex hormones in primary sexual differentiation and the similar effect of embryonic hormones and crystalline hormones. They prove that the hormones act directly on the gonadial rudiments and that the hormones act in the absence of all connections with other organs.

Using chick embryos, Weniger (53, 54) confirmed the results obtained on the duck embryos. He linked in parabiosis very young gonads of more than 5 days' incubation. In heterosexual parabiosis both left and right

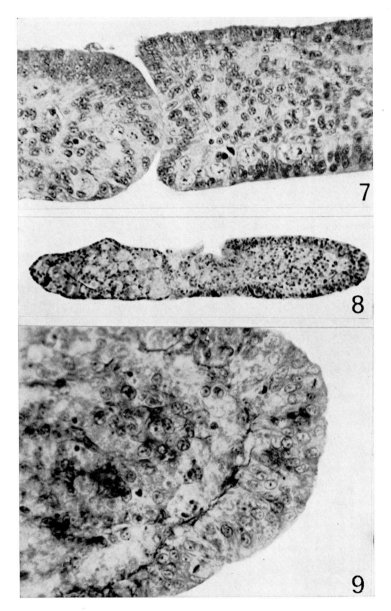

FIG. 7.   Heterosexual parabiosis between two left embryonic gonads of ducks, cultured for 5 days. The ovary is on the left and the feminized male gonad on the right. A thick fertile cortex encloses the two gonads. The medulla of the ovotestis has a poorly developed testicular structure. After Et. Wolff and K. Haffen.

FIG. 8.   Heterosexual parabiosis between a right female gonad and a left male gonad

female gonads had a strong feminizing effect on genetically male left gonads. This result indicates that hormone secretion by the gonads occurs very early. It is also interesting that a female gonad, although morphologically testicular, has the physiological activity of an ovary. Weniger (53) showed also that female gonads cultured for a long time *in vitro* (31 days) retained their secretory activity and were able to feminize young male gonads (Fig. 10).

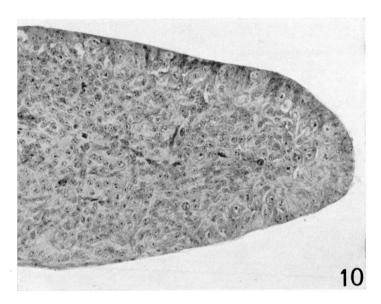

FIG. 10.   Left testis from a 6-day chick embryo showing gross feminization. It has been cultured for 4 days on a medium on which two female 8-day chick gonads had previously been cultured for 7 days. After Weniger.

3. Heterosexual Association of the Germinal Epithelium and the Medulla of Duck Gonads

The observation that male germinal epithelium taken at an early stage of embryonic development (less than $6\frac{1}{2}$ days) cannot undergo sexual differentiation led Haffen (19) to investigate the action of the medulla

---

from duck embryos. The female right gonad, vacuolated and lacking an ovarian cortex, has induced transformation of the left gonad into an ovotestis. After Et. Wolff and K. Haffen.

FIG. 9.   Detail of the lateral edge of a male embryonic duck gonad feminized by the addition of crystalline female hormone to the culture medium (estradiol benzoate at a concentration of 5 mg/ml). The germinal epithelium has reacted with an intense cortical proliferation. After Et. Wolff and K. Haffen.

on sexual differentiation and to ask whether, in the presence of a medulla from the opposite sex, the germinal epithelium differentiates according to its own genetic sex, or that of the medulla?

Haffen associated the undifferentiated germinal epithelium of gonads from 5–7 day duck embryos with ovarian or testicular medullas from sexually differentiated 9–13 day embryos.

In all these experiments the medulla always had a characteristic appearance.

a. Development of Female Germinal Epithelium. Female germinal epithelium developed and differentiated into ovarian cortex from the age of 5 days, independently of the origin of the medulla with which it was associated. Culture in close contact with a male medulla did not hinder the differentiation of the female germinal epithelium into an ovarian cortex.

b. Development of Male Germinal Epithelium. Development of male germinal epithelium was modified by the tissue with which it was in contact. This influence was especially marked when the germinal epithelium was taken from 5–6 day gonads. There was no differentiation when it was associated with mesonephric tissue.

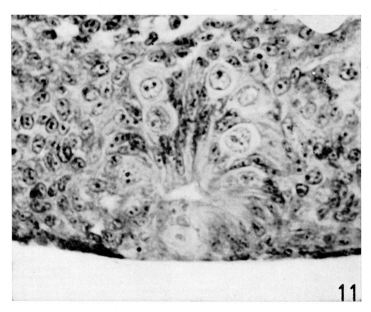

Fig. 11. Detail of an association between male germinal epithelium of a 6-day and ovarian medulla of an 11-day duck embryo cultured for 5 days. The structure of a cortex differentiated from male germinal epithelium can be seen. It is comparable to that of an ovarian cortex. After Haffen.

In the presence of testicular medulla the germinal epithelium gave rise to medullary cords more or less differentiated into testicular cords. The majority of these cords were in the process of organization. Remnants of the germinal epithelium persisted around the organ.

In the presence of an ovarian medulla male germinal epithelium differentiated into an ovarian cortex. There was an epithelium composed of many layers of tall, narrow, refractile cells, with germinal cells scattered among them or grouped in islets at the base of the cortex (Fig. 11).

Germinal epithelium from 7–9 day male embryos still gave rise to a cortex, but testicular cords developed at the same time. It appeared probable that once the epithelium was oriented toward male differentiation, it could be only partially affected. This orientation was first seen after $6\frac{1}{2}$ days of incubation.

These experiments show that the medulla is necessary to ensure differentiation of the male germinal epithelium in the early stages of development. They also show that it is possible to direct the differentiation of male germinal epithelium in the opposite direction until the 7th day of incubation.

Feminization of the germinal epithelium by the ovarian medulla, and feminization of male gonads by the female right gonad, confirm the experiments using grafts *in ovo* carried out by Et. Wolff (64), Et. Wolff and Em. Wolff (77), and B. Mintz and Et. Wolff (35, 36): the medulla is the tissue that secretes the feminizing hormone.

C. The Effect of Teratogenic Agents on the Development of Chick Embryo Gonads

In 1957, Salzgeber (41) showed the effect of various teratogenic agents on the development of chick embryo gonads cultured *in vitro*, after testing several chemical factors including mitotic poisons and metabolic inhibitors. It is known from the work of Et. Wolff and Haffen (72) that the female gonad of chick embryo differentiates into an ovotestis *in vitro*. This ovotestis has an ovarian cortex and a testicular medulla. Is this due to a metabolic disturbance, unbalanced nutrition, or the lack of a hormone?

Salzgeber's experiments related the morphological and histological development of the gonads to the selective sensitivity of their different constituents to teratogenic agents.

1. CHEMICAL SUBSTANCES

Gonads were taken from 9–10 day embryos and grown on Wolff and Haffen's medium (1952) with the chemical substance to be tested added to it. Three series of experiments were carried out (Fig. 12) to determine:

1. The effect of trypaflavine.

2. The effect of narcotine and colchicine.

3. The effect of nicotine.

a. The Effect of Trypaflavine. The effect was exerted essentially on the ovarian medulla and on the testicular structures of the male gonad. The ovary consisted of a normal lobed cortex, studded with germinal cells, but the medulla developed in an atypical fashion. It atrophied and many lacunas separated the testicular cords (Fig. 13).

The male gonad showed the same tissue involution. The seminiferous tubules degenerated and were replaced by vacuoles and lacunas (Fig. 14).

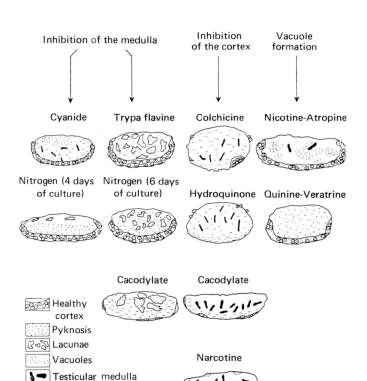

FIG. 12. Diagrammatic representation of the action of different teratogenic materials on female chick embryo gonads cultured *in vitro*. After Salzgeber.

The inhibition of the medullary zone in the ovary gave it a more normal structure. Under normal conditions the lacunar appearance occurred from the 10th day of incubation.

Thus trypaflavine exerts on the medulla an inhibitory effect resembling that of a hormone. The substance has little effect on the germinal elements.

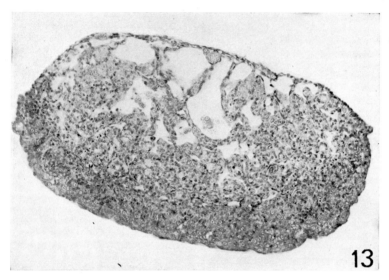

Fig. 13. Female gonad from 10-day chick embryo, cultured with trypaflavine for 5 days. There is a zone of large lacunae in the region of the hilum. The cortex is studded with gonocytes. After Salzgeber.

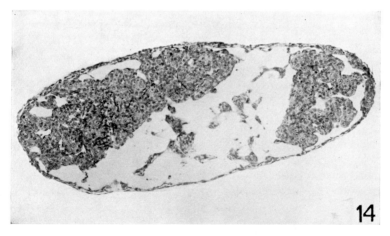

Fig. 14. Ten-day chick embryo testis cultured with trypaflavine for 4 days. The testicular structure of the explant has become disorganized. After Salzgeber.

Organs maintained under anaerobic conditions for 40–48 hours and then cultured under normal conditions for 2–3 days showed a change similar to that above. Nuclear pyknosis is another form of degeneration which occurs in the medullary zone. This type of inhibition was shown by gonads treated with potassium cyanide or exposed to a lack of oxygen.

b. *The Effects of Colchicine and Narcotine.*   Colchicine, sodium cacodylate, hydroquinone, and narcotine exerted effects opposite to that of trypaflavine. The cortex was destroyed and was replaced by a zone with a compact structure composed of diffuse cords. Nuclei with their divisions blocked at metaphase were scattered throughout the tissue. The testis developed normally, only differing from the controls by the presence of metaphase plates in the seminiferous tubules.

c. *The Effect of Nicotine.*   After culture for 24 hours in the presence of nicotine or quinine, both male and female gonads showed extensive vacuolation of both parts of the gonads. The action of nicotine was nonspecific.

Mitotic poisons used in these experiments exerted a differential inhibitory effect on the male and female chicken gonads. Depending on the material used, one or other tissue was modified selectively. It was suggested that the different poisons upset the metabolic pathways. The changes induced *in vitro* were irreversible.

2. X-Rays

Salzgeber (46) took gonads of both sexes from 9–10 day embryos and irradiated them in culture *in vitro*. The X-ray doses used varied from 2490 to 12,450 r. Irradiation induced complete disorganization of the gonad in both sexes. The medullary cords remained undifferentiated or degenerated. The cortex was grossly reduced or disappeared.

3. Physiological Activity of Gonads Affected by Toxic or Teratogenic Substances

Salzgeber attempted to determine whether gonads that had been treated *in vitro* with antimitotic agents (43) or X-rays (44) would continue to produce hormones when regrafted into a host embryo. Gonads treated with trypaflavine or narcotine continued to develop, but only those structures that had been protected from the treatment could differentiate.

Ovaries in which most of the medulla had been destroyed by trypaflavine continued to feminize male embryos. The same occurred where the gonads had been treated with narcotine, so eliminating the cortex.

These results show that in the first case the toxic material has not disturbed the secretory cells of the ovary and that in both cases the medulla alone is needed for the production of the female hormone.

In contrast, the testicular medulla is very sensitive to the action of trypaflavine. After treatment it does not cause regression of the Müller ducts in a host female, which is a very sensitive test for masculinizing hormone. The secretion of male hormone is much more sensitive to the action of these toxic substances than is the secretion of female hormone.

Salzgeber (44) showed that when irradiated ovaries were reimplanted into either male or female hosts, they retained their ability to produce female hormone, despite the morphological changes. When testes were regrafted immediately after irradiation, they retained their masculinizing effect on female Müller ducts. If they were cultured for 2–4 days before being grafted into the host, they could no longer affect the Müller ducts.

D. Differentiation of the Sexual Characteristics and Their Hormone Dependence

The secondary sex organs were cultured using Wolff and Haffen's method (70).

1. MÜLLER DUCTS OF CHICK EMBRYOS

Among the sex organs showing early sexual dimorphism we shall first turn our attention to the Müller ducts.

In chick embryos the development of the genital canal is the same in both sexes until the 10th day of incubation. After this time the male ducts remain thin, regress in a caudo-cephalic direction, and finally disappear, while in the female the left Müller duct continues to grow and develop into a functional oviduct in the adult. The right duct regresses in a caudo-cephalic direction to become a cloacal rudiment.

If the Müller ducts from chick embryos were explanted after the sexual differentiation of the gonads had occurred (9–9½ day), the male ducts regressed, became necrotic, and autolysed in culture (Fig. 15). The female ducts survived and developed (Fig. 16a). However, if the Müller ducts were explanted before sexual differentiation of the gonads (7–8 days), they all developed in the same way as female ducts taken at 10 days, whatever the initial genetic sex (Fig. 16b). In the first case, the male ducts had already been subjected to the secretions of the differentiating testes. In the second, they developed the neutral condition, corresponding to a female differentiation (82).

a. Effect of Male Hormone. The following experiments will demonstrate

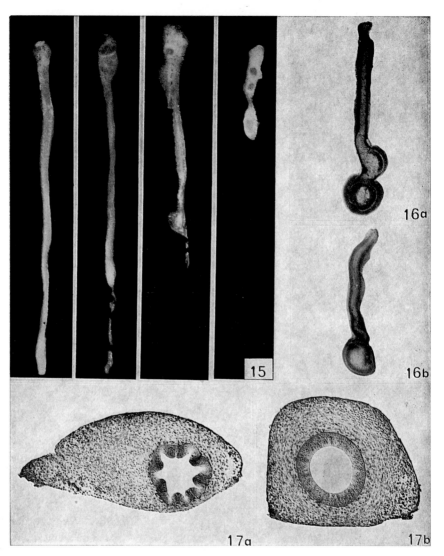

FIG. 15. Müller ducts from 9½-day male. From left to right: (1) At the time of explantation. (2–4) Three stages of regression during culture of the organ.

FIG. 16. Culture and differentiation of the Müller duct of chick embryo. Differentiation into an oviduct with a swollen shell gland in the cloacal region. (a) Development of a 9-day female duct, following the normal pattern. (b) Development of a male duct taken at 7 days (undifferentiated stage) which normally regresses in the male embryo after this time. It differentiates into the female form in the absence of hormone. After Et. Wolff and Y. Lutz-Ostertag.

FIG. 17. (a) Right Müller duct from an 8-day female, grown for 7 days 3 mm away from two female gonads of the same age. Histological section to show the epithelial folds. (b) Left Müller duct cultured as a control for 7 days. After Weniger.

136

the atrophying effect of the male hormone. Undifferentiated 7-day Müller ducts, or 9-day differentiated female Müller ducts were explanted onto a medium containing crystalline male hormone (aqueous suspension of testosterone propionate at a concentration of 1–1.6 mg/ml). The ducts became necrotic and autolysed more or less completely depending on the dose of hormone used. This necrosis was a specific reaction of the Müller ducts to male hormone, since other organs, such as the Wolff ducts or the gonads are not sensitive.

The same effect was produced if embryonic testis and Müller duct were cultured parabiotically (83).

These results confirm those of Et. Wolff (65), who showed that in the absence of male hormone, the spontaneous development of the Müller ducts corresponded to the female form, realizing the type without hormone. It was the male hormone from the differentiating testes which was directly responsible for the regression of the Müller ducts (64).

In addition, Scheib-Pfleger (49) showed that a proteolytic enzyme was involved in this regression.

b. Protective or Stimulating Effect of Female Hormone on the Müller Ducts. If Müller ducts from 9½-day male embryos were grown in the presence of female hormone (aqueous suspension of 0.5 mg/ml of estradiol propionate), the hormone had a protective effect. Living tissue survived in the ducts. The parts that escaped necrosis formed a chain of vesicles alternating with the thin duct (28).

Scheib-Pfleger (49) used the Kjeldahl micromethod for the estimation of total nitrogen to show that undifferentiated Müller ducts or differentiated female Müller ducts maintained themselves in organ culture but did not grow. Growth occurred only when female hormone was present.

Weniger (55) cultured undifferentiated Müller ducts in contact with embryonic female gonads and found that this stimulated their development. This was seen in the epithelium of the canal, which showed many folds around an enlarged lumen (Fig. 17a,b).

c. The Effect of Physical Agents on the Müller Ducts.   Lutz and Lutz-Ostertag (29) showed that 6½–7 day Muller ducts could be maintained in culture if they were exposed to ultrasonics immediately before being associated with 9½–10 day male gonads. These authors suggested that there was a direct inactivation of the proteolytic enzyme produced by the duct in the male embryo. Salzgeber (42) used a raised temperature or X-rays (46) on 7–9 day ducts cultured *in vitro* either alone or in association with testes, and showed that these agents had a direct action on the Müller ducts which did not regress even in the presence of male hormone.

2. Duck Embryo Syrinx

The syrinx is the organ of phonation in birds, situated at the junction of the bronchi and the trachea. In the duck the syrinx shows marked sexual dimorphism.

The syrinx has been explanted both before and after sexual differentiation of the gonads (81).

a. Explantation after the Stage of Sexual Differentiation ($9\frac{1}{2}$–12 *days*). The male syrinx showed a distinct asymmetry to the left at the time of explantation. Differentiation of the cartilaginous arches commenced and continued *in vitro* as in the intact embryo. Two well-marked narrow bands appeared on the left-hand side while only one, less swollen, band appeared on the right. Toward the middle of this ring a large ventral swelling constituted the mamillary tubercle.

In contrast, the female syrinx formed thin-walled vesicular ampullas with a pair of symmetric arches.

b. Explantation before the Stage of Sexual Differentiation. The syrinx was taken from 7–8 day embryos. At this stage, the syrinx appeared as a slight, transparent, almost symmetric swelling composed of connective tissue. The gonads of the donor embryo were cultured separately to determine the genetic sex. Each syrinx developed the male form (Fig. 18). The first pair of cartilaginous arches appeared 2 or 3 days after explantation, at a stage that corresponded to 11 days of incubation. That on the left was already better developed than that on the right. The longitudinal partition of the syrinx or pessulus developed at the same time, separating the chamber into two unequal parts; in most cases, the left side was more swollen than the right. The asymmetry of the syrinx became more marked between the 12th and 15th days of development. On the left side of the ventral surface, two cartilaginous arches developed and fused together at the midline. On the right side there was only one cartilaginous arch, much shorter and thinner than that on the left.

When the asymmetry was not well marked, the male syrinx could still be identified by a large ventral swelling, the mamillary tubercle, which developed on the midline at the meeting point of the right and left cartilages (Fig. 18).

These results verified the results obtained with castrated embryos. The so-called masculine form of the syrinx developed in the absence of hormones, into a neutral or asexual form (76, 62).

Differentiation of the syrinx into the female form depended on the presence of female hormone from the embryonic ovary. This has been confirmed by using injections of crystalline hormones (62).

The following experiments verified this hypothesis. Et. Wolff and Em. Wolff (79) explanted undifferentiated syringes and cultured them for 6–10 days, in contact with drops of an oil solution of estradiol benzoate (5 mg/ml) added to the medium.

All the syringes cultured with female hormone differentiated into the female type.

The results were the same when the undifferentiated syrinx was cultured with ovaries from 12–16 day duck embryos (63).

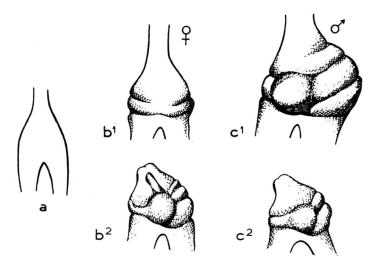

Fig. 18. Diagrammatic representation of the differentiation of the syrinx after explantation at the undifferentiated stage. (a) Syrinx at the time of explantation (7 days). There is a slight, symmetric swelling at the junction of the trachea and the bronchi. (b¹, c¹) This shows the normal differentiation of the syrinx in a female embryo (b¹) and a male embryo (c¹) between 12 and 14 days of incubation. (b², c²) Explants from a female embryo (b²) and a male embryo (c²) after 6 days of culture. Both resemble the male (neutral) type of differentiation. After Et. Wolff and Em. Wolff.

3. The Genital Tubercle of Duck Embryos

The genital tubercle also shows sexual differences in the duck embryo. Em. Wolff (62) showed that the male form corresponds to the neutral or asexual type at the beginning of its development, as does the syrinx.

This was confirmed by Et. Wolff and Em. Wolff (78) using organ culture techniques. The genital tubercles were taken both before and after sexual differentiation of the gonads and were cultured until the 15th or 16th day of incubation, at which time sexual differences in the genital tubercle become very marked in the normal embryo.

At this stage, the genital tubercle in the male is an elongated cylindrical organ. It is coiled in a helix and is traversed by a helical furrow that is the forerunner of the seminal gutter. The genital tubercle in the female, in the process of regression, is reduced to a small mass resting on two symmetric swellings separated by a straight gutter. Neither the organ nor the gutter shows any tendency to twist.

At the time of explantation (7–11 days), the genital tubercle was identical in the two sexes. It was a simple bulbous swelling in the oral margin of the anal fold. When cultured, it grew, elongated, and acquired a pedicle. Although the differentiation was slower in the culture it was often possible to recognize into which sexual type the tubercle was developing.

Explanted after 10 days of incubation, male genital tubercles developed into the male type and female genital tubercles developed into the female type. Thus at this stage of development the hormone from the female gonads has already affected the development of the genital tubercle.

If the genital tubercles were explanted after 7–9 days of incubation they differentiated into the male type, whatever the original genetic sex of the embryo. They showed a swollen base, a long pedicle, and a helical gutter.

Male differentiation of the genital tubercle corresponded to the neutral type. Hormone from the female gonads determined female differentiation and induced atrophy of the genital tubercle.

E. Diffusion of Embryonic Sex Hormones in the Culture Medium

In 1962, Weniger (55) showed that hormones produced by embryonic gonads diffuse in the culture medium, by observing that the left testes of chick embryos were feminized when they were cultured at a distance from female gonads so that the only connection between the two organs was that provided by the culture medium. When the Müller ducts were used as the target organ, their development was stimulated.

That ovarian hormone can diffuse into the culture medium was shown by Weniger in another way. He substituted the receptor organs for the female gonads, or even implanted an extract of the medium into castrated mice. In the latter case, Allen and Doisy's test was positive (59).

On media into which testicular hormone had diffused the Müller ducts regressed and died.

Hormones secreted by the embryonic gonads retained their physiological activity even if the medium into which they had diffused was incubated for 5–7 days at 38°C.

F. Conclusions

The following conclusions can be drawn from the experiments using *in vitro* culture of the sex organs of birds.

1. The gonads develop outside the organism into testes or ovaries according to their genetic sex.

2. Male or female development of a gonad precursor is an example of autodifferentiation.

3. The gonads possess the factors necessary for differentiation at an early stage in their development. When the germinal epithelium is explanted alone it can give rise to tissues analogous to those developed from a whole gonad.

4. Natural and synthetic hormones act directly on the target organ (testis, Müller duct, syrinx) without the intervention of any other gland in the embryo.

5. The similarity of the effects exerted by natural and steroid hormones speaks in favor of the identity or at least a close relationship between the two groups of materials.

6. The gonads produce hormones early in their development, prior to, or at the onset of sexual differentiation.

7. The medulla of the female gonads is all that is necessary for the production of female hormone.

8. Teratogenic agents act selectively on certain parts of the genital apparatus. Effects similar to those produced by hormones occur after treatment with X-rays, ultrasonic radiation, increased temperature, or trypaflavine.

III. MAMMALS

A. Culture of Mammalian Gonads

Mammalian gonads have been explanted both before and after sexual differentiation has occurred.

1. DIFFERENTIATED GONADS

Martinovitch (33, 34) cultured sexually differentiated gonads from 15–20 day rat and mouse fetuses and from the newborn animals. The ovaries of rats and mice behaved in an identical fashion. The cultures were carried out on Fell and Robinson's medium (6), composed of equal parts of embryo extract and chicken plasma. The most favorable temperature was 34°C. Gonads of both sexes survived for several weeks. In the testes, the seminiferous tubules were maintained and the spermatogonia continued to differentiate. The spermatogonia began the change into spermatocytes and were able to develop as far as the pachytene stage. They degenerated very often on the 20th day of culture.

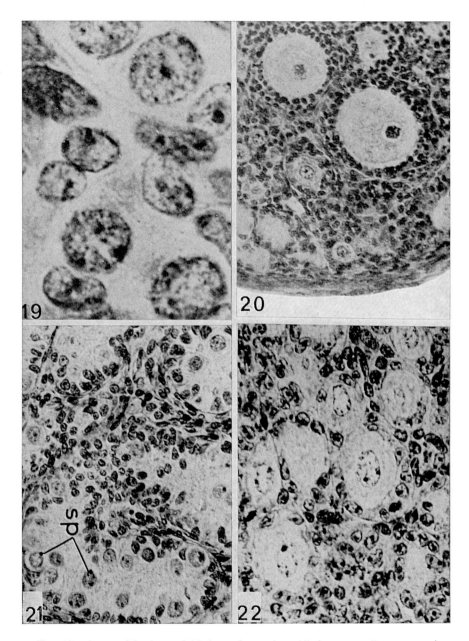

FIG. 19.   Ovary of fetal rat of 16 days of gestation. All the germ cells are oogonia.

FIG. 20.   Detail of 19–20 fetal rat ovary after 12 days of culture. Typical Graafian follicles have developed. After Martinovitch.

a. Development of the Ovaries of the 15- to 16-Day Rat Fetus. At this stage the oogonia are dividing mitotically and no meiotic figures are yet visible (Fig. 19). In explants studied after periods of between 19 hours and 8 days of culture, the nuclear chromatin was modified and passed through the stages of meiosis (leptotene, zygotene, pachytene, and diplotene). At the same time, the germinal epithelium disappeared from the surface of the ovary, which became covered by 3–4 layers of fibroblasts.

Between 8 and 30 days of culture, the oocyte nuclei in the diplotene stage returned to the resting phase. Some oocytes increased in size, reaching diameters of 50–55 μ, but they were not surrounded by Graafian follicles. Moreover, they did not migrate toward the center of the organ but remained massed together near the surface of the ovary. The center of the ovary was occupied by a fibrous stroma. Degeneration of the organ began after 26–28 days of culture.

b. Development of the Ovaries from Newborn Rats and 17- to 20-Day Fetuses. Ovaries taken at the end of gestation or after birth showed much better differentiation, especially of the follicles. Ovaries taken between 19 and 25 days showed almost normal young Graafian follicles after 3 weeks of culture (Fig. 20). These follicles had migrated to the center of the organ as in the normal ovary. Necrosis occurred in the center of the gonad soon after explantation, but these areas were resorbed after a few days. Some cultures were still healthy after 70–80 days.

Martinovitch's results showed that the entire process of oogenesis could occur *in vitro*. The stages that occurred *in vitro* were comparable to those occurring *in vivo*.

In 1959, Van de Kerckove (25) obtained similar results culturing gonads from 18- to 21-day mouse fetuses. However, he found that in cultures from 3-day old mice, the multilayered follicles already present had regressed. The granular layer showed signs of degeneration and the oocytes were surrounded only by a thin layer of flattened, follicular cells.

2. UNDIFFERENTIATED MOUSE GONADS

Et. Wolff (66) explanted 10- to 13-day fetal mouse gonads on Wolff and Haffen's medium (70). Taken at 12–13 days immediately after the beginning of sexual differentiation, further differentiation of the explants followed

FIG. 21. Continuing differentiation of mouse testes taken after 14 days of gestation. Spermatogonia (sp) are present in the seminiferous tubules. After Et. Wolff.

FIG. 22. *In vitro* development of a 14-day mouse ovary. Primary follicles have formed around the growing oocytes. After Et. Wolff.

its normal course (Figs. 21 and 22). In particular, after 5 days of culture most of the primary oocytes had begun to mature.

Undifferentiated gonads at the 10- to $11\frac{1}{2}$-day stage could not be cultured easily in the absence of the surrounding tissues, but they could be grown with the mesonephros. Sexual differentiation did occur, but the ovaries and testes that developed were more or less sterile.

a. Testicular Differentiation of Gonads Taken between 10 and $11\frac{1}{2}$ Days of Gestation. At the time of explantation, the gonadial precursor consisted of a block of undifferentiated epithelial cells. It was continuous with the epithelium of the genital ridge and many germ cells were present among the epithelial cells.

After 4–6 days of culture male gonads acquired the typical structure of testes with tubules converging toward the hilum. These were well-filled sinuous channels, lined with Sertoli epithelium. On one side the organ was bordered by a tunica albuginea composed of several layers of connective tissue; the other side was in contact with the mesonephros. Several tubules from this tissue came into close contact with the testicular tubules to form the rete testis.

b. Ovarian Differentiation of Gonads Taken between 10 and $11\frac{1}{2}$ Days of Gestation. Sterile ovaries differed in their general appearance from normal ovaries, which derived their characteristic appearance from the presence of developing oocytes.

Gonads definitely differentiating to form ovaries had a domelike appearance, formed by a mass of tissue continuous with the germinal epithelium. The latter showed areas of proliferation, which formed lobes separated by furrows from the remainder of the gonad. These formations illustrated the cortical nature of this part of the gland better than a normal ovary.

The medulla was composed of cell cords in close proximity to the mesonephric tubules. The latter represented the rete ovarii as in the normal ovary.

Borghese and Venini (2) cultured gonads from 13- to 18 day fetal mice, and their results confirmed those of Et. Wolff and of Martinovitch. In particular, they showed that testes taken at 13 days continued to develop. At the time of explantation, the testis primordia contained Sertoli cells and spermatogonia intimately mixed together. After culture for a few days, the latter separated from the Sertoli cells, and became concentrated around the axis of the tubules.

Asayama and Furusawa (1) explanted gonads immediately before and after sexual differentiation and cultured them for 24–48 hours. Their results seemed to show that the horse serum which they used had a retarding effect on sexual differentiation. In contrast, a medium consisting of Tyrode's solution with added glucose appeared to favor differentiation in short-term experiments.

3. HUMAN OVARIES

Gaillard (14) carried out systematic culture of human ovaries between 14 weeks of gestation and birth. He used a medium composed entirely of human tissue extracts and serum.

The composition of the medium was as follows:

Human blood plasma	2 volumes
Serum from a placental vein	1 volume
Gey's saline solution with streptomycin	1 volume (10 units)
Human fetal cerebrospinal fluid, eventually replaced by human ascitic fluid	2 volumes
Gey's saline solution	4 volumes

The work of Gaillard was in three parts:

1. Explantations from embryos between 14 and 21 weeks of gestation.
2. Explantations from embryos between 24 and 36 weeks of gestation.
3. Explantations from the fetus at term.

The survival of fragments of human ovary in culture depended principally on the presence of germinal epithelium. Polar fragments survived better than those from the medial region. Those that had no germinal epithelium died after a few days while those possessing even a small fragment of germinal epithelium survived. The epithelium proliferated and enclosed the explant completely. In explants from young ovaries the entire central parenchyma degenerated, including the young oocytes. In explants from older embryos the cells of the primary follicles survived. In all cases a reticular stroma persisted after the disappearance of the degenerating structures.

After 10–12 days of culture, cell cords regenerated from the covering epithelium, penetrated into the reticular stroma, and anastomosed (Fig. 23). The organ had the appearance of a young ovary. In some cases the new parenchyma completely filled the center of the explant (Fig. 24). New germ cells appeared in the cell cords. These passed through all the stages between undifferentiated gonocytes and completely differentiated oocytes (Fig. 25). All characteristic stages of the prophase of the first maturation division could be observed. In some cases this mitosis was completed and resulted in complete division of the initial cell. Such division was never seen at this stage in the normal ovary. Thus, the covering epithelium alone could regenerate the ovarian parenchyma, including the germinal cells. A second type of cell cord could be seen in explants from 24–36 week embryos. These

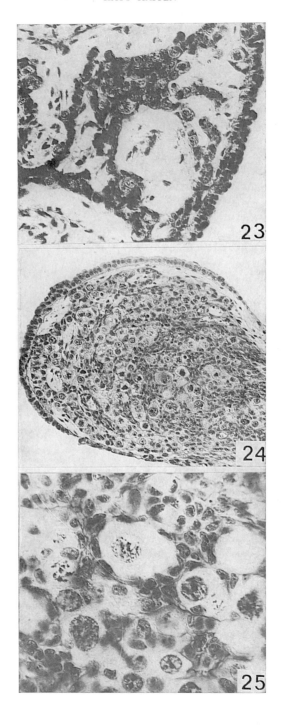

were regenerated from the follicular cells that did not degenerate although the oocytes already formed had all degenerated. Many new oocytes differentiated in these cords. In many explants these new oocytes were surrounded by a layer of flattened or cuboid cells. These follicular cells were derived from undifferentiated parenchyma cells.

These remarkable experiments demonstrate the great regenerative capacity of the ovary. The undifferentiated cells of the germinal epithelium can replace all the tissues of the ovarian cortex, including even the oocytes.

B. Modification of the Sexual Differentiation of Mammalian Gonads

The work of Lillie (26, 27) and of Keller and Tandler (24) on bovine freemartins was the starting point for many experiments on intersexuality in the vertebrates. Although many results have been obtained using amphibians, fish, birds, and reptiles, few experiments using mammals have been successful. The work of Burns (3) must be considered separately. The latter author showed that the sexual differentiation of male opossums could be modified by injecting estrogenic hormones. Among the placental mammals, hormone injections and gonad grafts can induce important modifications of the genital tract. Such injections have never achieved complete sexual reversal of the gonads, but some inhibition and intersexuality of the gonads have been obtained by grafting in parabiosis (MacIntyre, Holyoke, Beber, and Salzgeber).

1. PARABIOSIS *IN VIVO*

MacIntyre (30, 31) implanted pairs of associated organs from 16-day rat fetuses (ovary and testis) beneath the renal capsule of adult rats castrated 3 weeks before the operation. The grafts remained in place for 3 weeks. Ovarian differentiation was suppressed in some explants. Other grafts showed ovarian rudiments with degenerate follicles. The development of follicles was inhibited in most cases. MacIntyre also showed that ovarian tissue was transformed into the male type. In 7 cases out of 23 he observed tubular formations containing oocytes.

FIG. 23. Fragment of ovarian cortex from a 16-week human fetus, cultured *in vitro*. After 13 days, the cell cords have regenerated from the covering epithelium. They penetrate into the central reticular stroma and anastomose. After Gaillard.

FIG. 24. Fragment of ovarian cortex from a 20-week human fetus, cultured *in vitro*. After 12 days of culture, new parenchyma fills the interior of the explant. The organ resembles a young ovary. After Gaillard.

FIG. 25. Detail of the regenerated cell cords. New germ cells can be seen and these pass through all the intermediate stages between morphologically undifferentiated gonocytes and completely differentiated oocytes. After Gaillard.

Holyoke (20) obtained similar results with 17–24 day rabbit fetuses.

MacIntyre *et al.* (32) showed that the tissues had to fuse intimately to obtain an inhibitory effect. They grafted the male and female gonads at varying distances from one another (1–10 mm) and showed that when the two gonads were more than 8 mm apart the male gonad no longer affected the female one.

Turner and Asakawa (50) took testes and ovaries from $12\frac{1}{2}$–$14\frac{1}{2}$ day fetal mice and grafted them beneath the renal capsule of castrated adult male mice. They showed that in ovaries that had been masculinized by the testes the oogonia could develop into spermatocytes.

2. Parabiosis *in Vitro*

Experiments using parabiosis *in vitro* were carried out by Holyoke and Beber (21) and by Salzgeber (45, 47, 48).

Holyoke and Beber associated the gonads of fetal rabbits or fetal rats on a medium that was composed of plasma coagulum and 11-day chick embryo extract (only the anterior part of the embryo, excluding the gonads was used in preparing the extract). In heterosexual combinations the development of the ovaries was always retarded and they did not develop cortical elements. In three cases, structures resembling testicular cords were observed in the ovarian medulla.

Salzgeber combined parabiosis experiments *in vitro* with heteroplastic grafting. She associated the ovaries from 12–$21\frac{1}{2}$ day fetal mice with gonads from 6–10 day chick embryos. After culture for 2–6 days on Wolff and Haffen's medium (70), the associated explants were grafted into the coelomic cavities of young chick embryos where they developed until the hosts were killed (12–19 days). Salzgeber (47) showed that fetal mouse ovaries continued to develop when they were grafted into the coelom of chick embryos. The germinal cells passed through the stages of meiotic prophase. The oocytes developed into primary follicles. Culture of the organs before their implantation into the host embryo encouraged the acceptance of the heterograft. Blood vessels from the host perfused the mouse tissues. The grafts had no effect on the genital system of the host. The host had no influence on the implant unless the latter was grafted onto the testis of a male embryo, and under these conditions the development was aberrant. Proof of this inhibition was gained from association experiments on mouse ovaries and chicken gonads.

a. Associations between Mouse Ovary and Chicken Ovary.   In this combination the two organs fused intimately to produce chimeras. The mouse ovary was clothed by chick ovary cortex containing many gonocytes in the process of meiosis. The mouse tissue, populated by primary follicles, took the place of the chicken ovarian medulla. As the mouse cells were strongly basophilic, it was possible to distinguish between the tissues from the two species. The degree of development reached depended on the stage at which the mouse ovary was taken. Follicles were more numerous in gonads from 15–21 day embryos than in gonads from 13–14 day embryos. In those taken after only 11–12 days of gestation the development was difficult.

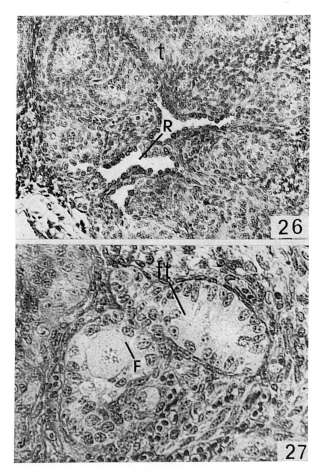

FIG. 26. Combination between a 13-day embryo mouse ovary and 2 fragments of testis from an 8-day chick embryo. Cultured for 3 days, then grafted into a host for 15 days. The rete ovarii (R) communicates with the testicular tubules of the chicken (t). After Salzgeber.

FIG. 27. Ovary from 14-day mouse embryo explanted between two pieces of 8-day chicken testis. Cultured for 2 days, then grafted into a host embryo for 12 days. The gonad contains two tubules reminiscent of testicular tubules (ft). An aberrant follicle (F) is seen in one of the tubules. After Salzgeber.

b. Associations between Mouse Ovary and Chicken Testis. In this type of association, the organs fused intimately. When taken at a late stage of their development (17–19 days of gestation), the ovaries developed follicles but their appearance was altered. The follicular cells were lacking in some cases and flattened in others. This change in the ovaries was even more marked if they were associated with chick testis at an earlier stage in their development. When taken at 13–14 days, the ovaries developed in an atypical fashion. They consisted of loose mesenchyme cells and the cortical and medullary zones could not be distinguished. A few isolated oocytes were able to persist in this undifferentiated tissue. In most of the inhibited ovaries the tubules of the rete ovarii could be clearly distinguished. They were sinuous hollow tubes with walls composed of a layer of irregularly arranged cells (Fig. 26), penetrating into the chicken tissue to form a mixed structure with the seminiferous tubules. In some explants a few cords seen in the vicinity of the rete had a testicular appearance, and these occasionally contained oocytes or degenerating follicles (Fig. 27).

This group of experiments by Holyoke, Beber, and Salzgeber shows that the testis has a profound action on the developing mammalian ovary. The effects seen can be interpreted as inhibition or—in certain cases—as sexual inversion.

C. *In Vitro* Culture of the Genital Tract of Mammalian Embryos

Experiments using injections of steroid hormones, grafts, and castration have shown the role of the sex hormones in the differentiation of the genital tract.

Jost and Bergerard (23) were the first to culture the genital tract *in vitro*. Subsequently Price and Pannabecker (39) explanted about 300 genital tracts from fetal rats of both sexes. The explants were taken after $14\frac{1}{2}$–$18\frac{1}{2}$ days of gestation and were cultured for 4–6 days at 34°C on a medium containing cockerel plasma and embryo extract. In some cases aqueous extracts of testosterone (0.1–153 μg/ml of medium) or estradiol (0.02–20 μg/ml of medium) were added. The genital tracts comprised the Wolff ducts, the Müller ducts, and the urogenital sinus.

Genital tracts taken at different stages, either before or after sexual differentiation were subjected to varying experimental conditions. They were cultured as follows:

1. Genital tract together with both gonads
2. Genital tract together with one gonad
3. Genital tract with no gonads

4. Genital tract together with gonads of the opposite sex

5 and 6. Genital tract with no gonads but with exogenous hormone.

The results of these experiments can be summarized as follows. The male genital trace developed normally when cultured for 4 days, the development being retarded by 1–2 days as compared to the normal development *in vivo*. The Wolff ducts developed and gave rise to the seminal vesicles, derived from dilatations of the Wolff duct, and to the prostatic buds derived from the epithelium of the urogenital sinus. The Müller ducts regressed anteriorly, the posterior parts forming the prostatic utriclulus by fusion of the two posterior trunks. Complete absence of the testis induced regression of the Wolff duct. The presence of a single testis assured the maintenance of both canals in the early stages but of only one canal in the later stages. These experiments show that the embryonic testis secretes a substance that diffuses in the culture medium and allows maintenance of the Wolff ducts and the development of the associated glands.

The same results were obtained if the testes were removed and testosterone added to the culture medium.

Normal development occurred when the female genital tract was cultured for 4 days. The Wolff ducts regressed, the Müller ducts developed, and the uretero-vaginal canal was formed by fusion of the posterior trunks. Removal of the ovaries did not affect the Müller ducts, which continued to develop. The Müller ducts were inhibited neither by testes placed near them nor by testosterone. Slight stimulation occurred in both instances. Female Wolff ducts were slightly stimulated by testes or testosterone, but their regression was not completely inhibited and no seminal vesicles were formed.

It seems probable that sexual differentiation of the genital tracts of fetal rats depends on the presence of testicular hormone in the male, and on the absence of such a hormone in the female.

These results support those obtained by Jost (22), by Wells (51), and by Raynaud and Frilley (40). These workers used embryonic castration followed by grafting of gonads into the castrated embryos.

D. Interspecific Associations between Embryonic Gonads and Genital Tracts

Weniger (57) cultured ovaries from 12- to 19-day fetal mice in contact with undifferentiated gonad rudiments from male chick embryos and found that the ovaries had no hormonal activity. On the other hand, fetal mouse ovaries could stimulate the Müller ducts of 8-day female chick embryos without direct contact.

Testes from 12- to 19-day fetal mice produced a hormone with a feminizing action on chicken testis. This was shown in experiments where testes from

15- to 18-day mice were associated with undifferentiated chicken testes (56). This feminizing action occurred both on the Müller ducts of 8-day female chick embryos, where development was stimulated, and on those of 8-day male embryos, where regression was inhibited. Direct contact was not necessary. The hormone produced by the fetal mouse testis could diffuse into the medium, as was shown in experiments where the Müller ducts were substituted for fetal mouse testes (57).

Chick embryo testis caused regression of the Müller ducts of fetal mice but it could maintain the Wolff duct.

In contrast fetal mouse testis stimulated development of the Wolff duct but could not induce regression of the Müller duct (see Table I).

Confronted *in vitro* with the same receptor organs, embryonic testes from chickens and mice did not have the same actions and they did not appear to secrete the same hormone (58). The question is whether the hormone secreted by fetal mouse testis is different *in vitro* from what it is *in vivo*. Weniger interpreted these results as a gradual denaturation of the secretion under the conditions of culture.

Conclusions

Experiments on the culture of the sex organs of mammals lead to the following conclusions:

1. When explanted at an undifferentiated stage, the gonads achieve their normal sexual differentiation. Explanted after sexual differentiation, the ovaries and testes continue to differentiate up to the stage of gametogenesis.

2. Experiments using *in vitro* culture of differentiated human fetal ovaries show that after a phase of extreme degeneration sex cords regenerate from the germinal epithelium and undifferentiated gonocytes reappear in these cords.

3. *In vitro* and *in vivo* parabiosis of heterosexual gonads using homoplastic and xenoplastic combinations induces both inhibition and intersexuality. The mammalian ovary reacts when it is paired with a male partner (mouse or chicken). The cortex is more or less completely inhibited, and the medulla shows varying degrees of masculinization. In some cases young oogonia may differentiate into spermatogonia or even spermatocytes in the testicular tubules of an ovary.

4. Experiments using *in vitro* culture of the genital tract lead to the same conclusions as those using castration *in vivo*. They show that the neutral organism starts its development in the female pattern. Testicular hormone induces regression of the female ducts and is also necessary for the maintenance of the Wolff ducts and associated glands of the male genital tract.

TABLE I

Interspecific Associations between Embryonic Gonads and Genital Ducts

Organs used for testing hormone action	Target organs				
	Chicken testis (5–7 days of incubation)	Female chick Müller ducts (8 days of incubation)	Male chick Müller ducts (8 days of incubation)	Male mouse Wolff ducts (15–18 days of gestation)	Female mouse Müller ducts (15–18 days of gestation)
Mouse testis (12–19 days of gestation)	Feminization	Stimulation	Maintenance	Development (normal)	Development (stimulated)
Mouse ovary (12–19 days of gestation)	Development (normal)	Stimulation	Maintenance	Degeneration (normal)	Development
Chicken testis (7–11 days of incubation)	—	Regression[a]	Regression[a]	Degeneration (abnormal)	Regression ± complete
Neutral tissue (segment of intestine)	—	Maintenance	—	Degeneration (normal)	Development
No associated organ	—	Maintenance	Maintenance	Degeneration	Development

[a] See Ref. (28).

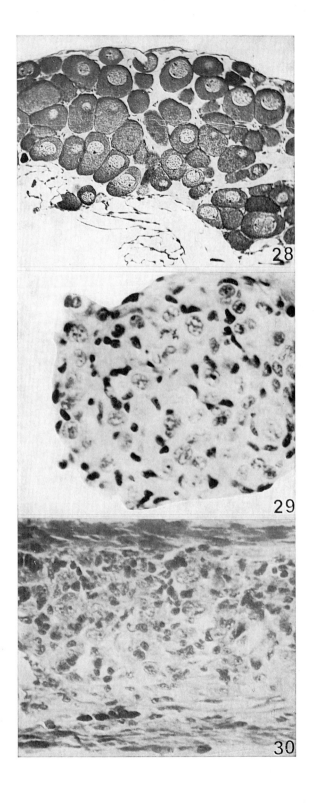

5. When confronted *in vitro* with the same receptor organs, embryonic testes from chickens and mice do not have the same actions. These results can be interpreted as due to a denaturation of the hormonal secretion under culture conditions.

IV. AMPHIBIANS

The culture of undifferentiated gonads from amphibians has proved more difficult than the culture of undifferentiated gonads from birds and mammals. Ch. Foote and F. Foote (7–13) have been successful in organ culture of differentiated gonads from larval and adult amphibians.

A. Gonad Culture

The above workers explanted gonads from *Rana clamitans* (7) and *Rana catesbeiana* (10) during the second year of larval life. At this stage the gonads were already sexually differentiated. Two media were found to be favorable for organ culture of amphibian gonads. The first was based on the technique of Fell and Robinson (6).

Gonads cultured on this medium at 26°C survived for several weeks (37 days). Considerable fibroblastic proliferation of somatic elements occurred in the gonads of both sexes. In the ovaries the auxocytes (more differentiated germ cells) degenerated while the oogonia and young oocytes became fibroblastic, as did the germinal elements of the testes.

Similar results were obtained with adult ovaries and testes from *Triturus cristatus* (9).

The second culture medium used by Foote and Foote was that of Et. Wolff and Haffen (70). This medium was more favorable for the maintenance of the structural integrity of the explants. The large oocytes (auxocytes) degenerated, but the young oocytes survived and the oogonia and spermatogonia multiplied (Figs. 28 and 29).

Gonads from *Xenopus laevis* (8) did not differentiate when they were taken before or at the stage of sexual differentiation [stage 49–50 of Nieuwkoop

---

FIG. 28.   Larval ovary from *Rana catesbeiana*, cultured for 9 days on a medium based on agar and chick embryo extract. After Ch. L. Foote and F. M. Foote.

FIG. 29.   Larval testis from *Rana catesbeiana*, cultured for 28 days on a medium based on agar and chick embryo extract. After Ch. L. Foote and F. M. Foote.

FIG. 30.   Detail of a gonad from a female larva of *Rana catesbeiana* cultured *in vitro* on a medium based on cockerel plasma and chick embryo extract with the addition of 10 γ of Su-61. All the auxocytes have degenerated and the structure is testicular in appearance. After Ch. L. Foote and F. M. Foote.

and Faber (38)]. Neither somatic tissues nor germinal cells were identifiable. When they were explanted at a more advanced stage preceding metamorphosis, the gonads retained their ovarian or testicular structure. The germinal cells survived and multiplied.

In 1962, Ch. Foote and F. Foote (13) cultured the following tissues in the vitelline membrane of nonincubated hen egg, using the technique of Et. Wolff (67):

1. Fragments of the trunk from hatching larvae of *Pleurodeles waltlii* (stages 37–38 of Gallien and Durocher (18)).

2. Gonads from $4\frac{1}{2}$-month larvae (this stage corresponded to metamorphosis and sexual differentiation).

3. Testes from adult animals. Culture was continued for 21–57 days.

In the first case none of the gonads were differentiated but primary germinal cells were seen in some explants. In the second case the gonads survived and the germinal cells were in the premeiotic phase. In the third case the testes could be cultured more easily than those from other amphibian species. Only the spermatogonia survived.

B. Effect of Sex Hormones

Since 1936 many workers have induced sex inversion in the Amphibia by using crystalline sex hormones. This work has been reviewed by Gallien (16, 17) and Witchi (61).

1. THE EFFECT OF MALE HORMONE

Ch. Foote and F. Foote (11) demonstrated the action of testosterone Su-61 (17β-diethylaminoethyl carbonate hydrochloride) both *in vivo* and *in vitro*. When injected into larvae of *Rana catesbeiana* this hormone induced sexual inversion. Females changed into males after 42 days. The same hormone did not induce sex inversion in *Xenopus laevis* but the development of the females was retarded as compared to control animals.

Ovaries and testes from larvae of *Rana catesbeiana* were grown for 17–42 days in the presence of testosterone Su-61 at a concentration of 10–100 γ in the medium. The ovaries transformed partially or totally into testes (Fig. 30). Histological examination of the controls showed that the transformed ovaries came from young animals where the gonads contained few auxocytes but many oogonia.

Gonads from *Xenopus laevis* (taken at stages 55–56 of Nieuwkoop and Faber (38)) were cultured for 22 days in the presence of Su-61, using a dose of 10 γ in the medium. The gonads survived but differentiation was retarded as compared to the controls. There was no sexual inversion (11).

2. THE EFFECT OF FEMALE HORMONE

Gallien (15) and Chang and Witchi (4) induced sexual inversion of male *Xenopus laevis* larvas by treating them with estradiol at the moment of sexual differentiation (stages 48–55 of Nieuwkoop and Faber (38)).

Ch. Foote and F. Foote (12) cultured *Xenopus laevis* gonads in the presence of estradiol. This hormone did not induce sexual inversion of testes grown *in vitro*. Gonads taken before the sexual differentiation had occurred did not differentiate. Sexually differentiated gonads, both ovaries and testes (stages 55–56) continued to develop on culture. It is thought that the absence of a reaction in culture may be due to the fact the gonads had not differentiated at the time of explantation to a stage favorable for sexual inversion.

C. Conclusions

Gonads from sexually undifferentiated Amphibian larvae survived in culture but did not differentiate.

Sexual inversion in culture was obtained only in *Rana catesbeiana*. Gonads from larval females were transformed into testes by the action of testosterone (Su-61).

The same hormone had no effect on the female gonads of *Xenopus laevis*.

BIBLIOGRAPHY

1. Asayama S. and Furusawa M.   Sex differentiation of Primordial Gonads of the Mouse embryo after cultivation *in vitro*. *Japan. Journ. exp. Morphol.*, 1961, **15**, 34–47.
2. Borghese E. and Venini M. A.   Culture *in vitro* de gonades embryonnaires de Mus musculus. *Symposia genetica*, 1956, **5**, 69–83.
3. Burns R. K.   Effects of female sex hormones in young Opossums. *Proc. Soc. exp. Biol. and Med.*, 1939, **41**, 270–272.
4. Chang C. Y. and Witschi E.   Breeding of sex reversed male of *Xenopus laevis Daudin*. *Proc. Soc. exp. Biol. Med.*, 1955, **89**, 150.
5. Dantchakoff V.   Sur l'inversion sexuelle expérimentale de l'ébauche testiculaire chez l'embryon de Poulet. *C. R. Acad. Sci.*, 1935, **200**, 1983–1985.
6. Fell H. B. and Robison R.   The growth, development and phosphatase activity of embryonic avian femora and limb buds cultivated *in vitro*. *Biochem. Jour.*, 1929, **23**, 767–784.
7. Foote Ch. L.   Growth of amphibian gonads in organ cultures. *Amer. Philosophical Society*, 1957, 246–248.
8. Foote Ch. L. and Foote F. M.   Maintenance of gonads of frog larvae in organ culture. *Transactions of the Illinois State. Academy of Science.* 1957, **50**, 243–246.
9. Foote Ch. L. and Foote F. M.   *In vitro* cultivation of gonads of adult amphibia. *Anat. Rec.*, 1957, **127**, 415.
10. Foote Ch. L. and Foote F. M.   *In vitro* cultivation of gonads of Larval Anurans. *Anat. rec.*, 1958, **130**, 553–565.
11. Foote Ch. L. and Foote F. M.   Effects *in vivo* and *in vitro* of a water soluble testost-

erone on gonads of two species of anurans. *Arch. Anat. micr. Morph. exp.*, 1959, **48** *bis*, 71–82.

12. Foote Ch. L. and Foote F. M. Maintenance of gonads of Xenopus laevis in organ cultures. *Proc. Soc. exp. Biol. Med.*, 1960, **105**, 107–108.

13. Foote Ch. L. and Foote F. M. The culture *in vitro* of Urogenital Organs of Pleurodeles waltlii. *J. Embryol. exp. Morph.*, 1962, **10**, 465–470.

14. Gaillard P. J. Sex cell formation in explants of the foetal human ovarian cortex I et II. *Kon. Ned. Akad. v. Wetensch.*, 1950, **53**, 1300–1347.

15. Gallien L. Inversion totale du sexe chez *Xenopus laevis Daud*, à la suite d'un traitement gynogène par le benzoate d'œstradiol administré pendant la vie larvaire. *C. R. Acad. Sci.*, 1953, **237**, 1565.

16. Gallien L. Hormones sexuelles et différenciation du sexe chez les Amphibiens. *Rev. Suisse Zool.*, 1954, **61**, 349–374.

17. Gallien L. Analyse des effets des hormones stéroïdes dans la différenciation sexuelle des Amphibiens. *Arch. Anat. micr. Morph. exp.*, 1959, **48** *bis*, 83–100.

18. Gallien L. and Durocher M. Table chronologique du développement chez Pleurodeles Waltlii. *Bull. Biol.*, **91**, 97–114.

19. Haffen K. La culture *in vitro* de l'épithélium germinatif isolé des gonades mâles et femelles de l'embryon de Canard. 2. *J. Embr. exp. Morph.*, 1960, **8**, 414–424.

20. Holyoke E. A. The differentiation of embryonic gonads grafted to adult gonads in the rabbit. *Anat. Rec.*, 1957, **127**, 470.

21. Holyoke E. A. and Beber B. A. Cultures of gonads of Mammalian embryos. *Science*, 1958, **128**, 1082.

22. Jost A. Castration de l'embryon femelle de Lapin. *C. R. Soc. Biol.*, 1946, **140**, 774–775.

23. Jost A. and Bergerard Y. Culture *in vitro* d'ébauches du tractus génital du fœtus de Rat. *C. R. Soc. Biol.*, 1949, **143**, 608–609.

24. Keller K. and Tandler J. Ueber das Verhalten der Eihäute bei der Zwillingsträchtigkeit des Rindes. *Mschr. Ver. Tierärz. Ust.*, 1916, **3**, 513–526.

25. Van de Kerckove. L'ovaire périnatal de la Souris blanche en culture organotypique. *C. R. Ass. Anatomistes*, 1959, **104**, 754–759.

26. Lillie F. R. The theory of the Free-Martin. *Science*, 1916, **43**, 611.

27. Lillie F. R. The Free-Martin: a study of the action of sex hormones in the foetal life of cattle. *J. exp. Zool.*, 1917, **23**, 371–452.

28. Lutz-Ostertag Y. Contribution à l'étude du développement et de la régression des canaux de Müller chez l'embryon d'Oiseau. *Bull. Biol.*, 1954, **88**, 333–412.

29. Lutz H. and Lutz-Ostertag Y. Contribution à l'étude du maintien des canaux de Müller de l'embryon de Poulet mâle par l'action des ultra-sons. *Arch. Anat. micr. Morph. exp.*, 1956, **45**, 218–234.

30. Mac Intyre M. N. Effect of the testis on ovarian differentiation in heterosexual embryonic Rat gonad transplants. *Anat. Rec.*, 1956, **124**, 27–45.

31. Mac Intyre M. N., Baker J. and Wykoff J. W. Effect of the ovary, on testicular differentiation in heterosexual embryonic Rat gonad transplants. *Arch. Anat. micr. Morph. exp.*, 1959, **48** *bis*, 141–154.

32. Mac Intyre M. N., Hunter G. E. and Morgan A. H. Spatial limits of activity of foetal gonadal inductors in the rat. *Anat. Rec.*, 1960, **138**, 137–148.

33. Martinovitch P. N. The development *in vitro* of the Mammalian gonad. Ovary and ovogenesis. *Proc. Roy. Soc. London.*, 1938, **125**, 232–249.

34. Martinovitch P. N. The effect of subnormal temperatures on the differentiation and survival of cultivated *in vitro* embryonic and infantile rat and mouse ovaries. *Proc. Roy. Soc. London. Série B*, 1939, **128**, 138–143.

35. Mintz B. and Wolff Et. Sur les greffes cœlomiques de la médullaire ovarienne d'embryons de Poulet. L'évolution des greffons et leur action féminisante sur les hôtes mâles. *C. R. Soc. Biol.*, 1951, **146**, 494–495.

36. Mintz B. and Wolff Et. The development of embryonic chick ovarian medulla and its feminizing action in intracoelomic grafts. *J. exp. Zool.*, 1954, **146**, 494–495.

37. Moscona A. Cell suspensions from organ rudiments of chick embryos. *Exp. Cell Res.*, 1952, **3**, 535–539.

38. Nieuwkoop P. D. and Faber J. Normal table of Xenopus laevis (Daudin). *North Holland. Publ. Co. Amsterdam*, 1956.

39. Price D. and Pannabecker R. La différenciation du sexe chez l'embryon de Rat. Comparaison entre le comportement des tractus génitaux ♂ et ♀ en culture. *Arch. Anat. micr. Morph. exp.*, 1959, **48** *bis*, 223–243.

40. Raynaud A. and Frilley M. Destruction des glandes génitales de l'embryon de Souris par une irradiation au moyen des rayons X, à l'âge de 13 jours. *Ann. Endocr.*, 1947, **8**, 400–419.

41. Salzgeber B. Influence des facteurs tératogènes sur l'évolution des organes sexués de l'embryon de Poulet. I: Action des facteurs physiques. II: Action des facteurs chimiques. *Bull. Biol.*, 1957, **91**, 355–438.

42. Salzgeber B. Contribution à l'étude de l'action d'une température élevée d'incubation sur les canaux de Müller cultivés *in vitro. C. R. Acad. Sci.*, 1959, **248**, 1707–1709.

43. Salzgeber B. Greffe dans l'embryon de Poulet de Gonades préalablement soumises en culture à l'influence de poisons mitotiques. *Arch. Anat. micr. Morph. exp.*, 1960, **49**, 261–280.

44. Salzgeber B. Évolution des gonades d'embryon de Poulet greffées dans un embryon hôte après traitement en culture par les rayons X. *Acta anat.*, 1961, **47**, 388.

45. Salzgeber B. Action inhibitrice du testicule de l'embryon de Poulet sur le développement de l'ovaire embryonnaire de Souris. *C. R. Acad. Sci.*, 1960, **251**, 1576–1577.

46. Salzgeber B. Évolution des gonades et conduits génitaux de l'embryon de Poulet soumis en culture à l'action des rayons X. *Bull. Biol. Fr. Belg.*, 1961, **45**, 645–664.

47. Salzgeber B. Étude du développement de l'ovaire de Souris greffé dans l'embryon de Poulet après culture *in vitro. Arch. Anat. micr. Morph. exp.*, 1962, **51**, 1–10.

48. Salzgeber B. Modification expérimentale du développement de Souris sous l'influence du testicule embryonnaire de Poulet. *J. Embryol. exp. Morph.*, 1963, **11**, 91–105.

49. Scheib-Pfleger D. Contribution biochimique à l'étude des processus de différenciation des canaux de Müller chez l'embryon de Poulet. *Thèse Doct. Sciences. Bull. Biol. France et Belgique*, 1955, **89**, 404–499.

50. Turner C. D. and Asakawa H. Experimental Reversal of germ Cells in Ovaries of Fetal Mice. *Science*, 1964, **143**, 1344–1345.

51. Wells L. J. Effects of androgen upon reproductive organs of normal and castrated fetuses with note on adrenalectomy. *Proc. Soc. Exp. Biol. Med.*, 1946, **63**, 417–419.

52. Weniger J. P. Culture *in vitro* et différenciation de très jeunes gonades d'embryon de Poulet. *C. R. Soc. Biol.*, 1958, **152**, 647–649.

53. Weniger J. P. Persistance de la sécrétion hormonale de l'ovaire gauche de l'embryon de Poulet après culture *in vitro. C. R. Soc. Biol.*, 1958, **52**, 515–517.

54. Weniger J. P. Activité hormonale des gonades morphologiquement indifférenciées de l'embryon de Poulet. *Arch. Anat. micr. Morph. exp.*, 1961, **50**, 269–288.

55. Weniger J. P. Diffusion des Hormones gonadiques de l'embryon de Poulet dans le milieu de culture. *Arch. Anat. micr. Morph. exp.*, 1962, **51**, 325–336.

56. Weniger J. P.   Action stimulatrice exercée en culture *in vitro* par le testicule de l'embryon de Souris sur le canal de Müller de l'embryon de Poulet. *C. R. Soc. Biol.*, 1962, **156**, 162–163.

57. Weniger J. P.   Associations de gonades embryonnaires de Souris et de canaux de Müller d'embryon de Poulet. Étude des actions hormonales. *C. R. Acad. Sci.*, 1963, **52**, 497–506.

58. Weniger J. P.   Les testicules embryonnaires de Souris et de Poulet ne sécrètent pas la même hormone *in vitro*. *C. R. Soc. Biol.*, 1963, **157**, 1057–1059.

59. Weniger J. P.   L'ovaire de l'embryon de Poulet cultivé *in vitro* sécrète une hormone œstrogène. *C. R. Soc. Biol.*, 1964, **158**, 175.

60. Willier B. H., Gallagher T. F. and Koch F. C.   Sex modification in the chick embryo resulting from injections of male and female hormones. *Proc. Nat. Acad. Sci.*, 1935, **21**, 625–631.

61. Witschi E.   The inductor theory of sex differentiation. *Jour. Fac. Sci. Hokkaido Univ. Serv. VI. Zool.*, 1957, **13**, 428–439.

62. Wolff Em.   La différenciation sexuelle normale et le conditionnement hormonal des caractères sexuels somatiques précoces: tubercule génital et syrinx chez l'embryon de Canard. *Bull. Biol. France et Belgique*, 1950, **84**, 119–193.

63. Wolff Em. and Lutz-Ostertag Y.   Free-martinisme spontané et expérimental chez l'embryon de Canard. *Arch. Anat. micr. Morph. exp.*, 1962, **50**, 439–468.

64. Wolff Et.   Recherche sur l'intersexualité expérimentale produite par la méthode des greffes de gonades à l'embryon de Poulet. *Arch. Anat. micr. Morph. exp.*, 1946–1947, **36**, 69–90.

65. Wolff Et.   L'évolution des canaux de Müller de l'embryon d'Oiseau après castration précoce. *C. R. Soc. Biol.*, 1949, **143**, 1299.

66. Wolff Et.   Sur la différenciation sexuelle des gonades de Souris explantées *in vitro*. *C. R. Acad. Sci.*, 1952, **234**, 1712–1714.

67. Wolff Et.   Sur une nouvelle modalité de la culture organotypique. *C. R. Acad. Sci. Paris*, 1960, **250**, 3881–3882.

68. Wolff Et. and Ginglinger A.   Sur la transformation des Poulets mâles en intersexués par injection d'hormone femelle (folliculine) aux embryons. *Arch. Anat. Hist. Embryol.*, 1935, **20**, 219–278.

69. Wolff Et. and Haffen K.   Sur la culture *in vitro* des glandes génitales des embryons d'Oiseau: obtention de la différenciation sexuelle normale et de l'intersexualité expérimentale des gonades explantées. *C. R. Acad. Sci.*, 1951, **233**, 439–441.

70. Wolff Et. and Haffen K.   Sur une méthode de culture d'organes embryonnaires *in vitro*. *Texas Rep. Biol. Med.*, 1952, **10**, 463–472.

71. Wolff Et. and Haffen K.   Sur le développement et la différenciation sexuelle des gonades embryonnaires d'Oiseau en culture *in vitro*. *Jour. exp. Zool.*, 1952, **119**, 381–399.

72. Wolff Et. and Haffen K.   Sur la différenciation sexuelle des gonades embryonnaires de l'embryon de Poulet en culture *in vitro*. *Ann. Endocr.*, 1952, **13**, 724–731.

73. Wolff Et. and Haffen K.   Sur l'intersexualité expérimentale des gonades embryonnaires de Canard cultivées *in vitro*. *Arch. Anat. micr. Morph. exp.*, 1952, **41**, 184–207.

74. Wolff Et. and Haffen K.   Action féminisante de la gonade droite de l'embryon femelle de Canard en culture *in vitro*. *C. R. Soc. Biol.*, 1952, **146**, 1772–1774.

75. Wolff Et. and Haffen K.   La culture *in vitro* de l'épithélium germinatif isolé des gonades mâles et femelles de l'embryon de Canard. *Arch. Anat. micr. Morph. exp.*, 1959, **48** *bis*, 331–346.

76. Wolff Et. and Wolff Em. The effects of castration on bird embryos. *J. exp. Zool.*, 1951, **116**, 1, 59–97.
77. Wolff E. and Wolff Em. Mise en évidence d'une action féminisante de la gonade droite chez l'embryon femelle des Oiseaux, par les expériences d'hémicastration. *C. R. Soc. Biol.*, 1951, **145**, 1218–1219.
78. Wolff Et. and Wolff Em. Sur la différenciation *in vitro* du tubercule génital de l'embryon de Canard. *C. R. Soc. Biol.*, 1951, **146**, 492–493.
79. Wolff Et. and Wolff Em. Le déterminisme de la différenciation sexuelle de la syrinx de Canard en culture *in vitro*. *Bull. Biol. Fr. et Belg.*, 1952, **86**, 325–350.
80. Wolff Et. and Wolff Em. Action de l'hormone femelle sur la différenciation sexuelle de la syrinx de Canard, cultivée *in vitro*. *C. R. Soc. Biol.*, 1952, **146**, 111–113.
81. Wolff Et., Wolff Em. and Haffen K. Sur la différenciation *in vitro* de la syrinx chez l'embryon de Canard. *C. R. Acad. Sci.*, 1951, **233**, 500–502.
82. Wolff Et., Lutz-Ostertag Y. and Haffen K. Sur les structures *in vitro* des canaux de Müller de l'embryon de Poulet. *C. R. Soc. Biol.*, 1952, **146**, 1791–1793.
83. Wolff Et., Lutz-Ostertag Y. and Haffen K. Sur la régression et la nécrose *in vitro* des canaux de Müller de l'embryon de Poulet sous l'effet de substances hormonales. *C. R. Soc. Biol.*, 1952, **146**, 1793–1795.

ADDENDUM

This addendum deals with investigations carried out since publication of the previous work in 1965. The research is confined exclusively to birds and mammals. As a very large number of the experiments were carried out using Wolff and Haffen's culture method (see Ch. IV, Ref. 70), the method used will be specified only when it was different.

I. BIRDS

A. Culture of Embryonic Gonads

1. Sexual Differentiation and Intersexuality in the Quail

Embryonic gonads of quail were cultured either alone or in heterosexual parabiosis (13). In the latter instance, the gonads were placed either in direct contact or else separated by the vitelline membrane from a nonincubated hen's egg, using Wolff's technique (50; also see Ch. IV, Ref. 67). Comparison of the results obtained with quail embryos with those already obtained for duck and chick embryos has shown one new fact, i.e., the rapid differentiation of the germinal elements, particularly in the ovaries and ovotestes. In ovaries removed at an undifferentiated stage (5 days' incubation), the oogonia were in the early stages of meiosis after 6 days of culture. The same is found for germinal cells located in the cortex of feminized male gonads. In ovaries removed after the stage of sexual differentiation (9–11 days) and cultured for 2 weeks the oocytes had grown and had become surrounded by primary follicles.

2. Hormonal Action of Male Gonads Feminized by Diethylstilbestrol

Wolff and Haffen's experiments (51) have shown that a feminized male gonad of chick embryo exercized a feminizing action on an undifferentiated genetically male duck gonad when associated in *in vitro* culture, and Asayama and Maruoka (1) obtained the same result when a vitelline membrane was interposed between the two organs.

3. Culture of Testes from Hybrid Duck Embryos

Testes of hybrid duck embryos (obtained by crossing *Cairina moschata* L. male × *Anas plathyrhynchos* L. female) were removed before and after sexual differentiation ($7\frac{1}{2}$–$8\frac{1}{2}$ days' incubation and 8, 11, 17, and 24 days'

163

incubation, respectively) and were cultured for 12–14 days (16). In many cases the explanted gonads showed characteristics of weak intersexuality (small cortical border). It is also interesting that in these cultured hybrid gonads the same phenomena were found as in testes developed *in situ*, i.e., mitotic anomalies of the germinal cells, which occurred more frequently and at an earlier stage in the cultured gonads.

B. Influence of Teratogenic Factors on the Development of Embryonic Gonads

1. ACTION OF PARATHION

Lutz-Ostertag and Meiniel (18, 19) studied the action of a pesticide, parathion (o,o-diethyl-o,p-dinitrophenyl thiophosphate) on gonads from quail embryos (7–16 days) and from chick embryos (9–18 days of incubation). The gonads were cultured for 1–8 days.

An aqueous suspension of parathion in the culture medium caused selective destruction of the gonocytes and the Sertoli cells in testes from quail embryo. In chick testes, the Sertoli cells were not destroyed, only the germinal cells being affected.

In female gonads, parathion destroyed the cortex; the destruction could be total in quail ovaries. The medulla was unaffected.

2. ACTION OF MELPHALAN

Melphalan (p-dichloroethylamino-L-phenylalanine) is one of the group of alkylating agents used in cancer chemotherapy. Simpson (34) compared the effect of this substance on 10-day chick embryo gonads and on fragments of human cancers. We shall deal only with the results using gonads. After culturing for 7 days, and depending on the dose, there was an inhibition of growth, a reduction in the number of mitoses, and a very marked effect on the formation of germinal cells. Melphalan destroyed the germinal cells but had no effect on the somatic cells at doses that are lethal for tumors. Counts carried out on the surviving germinal cells showed that oogonia are more sensitive than spermatogonia.

C. Action of Gonadotropic Hormones on Differentiation of Embryonic Gonads

Narbaitz and Adler (22) cultured male gonads of 8–10 days' incubation with 8- to 13-day-old ovaries in both the presence and absence of FSH and LH. The gonadotropins were found to have no effect on differentiation of germinal cell in the gonads of either sex. The oogonia of the ovarian cortex entered meiotic prophase after 7, 6, or 4 days, depending on whether the ovary had been removed at 8, 10, or 13 days of incubation.

Preda *et al.* (27) cultured the left gonads from 7- to $7\frac{1}{2}$-day-old chick embryos for 7 days in the presence of 10 to 20 I.U. of Coripan (a Rumanian preparation of chorionic gonadotropic hormone). All 20 gonads developed into typical ovaries. The author concluded from this that the chorionic gonadotropic hormone exercizes a feminizing effect in *in vitro* culture, which is capable of reversing the sexual differentiation of male gonads, while the same hormone injected into embryos only gives rise to a condition of intersexuality or testicular agenesis. It is interesting to note that pituitary gonadostimulating hormones administered to amphibian or reptilian embryos caused various degrees of feminization in male individuals (12).

Manelli and Milano-Crassi (21) found that when gonads from 6-day-old chick embryos were cultured in contact with hypophyses from embryos of 17–18 days' incubation, the latter stimulated organ growth and multiplication of germinal cells.

D. Study of DNA Synthesis in the Germinal Cells of Chick Embryo Ovary

Callebaut and Dubois (4) studied the *in vitro* incorporation of ^{3}H-thymidine by embryonic ovarian germinal cells during the period between 9 days of incubation and hatching. Transverse strips were taken from the midportion of the gonad and were cultured for 18–20 hours on a medium containing ^{3}H-thymidine.

The authors found that ^{3}H-thymidine was strongly incorporated on Days 9, 10, 11, and 12, which is explained by the replication of DNA required for the numerous mitoses during oogonial multiplication, which lasts until Day 13. The plateau found between Days 13 and 14 corresponded to a period in which there was little numerical fluctuation in the germinal population. The "vesicular nuclei" that characterize oogonia at the 14-day stage did not incorporate ^{3}H-thymidine. On Day 17, the authors recorded a considerable peak of incorporation. Numerous leptotene figures of the meiotic prophase appeared on Day 18. The authors suggested that this late peak of incorporation reflects the replication of DNA in a large number of premeiotic oocytes. After 18 days the level of incorporation of the DNA precursor decreased rapidly, while numerous oocytes entered into meiosis.

E. Colonization of Gonad Rudiments by Chick Embryo Germinal Cells

Dubois' experiments (10, 11) consisted of various *in vitro* associations, using as the host tissue the gonadal region of an embryo sterilized at an early stage, which had differentiated 27 to 35 pairs of somites. Early sterilization of embryos was achieved either *in vitro*, by excising the germinal crescent at stages between 0 and 10 pairs of somites [Simon's technique (33) or *in ovo* by means of double X-ray irradiation of the anterior extraembryonic area (9)].

The grafts were of various types: fertile germinal crescent from an embryo with 10–12 pairs of somites; left gonad from 5-, 6-, $7\frac{1}{2}$-, 8-, 12-, or 13-day embryos: radioactive embryonic gonad.

The two tissues were cultured in direct contact or separated by a vitelline membrane for a maximum of 48 hours.

The principal results obtained by these experiments were as follows:

1. The young gonadal region exerted an attractive effect on the primordial germinal cells (PGC) of the germinal crescent in an *in vitro* association that completely excluded any action of the vascular system. The PGC of the graft migrated by autonomous and oriented movements to colonize the previously sterilized host germinal epithelium. These experiments refute the hypothesis that the vascular system plays a fundamental role in the mechanism of CGP fixation in reproductive regions.

2. The attractive stimulus also provoked *in vitro* emigration of the primary gonocytes from a young morphologically undifferentiated gonad. Association of a young normal gonadal region with a radioactive gonad, resulted in colonization of the nonlabeled germinal epithelium by ^{3}H-thymidine-labeled gonocytes from the graft.

3. Spermatogonia showed the same migratory properties as the PGC and the primary gonocytes. They retained their migratory power and their ability to colonize an attractive germinal epithelium until at least Day 12 of incubation. On the other hand, from Day 8 of incubation the large majority of oogonia no longer responded to the attraction of the gonadal rudiments.

4. The attractive stimulus was exercized *in vitro* across a filtering barrier interposed between the host and the graft. The existence of a positive chemotaxis both selective and specific, is the most satisfactory explanation of these results.

F. Hormonal Secretion and Biosynthesis of Steroid Hormones from Radioactive Precursors by Chick Embryo Gonads

1. ANALYSIS OF HORMONAL SECRETION

Using the biological test of Allen and Doisy, Weniger (38, 40, 44) found estrogenic activity after extraction of media on which 7- to 10-day-old female gonads had been explanted. Negative results were obtained with male gonads and other organs.

2. BIOSYNTHESIS OF STEROID HORMONES FROM RADIOACTIVE PRECURSORS

The radioactive precursor was introduced into the nutrient medium on which a number of embryonic gonads had been cultured. Several hours or days later the radioactive hormones synthesized from the precursor by the embryonic gonads were extracted from the culture media, and the extracts were purified by serial chromatograpy and formation of derivatives. The radioactive substances isolated were compared against reference hormones. It is essential to ensure radiochemical purity of the synthesized hormones by crystallization to constant specific activity or to constant isotopic ratio.

a. Metabolism of DHA-4-^{14}C and Testosterone-6, 7α-^{3}H. Haffen and Cedard (5, 14) found that when DHA-4-^{14}C was introduced into the culture medium as a steroid precursor, labeled 17β-estradiol and estrone were identified in the medium after culturing *in vitro* for 3 days the undifferentiated gonads from 6-day embryos.

In addition to estrogens, labeled testosterone was formed during 1 day of *in vitro* culture of morphologically undifferentiated gonads of 7-day-old embryos.

Female gonads formed estrogens in increasing amounts as the gonads were taken from progressively older embryos ranging from 12 hours to 10$\frac{1}{2}$ days of incubation. All stages studied produced more 17β-estradiol than estrone. Male gonads from embryos in the same age range did not produce significant amounts of estrogens, but the production of labeled testosterone increased progressively with embryonic age in parallel with the appearance of $\Delta^4 - \Delta^5$-isomerase and 3β-ol-oxidoreductase.

Testosterone and 17β-estradiol have been obtained in a state of radiochemical purity. Among other products of DHA-4-^{14}C metabolism 5-androstene-3β,17β-diol, 5-androstene-3β,17α-diol, and etiocholanolone were detected. These products indicate that 17β,17α-oxidoreductases and 5β-reductase are present in the gonads of both sexes.

Male gonads, experimentally feminized by crystalline female hormone injection and explanted at 10 and 12 days' embryonic age, formed labeled estrone and 17β-estradiol but not labeled testosterone from DHA-4-^{14}C.

Female and feminized male gonads were similarly able to aromatize testosterone-6,7α-^{3}H to produce tritiated estrone and estradiol-17β, but the yield was somewhat smaller than that obtained from DHA-4-^{14}C.

b. Estrogen Biosynthesis from Sodium Acetate-1-^{14}C and from Progesterone-4-^{14}C. Weniger *et al.* (44, 45) studied estrogen formation from these two precursors in avian embryonic gonads cultured *in vitro* for at least 24 hours. They demonstrated the synthesis of both labeled estrone and estradiol from sodium acetate-1-^{14}C by the female gonads from 7- to 9-day-old chick embryos, by the ovaries from 12-day duck embryos, and also by the ovotestes from an 18-day-old embryo.

Sodium acetate is also transformed into estriol and epiestriol by 10- to 16-day female gonads.

When progesterone-4-^{14}C or sodium acetate-1-^{14}C (49) was supplied to 5- and 6-day-old undifferentiated gonads, labeled estrone and estradiol were found in the culture media after 24 hours.

c. *Action of Chorionic Gonadotropin on Steroid Biosynthesis from Sodium Acetate-1-*^{14}C. Cedard *et al.* (6) studied the influence of HCG on steroid metabolism from this same precursor using 10- and 18-day-old embryonic gonads cultured *in vitro* for 48 hours. When the gonadotropin was incorporated into the medium at the same time as the labeled precursor, it enhanced considerably the production of steroids or ether-soluble sterols, namely, cholesterol (unpublished results). Moreover, it stimulated estrogen synthesis by female gonads, particularly that of 17β-estradiol from labeled acetate or DHA.

Gonadotropic hormone had no influence on the biosynthesis of testosterone from sodium acetate-1-^{14}C by male gonads cultured *in vitro*, and this synthesis did not seem quantitatively significant.

G. Culture of Chick Embryo Müllerian Ducts

1. ACTION OF SEX HORMONES ON DIFFERENTIATION

Following the work of Wolff *et al.* (see Ch. IV, Refs. 28, 29, 49, 82, 83), Hamilton and Teng (15) studied the response of 8½-day-old müllerian ducts to varying doses of steroids, such as testosterone, androsterone, and 17β-estradiol, using *in vitro* culture, the culture technique being based on that of Chen (7). The müllerian ducts were explanted for 20 days in the presence or absence of the hormones. The results of these authors were not found to agree with those of Wolff *et al.* According to the former, the effect of hormones on the müllerian ducts cultured *in vitro* was different from the effect obtained *in vivo*. The female hormone did not produce maintenance of the müllerian ducts, and the male hormone did not cause regression. The authors explain these divergences by the fact that different culture techniques and different hormones were used. Hamilton and Teng (15) and Weniger (41) attempted to determine the exact time when the male müllerian duct regressed. Their results indicate that it occurs between 8 days and 8 days 11 hours.

Weniger (42) showed that the right müllerian duct from female embryos behaves differently *in vitro* from *in vivo*. When removed after 12–15 hours of incubation it did not regress in contact with either left or right female gonads.

2. DIFFERENTIATION OF THE SHELL GLAND

Lutz-Ostertag and Didier (17) determined the presumptive region of the shell gland in the embryonic female müllerian duct by culturing different-sized segments of both left and right ducts for 6–10 days. Their results showed that the presumptive region of the shell gland is localized in the posterior fifth of the müllerian duct, when removed between $8\frac{1}{2}$ and $9\frac{1}{2}$ days of incubation. The right müllerian duct developed and formed a shell gland that was analogous in appearance, size, and structure to that of the left müllerian duct.

The development of the shell gland removed at stage 9+ (see Ch. IV, Ref. 28) and cultured for 5–8 days, usually followed a normal pattern except with regard to the glandular epithelium (8).

II. MAMMALS

A. *In Vitro* Differentiation of Embryonic Gonads from the Muskrat

Embryonic ovaries and testes of the muskrat (*Galemys pyrenaicus*) were explanted shortly after the stage of sexual differentiation and were cultured for 4 days (25). The results obtained suggest the following interpretations: the potentiality of the testis to an ovotestis is not manifested in culture. The germinal epithelium undergoes rapid involution. When associated with the ovary, the testis does not become feminized. The ovary develops normally and shows no aberrant formation either in control culture or in association with the testis. There is no masculinization of the ovary at this stage.

B. Interspecific Association of Mouse and Chick Testes

In 1961, Weniger (36) showed that the embryonic mouse testis feminized the testicular rudiment from a 5-day chick embryo when they were associated *in vitro*.

In 1965, Weniger (43) showed that the feminizing effect of embryonic mouse testis was sufficiently potent to be exercized on the 7- or 8-day-old morphologically differentiated testis, stimulating differentiation of the germinal epithelium into ovarian cortex.

C. Organ Culture Studies of Hormone Secretion in Fetal Gonads

Price, Ortiz, and Zaaijer (29) developed a new and highly sensitive method for detecting the presence of androgens. Briefly, this method consists of explanting fragments of rat ventral prostate gland and placing them in contact with the fetal organs to be tested. The combined explants are then cultured for a few days. The prostatic tissue remained histologically normal if androgen were present in the fetal organ, but it regressed, as it does *in vivo*, if androgen were not available. Testis and adrenal gland of both male and female guinea pig fetuses at 30, 31, 32, 34, and 36 days of gestation secreted androgens that maintained the normal histological structure of the prostate explants during the 5-day culture period. Prostate tissue cultured with ovaries or bladder, or cultured alone, showed total histological regression (54).

Using the bioindicator method, Ortiz, Price, and Zaaijer (23) explored the problem of androgenic secretion by the testis and adrenals during the much earlier stages of differentiation, beginning with the early formation of the gonad and the cortical primordium of the adrenal gland. The method was used with organs from 22- to 30-day-old fetal guinea pigs. The fetal organs were cultured for 5–6 days in contact with rat prostatic tissue. They secreted androgens at all stages.

The androgens from fetal testis, adrenals, and ovaries and their influence on sexual differentiation were studied by Price, Ortiz, and Zaaijer (30) and by Ortiz, Zaaijer, and Price (24).

Organs from 41-, 46-, and 62-day-old guinea pig fetuses were tested by placing them in contact with rat ventral prostate for 5 days. The testis and the adrenal cortex were highly androgenic at all three ages, while the ovary was mildly androgenic at 41 and 46 days of age and markedly so at 62 days.

Reproductive tracts of 26- to 30-day-old male and female fetuses were explanted with or without gonads, or with adrenal glands, and cultured for 9–11 days.

The müllerian ducts developed in all female-tract explants and regressed in all male-tract explants. The male and female wolffian ducts were maintained in tracts cultured with testis or adrenal cortex, or with fragments of 60-day-old fetal ovary. There were strong indications that the wolffian ducts of males are more androgen-dependent and that those of females are more androgen-responsive at 26–27 days than at 29–30 days of age. Comparison of the results of explanting male tracts without androgen-secreting organs at both ages, showed that complete regression of the wolffian ducts occurred in all cases in the younger group but in only 50% of the cases in the older group. As suggested by the authors in a previous paper, the wolffian ducts in 29- to 30-day-old male fetuses are approaching a state of stabilization and are beginning to lose their dependence on male hormone. The ducts in females of this age are losing their ability to respond to male hormone, i.e., regression is already determined. These results are in agreement with those reported for fetal rats (see Ch. IV, Ref. 39) and mice (3, 28).

The question of whether female müllerian ducts can be inhibited by testicular androgens has been studied in guinea pigs by Price, Ortiz, and Zaaijer (30, 31), and in mice by Brewer (3) and Weniger (37). Only Weniger reported partial degeneration of female müllerian ducts explanted imme-diately after their first appearance and cultured with testes.

The early secretion of androgenic hormones by human fetal gonads and adrenal glands in organ culture has been studied by Zaaijer (52) and by Zaaijer and Price (53).

Explants of gonads and adrenal glands from four male fetuses between $9\frac{1}{2}$ and 20 weeks of age, and female fetuses between $7\frac{1}{2}$ and 13 weeks were grown in organ culture for 5–6 days in order to test, using the bioindicator method, their capacity to secrete androgenic hormone. The results showed that fetal testes were secreting biologically active androgenic hormone at all stages tested. Prior to 13 weeks, fetal ovaries did not secrete detectable amounts of androgens; explants from 13-week-old ovaries had a mildly androgenic effect on prostatic tissue, and with fetal adrenal glands the androgenic test was positive in both sexes at all stages tested.

From all these results, it can be concluded that undifferentiated guinea pig testes and testes from human fetuses, at the time of reproductive tract differentiation, secrete androgens in organ culture. Androgen secretion by adrenal glands from male and female human and guinea pig fetuses is apparent in organ culture. This androgen secretion may be limited *in vivo* through the presence of an enzyme-inhibiting factor.

D. Biosynthesis of Sex Hormones from Labeled Precursors by Fetal Gonads

1. FETAL TESTIS

The capacity of the human fetal testis to synthesize androgens from sodium acetate-1-^{14}C has been studied in organ culture by Rice *et al.* (32). The authors explanted the testes of a 21-cm human fetus, approximately $6\frac{1}{2}$ months old, that had died 12 days previously. Nine days after explantation onto a plasma clot with chick embryo extract and a nutrient medium consisting of Eagle's basic medium and 10% calf serum, sodium acetate-1-^{14}C was introduced into the medium. Analysis of the medium showed that more pregnenolone and 17α-hydroxyprogesterone was formed than androstenedione and testosterone.

DHA was not demonstrated with certainty. The authors infer a deficiency of 20α–desmolase, rather than of $\varDelta_{4-5}$ hydroxyoxidoreductase, under the experimental conditions.

The two male hormones (androstenedione and testosterone) formed from sodium acetate-1-^{14}C were detected in the culture media 24 hours after explantation of embryonic testes from $3\frac{1}{2}$-month-old calf embryos (48) and in the culture media of mouse testes (12–19 days of gestation) (47).

The results complement other established chemical data and appear to confirm the hypothesis that the mammalian fetal testis synthesizes the same type of androgenic hormones from radioactive precursors as the adult testis.

2. Fetal Ovary

Information on the biosynthesis of steroid sex hormones by fetal ovaries is still limited despite experiments on well-differentiated organs supplied with radioactive precursors.

Price *et al.* (see Section C of this chapter) showed that ovaries of fetal guinea pig and of human fetuses at a well-advanced stage of gestation had an androgenic effect on prostatic tissue in culture.

Eleven-week-old human fetal ovary has been explanted in organ culture by Bloch *et al.* (2). The fetal ovary carries out reduction of progesterone-4-^{14}C only at position 20. The authors used a modification of Trowell's technique (35) with a liquid medium consisting of CMRL 1066 (70%) and horse serum (30%).

3. Histochemistry of Δ^5-3β-ol-Steroid Dehydrogenase

Picon (26) cultured rat fetal testes on grids, using Trowell's method (35) with a synthetic medium (M 199). When explanted at $14\frac{1}{2}$, $15\frac{1}{2}$, and $16\frac{1}{2}$ days of gestation, the testes sometimes displayed on Day 21 some structural alterations, and the interstitial cells were well developed. Δ^5-3β-ol-steroid dehydrogenase activity was similar to that of control fetuses of the same age. However, the cytoplasm of the interstitial cells was less abundant.

III. CONCLUSIONS

Among the investigations reported here, those which concern the analysis of hormonal secretions by embryonic gonads are of prime importance.

The results show that:

1. The embryonic gonads of birds when cultured *in vitro* carry out biosynthesis of steroidal sex hormones from several radioactive precursors. Female gonads, in particular, synthesize estrogens at a very early stage, as shown by experiments carried out with undifferentiated gonads at 5 and 6 days of incubation.

2. In mammals the most important results have been obtained in males: the fetal testis *in vitro* secretes androgens, which play a determining role in differentiation of the male reproductive tract.

3. *In vitro* culture of embryonic gonads reveals, in certain cases, an unexpected functional activity, i.e., androgenic activity of the ovary and a feminizing action of the testes.

BIBLIOGRAPHY

1. Asayama S. and Maruoka C. Sex modifying capacity of the feminized gonads of DES-treated chick embryos. *Zool. Mag.*, *Tokyo*, 1967, **76**, 265–270.
2. Bloch E., Romney S. L., Klein M., Lipiello L., Cooper P. and Goldring I. P. Steroid synthesis by human fetal adrenals and ovaries maintained in organ culture. *Proc. Soc. exp. Biol. Med.*, 1965, **119**, 449–452.
3. Brewer N. L. Sex differentiation of fetal mouse *in vitro*. *Ph.D. Thesis*, University of Chicago, 1962.
4. Callebaut M. and Dubois R. Sur l'incorporation de thymidine tritiée par les cellules germinales de l'ovaire embryonnaire de Poulet, en culture *in vitro*. *C. R. Acad. Sci.*, 1965, **261**, 5215–5218.
5. Cedard L. and Haffen K. Transformations de la déhydroépiandrostérone par les gonades embryonnaires de Poulet, cultivées *in vitro*. *C. R. Acad. Sci.*, 1966, **263**, 430–433.
6. Cedard L., Haffen K. and Guichard A. Influence de l'hormone gonadotrope chorionique sur la production d'oestrogènes à partir d'acétate de Na et de déhydroépiandrostérone radioactifs par les gonades embryonnaires de Poulet, cultivées *in vitro*. *C. R. Acad. Sci.*, 1968, **267**, 118–120.
7. Chen J. M. The cultivation in fluid medium of organized liver, pancreas and other tissues of fetal rats. *Exp. Cell Res.*, 1954, **7**, 518–529.
8. Didier E. Étude comparée de la différenciation histologique de la glande coquillière de l'embryon d'Oiseau au cours du développement normal et en culture *in vitro*. *C. R. Soc. Biol.*, 1965, **12**, 2353–2357.
9. Dubois R. Sur la stérilisation de l'embryon de Poulet par irradiation aux rayons X du croissant germinal extraembryonnaire. *Arch. Anat. micr. Morph. exp.*, 1962, **51**, 85–94.
10. Dubois R. Sur l'attraction de cellules germinales primordiales par la jeune région gonadique chez l'embryon de Poulet. *C. R. Acad. Sci.*, 1964, **258**, 3904–3907.
11. Dubois R. La colonisation des ébauches gonadiques par les cellules germinales de l'embryon de Poulet, en culture *in vitro*. *J. Embryol. exp. Morph.*, 1968, **20**, 189–213.
12. Dufaure J. P. Recherches descriptives et expérimentales sur les modalités et facteurs du développement de l'appareil génital chez le Lézard Vivipare *(Lacerta vivipara Jacquin)*. *Arch. Anat. micr. Morph. exp.*, 1966, **55**, 437–537.
13. Haffen K. Sur la culture *in vitro* des glandes génitales des embryons de Caille *(Coturnix coturnix)*. Obtention de la différenciation sexuelle normale et de l'intersexualité expérimentale des gonades explantées. *C. R. Acad. Sci.*, 1964, **259**, 882–884.
14. Haffen K. and Cedard L. Étude, en culture organotypique *in vitro*, du métabolisme de la déhydroépiandrostérone et de la testostérone radioactives, par les gonades normales et intersexuées de l'embryon de poulet. *Gen. comp. Endocrinol.*, 1968, **11**, 220–234.
15. Hamilton T. H. and Teng C. Sexual stabilization of Mullerian ducts in the chick embryo. *In* "Organogenesis" (R. L. De Haan and H. Ursprung, eds.), pp. 681–697. Holt, Rinehart & Winston, New York, 1965.
16. Lutz-Ostertag Y. Culture organotypique du testicule embryonnaire de l'hybride *Cairina moschata* L. mâle × *Anas plathyrhynchos* L. femelle. *C. R. Acad. Sci.*, 1966, **262**, 1734–1736.
17. Lutz-Ostertag Y. and Didier E. Localisation de la zonz présomptive de la glande coquillière du canal de Müller cultivé *in vitro* chez l'embryon de Poulet femelle. *C. R. Soc. Biol.*, 1965, **159**, 648–651.

18. Lutz-Ostertag Y. and Meiniel R.   Action stérilisante du *O,O*-diéthyl-*O*-paranitro-phényl thiophosphate sur les testicules de l'embryon de Caille *(Coturnix coturnix japonica)* en culture *in vitro. C. R. Acad. Sci.*, 1968, **267**, 96–97.

19. Lutz-Ostertag Y. and Meiniel R.   Action stérilisante du Parathion sur l'ovaire de l'embryon de Caille et de Poulet en culture *in vitro. C. R. Acad. Sci.*, 1968, **267**, 2178–2180.

20. Lutz-Ostertag Y. and Meiniel R.   Différences de sensibilité à l'action stérilisante du *O,O*-diéthyl-*O*-paranitrophényl thiophosphate des testicules embryonnaires de Caille et de Poulet en culture *in vitro. C. R. Soc. Biol.*, 1968, **162**, 1471–1472.

21. Manelli H. and Milano-Crassi, E.   Ipofisi e gonadi embrionali di pollo associate *in vitro. Arch. zool. ital.*, 1966, **51**, 855–862.

22. Narbaitz R. and Adler R.   Germ cell differentiation in embryonic gonads cultured in heterosexual pairs. *Experientia*, 1966, **22**, 677.

23. Ortiz E., Price D. and Zaaijer J. J. P.   Organ culture studies of hormone secretion in endocrine glands of fetal guinea pigs. II. Secretion of androgenic hormone in adrenals and testes during early stages of development. *Kon. Ned. Akad. v. Wetensch., Proc., C*, 1966, **69**, 400–408.

24. Ortiz E., Zaaijer J. J. P. and Price D.   Organ culture studies of hormone secretion in endocrine glands of fetal guinea pigs. IV. Androgens from fetal adrenals and ovaries and their influence on sex differentiation. *Kon. Ned. Akad. v. Wetensch., Proc., C*, 1967, **70**, 475–488.

25. Peyre A.   Culture *in vitro* de gonades embryonnaires de Desman (*Galemys pyrena icus G.*, Mammifère-Insectivore). *C. R. Acad. Sci.*, 1960, **252**, 605–607.

26. Picon R.   Activité Δ^5-3β-hydroxy stéroide deshydrogénasique du testicule foetal de Rat *in vitro. Arch. Anat. micr. Morph. exp.*, 1967, **56**, 281–290.

27. Preda V., Cracium O. and Cimpianu A. P.   L'action de l'hormone gonadotrope choriale sur les cultures de longue durée d'organes embryonnaires. II. L'action de l'hormone sur la gonade embryonnaire de poulet, cultivée dans le milieu de Wolff et Haffen. *Rev. Roum. Embryol. Cytol.*, 1966, **3**, 113–115.

28. Price D. and Ortiz E.   The role of fetal androgen in sex differentiation of the mammalian fetus. *In* "Organogenesis" (R. L. De Haan and H. Ursprung, eds.), pp. 629–652. Holt, Rinehart & Winston, New York, 1965.

29. Price D., Ortiz E. and Zaaijer J. J. P.   Secretion of androgenic hormone by testes and adrenal glands of fetal guinea pigs. *Amer. Zool.*, 1963, **3**, 553–554.

30. Price D., Ortiz E. and Zaaijer J. J. P.   Organ culture studies of hormone secretion in endocrine glands of fetal guinea pigs. III. The relation of testicular hormone to sex differentiation of the reproductive ducts. *Anat. Rec.*, 1967, **157**, 27–41.

31. Price D., Ortiz E. and Zaaijer J. J. P.   *In vitro* studies of the relation of fetal sex hormones to sex differentiation in the guinea pig. *Conference on Hormones in Development*, Nottingham, 1968, in press.

32. Rice B. F., Johanson C. A. and Sternberg W. H.   Formation of steroid hormones from acetate-1-^{14}C by a human fetal testis preparation grown in organ culture. *Steroids*, 1966, **7**, 79–90.

33. Simon D.   Contribution à l'étude de la circulation et du transport des gonocytes primaires dans les blastodermes d'Oiseau, cultivés *in vitro. Arch. Anat. micr. Morph. exp.*, 1960, **40**, 93–176.

34. Simpson P.   La sensibilité différentielle d'une tumeur humaine et des tissus somatiques et germinaux des gonades embryonnaires en culture *in vitro. European J. Cancer.*, 1969, **5**, 331–342.

35. Trowell O. A.   A modified technique from organ culture *in vitro*. *Exp. Cell Res.*, 1954, **6**, 246–248.
36. Weniger J. P.   Féminisation en culture *in vitro*, du testicule d'embryon de Poulet par le testicule embryonnaire de Souris. *C. R. Acad. Sci.*, 1961, **253**, 2410–2411.
37. Weniger J. P.   Régression du canal de Müller d'embryon de Souris mâle soumis *in vitro* à l'action de l'hormone testiculaire. *C. R. Acad. Sci.*, 1964, **259**, 1899–1901.
38. Weniger J. P.   L'ovaire de Poulet, cultivé *in vitro*, sécrète une hormone oestrogène. *C. R. Soc. Biol.*, 1964, **158**, 175–178.
39. Weniger J. P.   Extraction d'une substance oestrogène (test de Allen et Doisy positif) de milieux sur lesquels des gonades d'embryon de Poulet femelles de 7 jours furent cultivées pendant 24 heures. *C. R. Acad. Sci.*, 1965, **261**, 809–812.
40. Weniger J. P.   L'hormone sexuelle de l'embryon de Poulet femelle est-elle un stéroïde phénolique? *C. R. Acad. Sci.*, 1965, **261**, 1427–1429.
41. Weniger J. P.   Régression du canal de Müller d'embryons de Poulet mâles de 8 jours cultivé *in vitro* au contact de gonads femelles de même âge. *Z. Zellforsch.*, 1965, **66**, 155–160.
42. Weniger J. P.   Sur le mécanisme de la régression du canal de Müller doit chez l'embryon de Poulet femelle. *Experientia*, 1965, **21**, 523.
43. Weniger J. P.   Sur la puissance de l'effet féminisant du testicule embryonnaire de Souris, cultivé *in vitro*. *Ann. Endocrin.*, 1965, **26**, 267–471.
44. Weniger J. P.   Activité oestrogène de la fraction "oestrone-oetradiol" de milieux incubés avec des gonades d'embryons de Poulet femelle. *C. R. Acad. Sci.*, 1966, **262**, 578–580.
45. Weniger J. P.   Recherches sur la nature chimique des hormones sexuelles embryonnaires de Poulet. *Ann. Embryol. Morph.*, 1969, **2**, 433–444.
46. Weniger J. P., Ehrhardt J. D. and Fritig B.   Sur la formation d'oestrone et d'oestradiol par les gonades de l'embryon de Poulet femelle cultivées *in vitro*. *C. R. Acad. Sci.*, 1967, **264**, 838–341.
47. Weniger J. P., Ehrhardt J. D. and Fritig B.   Sécrétion de testostérone et d'androstène-dione par les testicules embryonnaires de Souris cultivés *in vitro*. *C. R. Acad. Sci.*, 1967, **264**, 1069–1071.
48. Weniger J. P., Ehrhardt J. D. and Fritig B.   Sécrétion de testostérone et d'androstène-dione par les testicules foetaux de Veau cultivés *in vitro*. *C. R. Acad. Sci.*, 1967, **264**, 1911–1912.
49. Weniger J. P. and Zeis A.   Formation d'oestrone et d'oestradiol radioactif à partir d'acétate de Na-1-^{14}C par les ébauches gonadiques d'embryons de Poulet de 5 à 6 jours. *C. R. Acad. Sci.*, 1969, **268**, 1306–1309.
50. Wolff Et.   Utilisation de la membrane vitelline de l'œuf de Poule en culture organo-typique. I. Technique et possibilités. *Dev. Biol.*, 1961, **3**, 767–786.
51. Wolff Et. and Haffen K.   Sur la féminisation induite par les gonades mâles intersexuées chez l'embryon de Poulet. *Arch. Anat. Histol. Embryol.*, 1961, **154**, Suppl., 274–302.
52. Zaaijer J. J. P.   Secretion of androgens by human fetal organs in culture, as demonstrated by a bioindicator test. *Acta Morph. neer.-scand.*, 1968, **7**, 102.
53. Zaaier J. J. P. and Price D.   Early secretion of androgenic hormones by human fetal gonads and adrenal glands in organ culture. *Conference on Hormones in Development*, Nottingham, 1968, in press.
54. Zaaijer J. J. P., Price D. and Ortiz E.   Organ culture studies of hormone secretion in endocrine glands of fetal guinea pigs. I. Androgenic secretion as demonstrated by a bioindicator method. *Kon. Ned. Akad. v. Wetensch., Proc.*, C, 1966, **3**, 389–399.

CHAPTER V

THE ACTION OF HORMONES AND INHIBITORS
ON ORGANS CULTURED *IN VITRO*

F. Dieterlen-Lièvre

INSTITUT D'EMBRYOLOGIE EXPÉRIMENTALE DU C.N.R.S.
ET DU COLLÈGE DE FRANCE
PARIS, FRANCE

It has been shown in the preceding chapters that many embryonic organs differentiate in an autonomous fashion in accordance with their normal development whether they are explanted onto natural or synthetic media. However, the development of some sex organs is subject to hormonal influence. Organ culture makes it possible to find if other humoral effects are likely or necessary during development. It is necessary to decide, first, when and how the endocrine glands become functional, and second, when the target organs become sensitive to their influence. This method makes it easier to determine which combinations of hormones are necessary for survival and functional activity of already differentiated organs. Explantation *in vitro* eliminates the complex interactions that occur *in vivo* and that may hide the effect of experimental intervention in the intact animal. For the same reason, the study of the effect of inhibitor substances added to the culture medium has resulted in much information on normal and pathological physiological mechanisms.

The field of such research is immense, and this chapter must be limited to the resolving of certain questions.

I. INTERACTIONS *IN VITRO* BETWEEN ENDOCRINE GLANDS AND TARGET ORGANS IN PARABIOSIS

Tixier-Vidal (83, 84) studied the effect of the hypophysis on the thyroid in chick embryos using Wolff and Haffen's technique in organ culture. Stimulation of the thyroid can be estimated by the presence of colloid droplets and the formation of follicles. He found that in the chick embryo thyrotrophic activity appeared during the 7th day of incubation. This is several days before PAS-positive cells appeared in the anterior pituitary (thyrotrophic and gonadotrophic cells). The thyrotrophic function of the pituitary differentiated in an autonomous fashion. Thyroid sensitivity to the thyrotrophic hormone appeared in the 6–7 day embryo. These results are difficult to interpret because the thyroid is capable of autodifferentiation, but according to Tixier-Vidal this capacity is limited. Thyroids from 7-day embryos never differentiated beyond the stage seen in normal 11-day embryos, when they were explanted onto Wolff and Haffen's standard medium. However, it has been shown that thyroid differentiation depends closely on the amount of nutritive material in the culture medium, and in particular on the concentration of amino acids (89). This is a striking example of how results vary with experimental conditions.

Schaberg (75–78) investigated the factors necessary for the structural and functional maintenance of the adrenal cortex in newly born rats and in fetal rats near term. The cortex was explanted according to Fell's technique onto a medium containing both human plasma and brain extract from human embryos. The cortex dedifferentiated, the fascicular cells disappeared, and only glomerular cells survived. However, if adrenocorticotrophic hormone (ACTH) was added to the medium, or if the adrenal was cultured in parabiosis with pieces of anterior pituitary, the glomerular cells were transformed into fascicular cells. Analyses showed that the production of corticosteroids was stimulated by the parabiosis or by ACTH. These experiments established several facts.

1. The adrenal cortex and the pituitary are capable of secretory activity in the fetal rat.

2. Under culture conditions, the anterior pituitary can produce corticotrophic hormones in the absence of hypothalamic stimulation.

3. In contrast, the adrenal cortex can only become active in the presence of stimulation by the pituitary.

4. There is no direct correlation between functional activity and morphological differentiation of the pituitary.

The last point was confirmed by Petrovic (71), who studied the potentialities of the pituitary of the adult guinea pig. Pieces of the gland were cultured for several weeks using either roller-tubes or Wolff and Haffen's method. Studies with the electron microscope showed that under these conditions the different cell types of the pars distalis retained their ultrastructural characteristics. Only the secretory granules disappeared almost entirely. Meanwhile, when the explants were reimplanted into the target organ, they stimulated the testis, the ovary, or the thyroid. When grafted into normal hosts, the explants regained the morphological characteristics which had been lost in culture. When grafted into hypophysectomized hosts, the explants remained poor in secretory granules because they liberated the hormones that were lacking in the host instead of accumulating them. Explants of adult guinea pig anterior pituitary stimulated the functional activity of fetal guinea pig adrenal cortex and 6-day chick embryo thyroid when they were cultured together for no longer than 6–8 days. These experiments established that when the adult pituitary was isolated from the animal, for an extended period, it underwent a limited functional involution which was reversed when the gland was reimplanted into the animal.

The above work shows that the anterior pituitary can exert its influence on many organs under the characteristically simple conditions of culture. It also demonstrates that functional activities known in the adult are also present in the embryo. Moreover, organ culture has made it possible to demonstrate the existence of previously unknown hormonal interrelationships. Thus, Guillemin and Rosenberg (42) showed that after 4 days of culture in roller-tubes the pituitary ceased to secrete the corticotrophic hormone. The ability to produce and secrete ACTH was restored to the pituitary, even after 31 days of culture, by the presence of additional hypothalamic tissue.

The role of the pineal gland was also established using organ culture (69, 70). The pineal is a diverticulum of the diencephalon, composed of neural and epithelial cells, attaining its maximum development in the young animal. That the pineal had an endocrine role was long suspected but could never be proved. Neither epiphysectomy nor transplantations had affected animals in any apparent way. By using Wolff and Haffen's method, Moszkowska was able to show in a striking way that there is an antagonism between the pineal and the pituitary in the chick embryo. She was also able to show that the anterior pituitary of the 16-day embryo has a gonadotrophic effect. The male gonad from a 16-day embryo showed definite stimulation of the sex cords when it was cultured for 3 days in parabiosis with several pituitaries. However, when a male gonad was associated in culture with several pituitaries and several pineals, the stimulating effect on the gonad was diminished or completely suppressed, according to the number of pineals used. Thus organ culture has indisputably shown that the pineal antagonizes the pituitary during embryonic life. This role probably persists in a more discrete way during the first few months of life. Other experiments have shown that this antagonistic effect is exerted mainly against the pituitary secretion of the luteinizing hormone (LH). Pineal glands from adult hens give negative results when used in implantation experiments.

Moszkowska's experiments show a curious interspecific difference. Pituitary taken from 16- or even 19-day duck embryos could not stimuatel embryonic gonads, whether these were derived from ducks or chickens. In contrast, the same pituitary showed strong thyrotrophic activity.

Parabiosis *in vitro* has already been used to study the organogenesis of the endocrine pancreas (8, 9). It is known that in the seed-eating birds, control of the glucose metabolism by pancreatic hormones is quite different from that found in mammals. In fact the most important hormone in the birds is glucagon or the hyperglycemia-glycogenolytic factor (HGF), the effects of which on the blood sugar level are the opposite to those of insulin. Total pancreatectomy, which is easily carried out, brought about death due to hypoglycemia (68). Biochemical analysis (86) showed that the bird pancreas was ten times richer in glucagon than the mammalian pancreas. A particular pancreatic anatomy corresponds to this type of physiology. The α-cells which secrete glucagon are very abundant. They form large islets localized

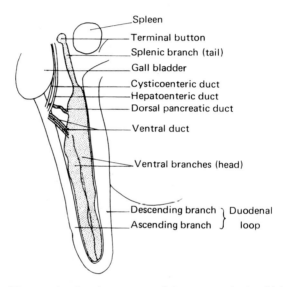

Fig. 1.   Diagram showing the anatomy of the pancreas in the chick embryo.

in the splenic lobe of the pancreas. The β-cells which secrete insulin are present in much smaller islets throughout the whole gland.

In the study of the embryonic pancreas, the activity of the islets can be tested by finding their effect on embryonic liver associated in the culture. When explanted *in vitro*, the embryonic liver produced glycogen during the first few days of organ culture, whatever the age of the donor embryo. The pancreas yielded several types of explant. In effect, the segregation of the two types of islets as described for adult birds was even more marked in the embryo. The exocrine tissue differentiated late, so that until the 15th day, the splenic lobe (or "tail" of the pancreas) was composed almost entirely of α-cells. The remainder ("head" or duodenal lobe) contained primitive tubules and islets of β-cells (Fig. 1). Various combinations of tissues were carried out in culture:

1. Liver from 6-day embryo with pancreatic "tail" from 14-day embryo.
2. Liver from 6-day embryo with pancreatic "head" from 14-day embryo.
3. Liver from 6-day embryo (no pancreas).

After 3 days of culture it could be shown that glycogen was present in liver that had been cultured alone or with the "head" of the pancreas (Fig. 2, top). In contrast, liver that had been cultured in association with the "tail" of the pancreas, that is, in contact with cells that produce glucagon, showed no glycogen (Fig. 2, bottom). Thus, in the "tail" of the pancreas there is a localized principle that inhibits the formation of glycogen. This inhibition was found in the "tail" of a pancreas from an embryo of only 7 days' incubation and before 7 days of incubation in the whole pancreas. At the latter time it was too small to be divided into separate zones. Finally, it was shown that only a few hours after it first appeared the dorsal bud of the pancreas in the 3-day embryo already concealed the glycogenolytic factor. This has been confirmed by observations using the electron microscope. The cells at the base of the dorsal pancreatic bud (Hamilton and Hamburger's stage 21) showed the characteristic granules of the α-cells.

A final example of a phenomenon that can be demonstrated by parabiosis is the accumulation of sex hormones by the syrinx of the duck embryo. It has been shown in another chapter that when the syrinx is explanted onto a medium lacking in hormones it develops into the asymmetric male form. The symmetrical female form develops in the presence of a female gonad or estrogen. Em. Wolff (87, 88) showed that syringes from 12–15 day female duck embryos feminized 7-day genetically male gonads that had been associated with them for 5–7 days in culture. A cortex composed of several layers of tall cylindrical cells appeared. The 12–15 day male syrinx exerted a similar effect, inducing the regression of Mullerian ducts from 7-day chick embryos when they were cultured together. It was known that when Mullerian ducts were explanted before sexual differentiation had occurred, they could maintain themselves in culture on a medium free of hormones, whatever their genetic sex. These experiments show that both male and female syringes accumulated hormone that is brought to them in the bloodstream. The mesonephros was also tested and found to have no effect on the differentiation of the associated sex organs.

In conclusion, it has been shown that the use of parabiosis is particularly well adapted to the study of the endocrine glands and embryonic receptors. The functional activity of these organs is quantitatively too small to be demonstrated by methods that do not put the two types of organs into direct contact. In some instances this method has been the means of proving the

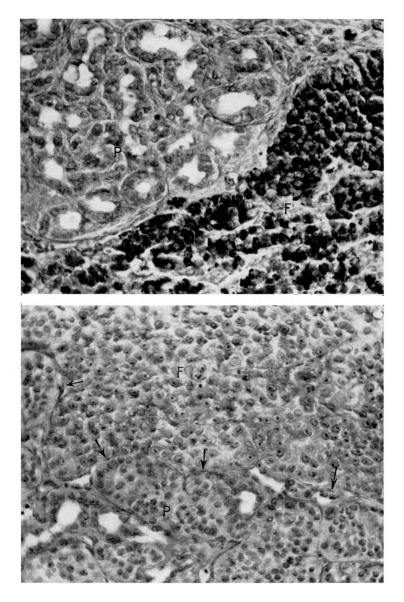

FIG. 2. The influence of chick embryo pancreas on the formation of hepatic glycogen *in vitro*. ×370. Top. Parabiosis between the "head" of a 14-day pancreas (P) and a 6-day liver (F) after 3 days of culture. There is abundant glycogen in the hepatic explant. Bottom. Parabiosis between the "tail" of a 14-day pancreas (P) (site of α-cell islets) and a 6-day liver (F). There is no glycogen in the liver explant. The arrows indicate the boundary between hepatic and pancreatic tissues.

existence of hormonal interrelationships, or of elucidating hitherto unknown functions of certain organs.

II. EFFECTS OF HORMONES AND INHIBITOR SUBSTANCES ADDED TO THE CULTURE MEDIUM

This study will be limited to two effector organs, the bone and the mammary gland, which have been studied from various aspects by many groups. These experiments bring together a number of results that shed light on the metabolic processes involved in bone growth and differentiation. The hormonal requirements of each stage of functional development in the mammary gland are also illustrated.*

A. Reactions of Embryonic Bone to Hormones and Inhibitor Substances Added to the Culture Medium

Considerable work has been done on the organ culture of embryonic bone in the presence of varying substances, the most prominent being that by Gaillard et al. on the action of parathormone, of Fell et al. on the actions of thyroxine, triiodothyronine, vitamin A, and papaine, and of Wolff and Kieny on the creeper factor.

Fell and Robinson (24) and Kieny (51) have shown that bone rudiments can grow and differentiate in the absence of hormones, both on synthetic and on natural media. The experiments to be discussed not only demonstrate the influences necessary for normal embryonic differentiation, but also indicate the mode of action of the substances tested. These substances normally act on organs further developed than in the embryo. Such experiments demonstrate the reactivity of the rudiments at a stage when they are not normally exposed to such influences. As a result of this reactivity it is possible to elucidate the functional activity of the embryonic endocrine glands.

1. INFLUENCE OF THE PARATHYROID AND OF PARATHORMONE ON EMBRYONIC BONE

Gaillard's culture medium is based on biological fluids (human plasma and human fetal brain extract). In a series of experiments (26–39) this author showed that the parathyroid from human newborn, young mice, fetal mice, or 9-day chick embryos induced the resorption of bone in the parietals of fetal mice that had been associated with the parathyroid in

---

* See the Chapter by K. Haffen for the results concerning the stimulating or inhibiting effects of sex hormones on the gonads and genital tract *in vitro*. The specific effects of other nonhormonal materials on the same organs are also discussed.

culture. This resorption was accompanied by proliferation of osteoclasts and disappearance of osteoblasts. In addition, the parathyroid tissue liberated a substance that was diffusible into the medium and could act on explanted bone when it was not in contact with the parathyroid.

In the same way, the addition to the medium of a commercial parathyroid extract (ETP) at concentrations of 0.04–4 units/ml induced lacunar resorption of the bone, stimulation of the osteoclasts, and inhibition of the osteoblasts. The action of the extract was studied on the parietal bone and on the radial rudiment in fetal mice. The hormone extract acted both on the cartilaginous tissue, where the cells dedifferentiated and "depolarized," and on the connective tissue, which proliferated and completely invaded the diaphysis (Fig. 3).

Hancox (43) carried out analogous experiments on the limb bone rudiments of chick embryos. In contrast to the fetal bones of mice, those of the chick embryo did not react to parathyroid extract by activation of the osteoclasts. It seems that only the osteoblasts dedifferentiated and proliferated.

In an attempt to elucidate the mechanism of the action of parathormone, Gaillard *et al.* approached the problem from several aspects:

1. The effect of parathyroid extract on the activity of several enzymes in the rudiments.

2. Reproduction of the effects of the hormone by chemical inhibitors.

3. Neutralization of the effects of the hormone by adding to the medium substances liable to inactivate it.

4. Influence of the parathyroid extract on the incorporation or liberation of labeled atoms.

The first type of experiment (48) showed that some enzymes were strongly inhibited. These were glucose-6-phosphate dehydrogenase, lactate dehydrogenase, isocitrate dehydrogenase, NAD- and NADP-diaphorases, and alkaline phosphatase. In contrast, the activities of succinate dehydrogenase, α-glycerophosphate dehydrogenase, and glutamate dehydrogenase were little affected.

In the second type of experiment, De Voogd van der Straatan found that dinitrophenol did not reproduce the effects of parathyroid extract, despite its effect on the oxidative processes essential to the production of energy-rich phosphate bonds. In contrast, fluoroacetate slightly stimulated the proliferation of the osteoclasts and induced a certain amount of bone resorption. This effect was limited to the bone. Cartilage and connective tissue were not affected.

Varying results were obtained in the third type of experiment.

Gaillard (34) found that ATP neutralized some of the effects of parathyroid hormone such as bone resorption, the appearance of osteoclasts, and the dedifferentiation of cartilaginous cells. It did not prevent the loss of basophilia in the ground substance of the cartilage, nor did it reestablish the formation of new bone.

Hekkelman (46) found that the addition of NADP to the medium prevented the inhibition of isocitrate dehydrogenase by the parathyroid extract. Thus

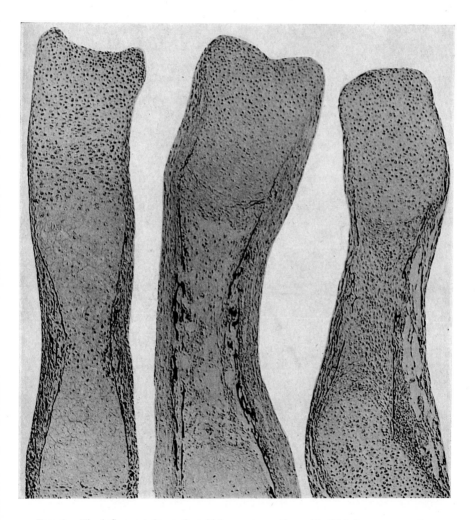

FIG. 3. The influence of parathyroid hormone on the radii of 15-day mouse embryos *in vitro.* ×77. After Gaillard (1960): Left. 15-day radius before culture. Beginning of ossification. Center. After 4 days of culture on the standard medium. Progressing ossification. Right. After 4 days of culture on a medium containing parathormone. The bone is lacunar and the diaphysis is filled with connective tissue.

perhaps the parathyroid extract acted by diminishing the amount of NADP available in the cells.

De Voogd van der Straaten (7) tested this hypothesis by studying the combined effects of materials on the explants. The combinations tested by this author were parathyroid extract and nicotinic acid (precursor of NADP); parathyroid extract and an analog of nicotinic acid, isonicotinic acid; and commercial parathyroid extract (ETP) and guanine monophosphate. These substances inhibited to a significant degree the effects of parathyroid extract on cultured bone. All these substances inhibited NADPase. Thus, these results seem to show that parathyroid extract acts on the bone by stimulating the activity of NADPase. This effect could be part of a general stimulation of the activity of the nucleotidases.

The fourth type of experiment has shown that the incorporation of labeled glycine into the proteins of the rudiments is greatly diminished by parathormone (31–37). De Voogd van der Straaten (5, 6) determined that the hormone first inhibited the incorporation of the amino acid, and then induced liberation of previously incorporated glycine into the medium. This inhibition of glycine incorporation was less pronounced if the glucose concentration in the medium was reduced from 100 to 15 mg/ml. The inhibition of glycine incorporation would thus be an indirect effect, resulting from disturbance of glucose metabolism by the parathyroid hormone.

Lastly, Raisz (74) showed the direct effect of parathyroid extract on the calcium metabolism of the rudiments. Fetal bones were labeled by injecting $^{45}CaCl_2$ into the mother 3 days before explantation. In the presence of parathyroid extract, labeled calcium was liberated into the culture medium at the same time that bone resorption was occurring. If the culture medium was rich in phosphates, or if the pH was raised above 7.5, the liberation of calcium was inhibited.

These results indicate the possibility of dissociating the different effects of parathyroid hormone, and show that:

1. The hormone can exert different effects on different cell types. The osteoblasts are inhibited whilst the osteoclasts are stimulated. Thus it is not only simply a toxic effect.

2. The hormone probably interferes with different metabolic pathways, particularly with the Krebs cycle.

2. The Influence of Thyroxine and Triiodothyronine on Bone in Vitro

A number of experiments have been carried out to find the effects of thyroid hormone on bone growth in vitro by Fell et al. Many clinical and experimental observations have shown the effect of thyroid disturbances on the growth or maintenance of the skeleton. Fell and Mellanby (21) tried to determine whether thyroid hormone could have a direct action on bone rudiments isolated *in vitro*. Two stages of differentiation could be distinguished in wing and claw rudiments taken from 4–7 day chick embryos. In the first stage, the limb buds were represented by simple condensations of mesenchyme which formed a single precartilaginous blastema. In the second stage the different bony rudiments were identifiable and cartilaginous hypertrophy occurred in the older explants. The whole bud was explanted in the first stage, and rudiments of each bone were cultured separately in the second stage. The dose of thyroxine was calculated on the basis of its levels in human plasma during hyperthyroid syndromes. Two types of reaction were induced by the hormone:

1. A stimulating effect on cartilaginous maturation.

2. A toxic effect that brought about a reduction in growth and cellular degeneration.

The remarkable characteristic of the effect of thyroid hormone was that it depended on the degree of bone differentiation that had occurred before the beginning of the experiment and on the origin of the bony rudiments.

Maturation of the cartilage was accelerated to varying degrees by the same hormonal concentration. It was greatest at the blastema stage, when the humerus responded best, while the ulna was unaffected. At a later stage, the stimulation was smaller and affected mainly the humerus, the radius, and the ulna.

The toxic effect was most marked in the older rudiments, and increased with the delay in culture. The bones of the foot were more affected than those of the wing; the femur was more sensitive than the tibia, and of the wing bones, the humerus was most sensitive and the radius most resistant.

Fell and Mellanby (22) carried out analogous experiments using triiodothyronine, the biological activity of which is much greater than that of thyroxine. These experiments showed that in the region of growth, maturation of the cartilage was accelerated in such a way that the growth in length of the explants was reduced.

Lawson (63–65) tried to define the mechanism of the differential response of the bony rudiments to triiodothyronine. Using bones cultured from 6-day chick embryos, she showed that the growth in length and weight of the tibia was decreased by triiodothyronine (T3) whilst that of the radius was increased. Also, rudiments of similar size (third metatarsal, radius, ulna, third metacarpal, and fourth metacarpal) reacted differently. Finally, the response of a single bone varied slightly according to its stage of development. Some bones, such as 5–$5\frac{1}{2}$ day tibia, could show a transient stimulation of growth followed by a delay.

Thus the kind of reaction is not determined by the size of the rudiment. Lawson was able to establish a correlation with the rate of growth of the rudiments. Some bones grew quickly and others more slowly. The rate of growth determined *in vivo* was maintained *in vitro*. It was suggested that triiodothyronine inhibited growth in bones with a rapid growth rate and stimulated those that grew slowly. Finally, by using concentrations of triiodothyronine varying from 0.01 to 0.32 μg/ml, Lawson was able to show that for any given rudiment the effect obtained with a small dose was a stimulation of growth, while above a certain dose the hormone caused inhibition. The differences between the sensitivity thresholds of different rudiments explain how the same dose of triiodothyronine can induce stimulation of growth in certain cases and inhibition of growth in others.

3. The Influence of Pituitary Growth Hormone on Bone *in Vitro*

Hay (45) cultured femur and tibia rudiments from 7-day chick embryos using Chen's method. In the presence of the somatotrophic (growth) hormone, there was a transient inhibition of growth during the first 2 days of culture. After this the explants increased in length faster than the controls, so that the length of both the control and the experimental explants was the same at the end of culture. Meanwhile, detailed analysis of the weight, total nitrogen, and water content of the explants showed that the hormone stimulated the protein synthesis. It is known that, *in vivo*, the anabolic effect of the growth hormone can only be manifested in the presence of insulin. Probably the serum used for the medium contained sufficient insulin to support the activity of the somatotrophic hormone.

Ito, Takamura, and Endo (49) and Ito and Endo (50) studied the influence of the growth hormone on the incorporation of labeled sulfate by 9-day chick embryo femurs. The rudiments were cultured using the roller-tube method in a medium composed of embryo extract, horse serum, and Gey's solution. At a high concentration (100 μg/ml) the somatotrophic hormone strongly inhibited the incorporation of labeled sulfate and decreased the elongation and increase in dry weight compared with the controls. The inhibition decreased with decreasing hormone concentration. At a low concentration (6.25 μg/ml) the incorporation of labeled sulfate increased significantly as compared with controls cultured without the hormone, and elongation was stimulated. The authors concluded that this concentration lay between the physiological limits (which were not known for the chicken). These results give a further example of the inversion of the effects of a hormone above a certain threshold.

4. Insulin

Landauer (56) and Zwilling (92) have shown that insulin injected into the chick embryo induced important skeletal defects (absence of rump, micromelia). It was interesting to see if insulin could have a direct effect on bone cultured *in vitro*. Chen (4) found that insulin at a concentration of 0.16 units/ml retarded growth in the diaphysis and induced deformations in the epiphyses. Zwilling (93) compared the effects of insulin on bone *in vivo* and *in vitro*. These effects were slightly different. In embryos treated with insulin the epiphyses of the long bones degenerated, while in bones cultured on an insulin-containing medium the epiphyses did not degenerate but were deformed and were composed of small-celled cartilage. However, nicotinamide protected bone rudiments *in vitro* from the teratogenic effect of insulin, just as it did *in vivo*. These results demonstrate that the micromelia induced by insulin injected into the embryo was due to a direct action of the hormone on the bone and not to the hypoglycemia induced by the treatment.

(Some work on the combined action of several hormones is also relevant to the actions of hormones on bones *in vitro*: 1. Insulin and growth hormone (45).   2. Thyroxine and parathormone (36, 38, 39)).

The results of these experiments are difficult to interpret.

5. VITAMIN A AND PAPAIN

A group of experiments was carried out by Fell *et al.* to find the effect of vitamin A on bone *in vitro*. These experiments led to the elucidation of the mode of action of vitamin A and to the precise localization of this action in the cells. Papain was used in these experiments because it has analogous effects on bone, and this has led to a new understanding of the mode of action of vitamin A.

In young animals an excess of vitamin A induced a generalized resorption of bone and cartilage, often accompanied by spontaneous fractures. Fell and Mellanby (20) showed that vitamin A added to the culture medium induced an analogous bony resorption. This bony resorption was even more rapid in the limb buds of fetal mice. In addition, the matrix of the terminal cartilage lost its capacity for metachromatic staining and then disintegrated, liberating still healthy chondrocytes. Almost identical observations have been described for the cartilaginous rudiments of the long bones of 6- to 7-day chick embryos cultured in the presence of vitamin A (Fig. 4.2). The effects of hypervitaminosis were partially reversible when the explants were returned to a normal medium after several days (47).

An early indication of the mode of action of vitamin A was obtained in a study of the incorporation of radioactive labeled sulfate into the bone rudiments of 6–7 day chick embryo limbs (23). Initially, the vitamin inhibited the incorporation of labeled sulfate, and then it induced liberation of the sulfate already incorporated. At the same time, there was a loss of metachromasia in the cartilage. From these results, the above workers concluded that it was possible that the vitamin affected an enzyme produced by the cartilage cells.

The next stage in the investigation was suggested by the strikingly analogous effects of vitamin A and papain. When papain was injected into young rabbits their ears drooped like those of a spaniel (81). The collapse of the ears was accompanied by histological changes in the cartilage throughout the body. There was a loss of basophilia and thinning of the intercellular partitions. These appearances corresponded closely to those seen with vitamin A. Moreover, high doses of vitamin A also caused rabbit ears to droop, though more moderately than after papain (82). The active fraction of crude papain is a protease (67).

(1)   (3)

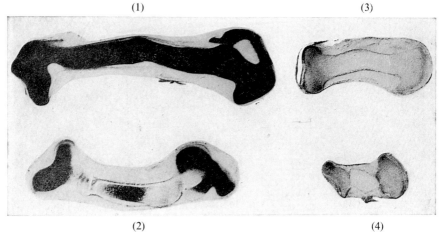

(2)   (4)

Fig. 4.   The effect of vitamin A and papain in culture on 7-day chick embryo humerus. ×12. After Fell (1960). (1) Humerus cultured for 8 days on the standard medium. The cartilaginous matrix is stained with toluidine blue. (2) Medium containing vitamin A. Metachromasia is reduced and the proliferating zones are deformed. (3). Medium containing papain. Complete disappearance of metachromasia. (4) Medium containing vitamin A and papain. The effects on the cartilage are additive.

Fell and Thomas (25) compared the effects of papain and vitamin A on the cartilaginous rudiments of chick embryo limbs and fetal mouse limbs near term. The two substances caused loss of metachromasia and reduced the intercellular partitions. However, papain had a relatively uniform effect throughout the explant, while vitamin A affected some zones more than others (Fig. 4.3). The histological appearance of the explant, particularly the cartilage cells, suggests that papain acts directly on the matrix, while vitamin A acts on the cells in the matrix. Vitamin A may act by activating a protease present in the chondrocytes. Vitamin A and papain together have a strong cumulative effect on the cartilage (Fig. 4.4). In contrast, differentiated bone in mouse rudiments disappears almost completely in a few days under the influence of vitamin A, but is not affected by papain. From this it must be concluded that the mode of action of vitamin A cannot be explained by the activation of a single enzyme analogous to the protease of papain.

Fell and Thomas (25) suggested that vitamin A stimulates the activity of several intercellular enzymes, one of which exhibits effects analogous to those of papain.

This hypothesis is supported by the observation that explants treated with vitamin A liquefied the medium much more than "normal" explants, and liberated into it an acid-soluble nitrogenous material (66). This is an indication of proteolytic activity in the medium. Finally, these workers were able to isolate a protease with an optimum pH of 3 from normal cartilage cells derived from the limb buds of 9-day chick embryos. This enzyme sedimented in a specific fraction on ultracentrifugation, showing that normal chondrocytes contain an enzyme or an enzyme system that is localized in specific cytoplasmic particles. This enzyme has an effect on the ground substance of cartilage similar to that of vitamin A.

Dingle (10) showed that vitamin A acting *in vitro* on rat liver lysosomes liberated a cathepsin. It remains to extend this observation to the cartilage itself.

The modes of action of papain on bone rudiments in chick embryos have also been studied in detail by Girard (40, 41) and Bazin, Girard, and Delaunay (2). Fell and Thomas (25) noted that embryonic cartilage resumed its growth and reconstituted its ground substance after it had been removed from the influence of papain *in vitro*. Girard confirmed that papain acted directly on the cartilaginous matrix and defined the conditions under which cartilage could be restored to normal. This restoration is better with a low concentration of papain, and it also depends on the richness of the medium in nutrient materials, notably glutamine, a substance that encourages cartilaginous growth. Meanwhile, the two processes that have been studied, that is, growth of the rudiment and acquisition of metachromasia by the cartilage, can be dissociated. They do not necessarily vary together, when the conditions for the action of papain and the composition of the medium are varied. Finally, papain seems to act differently on explants of varying ages, that is, on precartilaginous or cartilaginous cells. In an attempt to determine whether papain acted only on the matrix or on the chondrocytes as well, Bazin, Girard, and Delaunay (2) defined the biochemical effects of papain on cartilage. Destruction of the protein-chondroitin sulfate complex by the papain protease causes the disappearance of the ground substance. Mucopolysaccharides and collagen that have become soluble are released in addition to the chondroitin sulfate. Papain cannot attack the two former substances directly, but it destroys the nonfibrous protein part of the cartilaginous matrix. This causes rupture of the intermolecular bonds necessary for cohesion of the connective tissue framework.

6. THE CREEPER FACTOR

It has been shown above that many hormonal or inhibitor substances whose effect is known *in vivo* can act without an intermediate on embryonic bone rudiments explanted *in vitro*. Wolff and Kieny (90) applied this type of analysis to the study of a genetic mutation which affects the skeleton of chick embryos. The creeper mutation *Cp* (*courtes pattes*) is manifested as achondroplasia in the heterozygous state. The long bones, especially the tibia, become short and thick, with an abnormal curvature. These malformations are due to an irregularity in cartilage formation and precocious ossification. In the homozygous state (*Cp Cp*) the mutation is lethal, the embryos usually dying before the 3rd day of incubation. A few survive until the 18th day, by which time they show multiple defects, such as phocomelia, parrot beak, and retinal coloboma. The fact that the attenuated form occurs in the presence of a single gene (*Cp+*) and the severe form in the presence of two genes suggests that a quantitative factor may play a part in the determination of the two phenotypes. Ancel (1) has shown that a single teratogenic substance at different concentrations (54) (*p*-aminobenzene-sulfamide or eserine salts) can produce corresponding phenocopies.

The authors investigated whether a teratogenic substance could be demonstrated in the chain of reactions that leads from the gene to its phenotypic manifestation. Two hypotheses could be suggested to explain this external manifestation of a genetic character:

1. All the reactions may remain within the cell, the character being manifested in the cell in which the gene exerts its effect.

2. The character may be manifested in the cells of a target tissue under the influence of substances coming from other organs; that is, substances brought by the bloodstream (in the same way as hormones) that permeate the entire organism.

If such substances are formed outside the effector organ, it should be possible to demonstrate them by culture *in vitro*.

Several experiments by Wolff and Kieny (90, 91) and Kieny (52, 53) have been concerned with the effects of extracts from both normal and creeper embryos on the rudiments of the tibiotarsus from normal or creeper embryos.

The rudiments were taken from $6\frac{1}{2}$–$7\frac{1}{2}$ day embryos. The extracts were prepared from normal or Creeper embryos of $6\frac{3}{4}$–11 days' incubation. Creeper embryos *Cp+* can be distinguished from normal embryos only after $6\frac{3}{4}$ days. The two tibiotarsi from an animal, either normal or creeper, were cultured as follows. One was placed on a medium based on normal embryo extract, the other on a medium based on creeper embryo extract. In a preliminary series of experiments, culture of rudiments from the two types of embryo showed that the normal rudiments ($++$) developed like the control rudiments taken from the White Leghorn strain (Plate I, Fig. 1,N). Creeper rudiments (Cp^+) developed according to their genotype. They had a dumbbell shape, with massive epiphyses and a short poorly developed diaphysis with a central white cuff. This cuff was due to an already advanced ossification. The phenotype Cp^+ was maintained throughout the culture period and there was little growth in the rudiment (Plate I, Fig. 1,C).

Whereas the growth of tibias from 6–$6\frac{3}{4}$ day creeper embryos was minimal on the medium containing creeper embryo extract, it was much better on a medium containing normal embryo extract (Plate I, Fig. 3). Conversely, linear growth of normal tibias was considerably reduced on creeper embryo extract. Thus, the creeper embryo extract contained a factor that restricted growth, both in normal and creeper tibiotarsi, and normal embryo extract contained a factor that stimulated the growth of creeper tibias. It must be noted that variations in the growth of the rudiments were observed in all of these experiments, but the morphogenesis of the explant always conformed to the original genotype, whatever the nature of the embryo extract contained in the medium.

The distribution of the inhibitory creeper factor in the embryo has been determined. Extracts of the viscera of creeper embryos also had an inhibitory effect, not exhibited by the visceral extracts from normal embryos. Extracts of eviscerated creeper embryos had a smaller inhibitory effect than did extracts of whole creeper embryos. There was no difference in effect between extracts of whole normal embryos and extracts of eviscerated normal embryos. Thus the viscera of creeper embryos contained a significant fraction of the inhibitory substance.

Finally, the inhibitor substance could be found in the achondroplastic long bones, but an extract of creeper embryos that had had their limbs removed lost none of its inhibitor effects (Plate I, Fig. 4). Thus the creeper factor was not specially localized in the long bones.

Kieny and Abbot (personal communication) have shown that an extract prepared from embryos carrying a mutation that does not affect the skeleton (scaleless) stimulated the growth of both normal and creeper tibias in the same way as a normal embryo extract.

Certain questions remain to be resolved before genesis of the creeper malformation can be explained. According to our results, it has been shown that there is a factor present in the whole animal that affects the growth of the skeleton. However, morphogenesis of the explants appears to occur

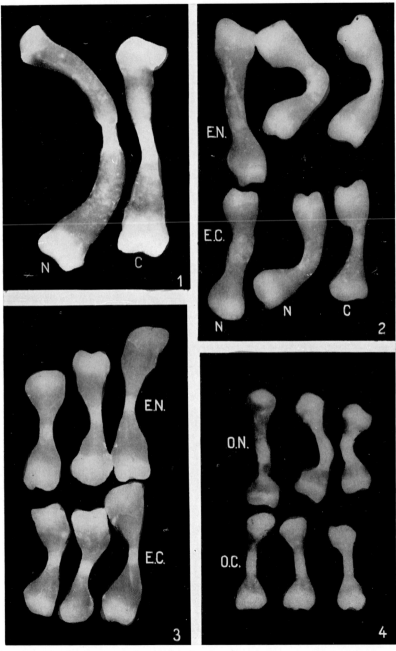

Plate I. *In vitro* development of normal and creeper long bones on media based on normal or creeper embryo extract. After Wolff and Kieny (1963). See opposite page.

according to an intrinsic pattern. It must be noted that the explants were taken at a relatively late stage for two reasons:

1. It is impossible to distinguish between the two phenotypes before 6 days.

2. Younger rudiments differentiate very poorly in culture, whether they are from normal or creeper embryos.

Wolff and Kieny are now trying to orient the differentiation of very young limb buds (3 days) from the White Leghorn strain, by grafting them into creeper embryo hosts of the same age. The results already obtained indicate that the creeper environment has an inhibitory effect on the growth of the normal grafted limb.

The nature of the "creeper factor" is not yet known. Is it an actual inhibitor substance or is the creeper embryo deficient in a substance present in the normal embryo? It can be suggested that the metabolism of creeper embryos is completely modified and that inhibition of growth by the "creeper factor" results in complex alterations of the embryonic medium. Biochemical experiments (53) have shown that the difference between the creeper embryo extract and the normal embryo extract lies in the protein constituents. It has not been possible to define the nature of the inhibition more precisely than this.

Kieny and Abbott (55) made an analogous study of the chicken mutation diplopode-4. This mutation is manifested in particular by supernumerary digits of the wing and foot, by shortening of the long bones, and by the exceptional length of the fibula, the only long bone that is not shortened. Kieny and Abbott showed that extracts of diplopode embryos reduced the growth of normal tibiotarsi even more than did creeper extracts. In the diplopode mutation, the tibiotarsus is even shorter than it is in the creeper mutation. Diplopode extract does not stimulate growth of the normal fibula.

Experiments devoted to the organ culture of embryonic bone have contributed a large amount of information from which it is possible to draw certain conclusions. Embryonic bone possesses the capacity for

---

FIG. 1.   Normal (N) and creeper (C) tibiotarsi from $7\frac{1}{2}$-day embryos, cultured for 7 days on the standard medium ($\times 9.5$).

FIG. 2. $6\frac{1}{2}$-day normal (N) and creeper (C) tibiotarsi, cultured for 7 days on (1) a medium containing normal embryo extract (upper row, E.N.) and (2) a medium containing creeper embryo extract (lower row, E.C.). $\times 9.5$.

FIG. 3. $6\frac{1}{2}$-day creeper tibiotarsi (1) on a medium based on normal embryo extract (upper row, E. N.); (2) on a medium based on creeper embryo extract (lower row, E.C). $\times 9.5$.

FIG. 4. $6\frac{1}{2}$-day normal tibiotarsi cultured on media based on (1) a medium containing extract from long bones of normal embryos (upper row, O.N.) and (2) extract from long bones of creeper embryos (lower row, O.C.). $\times 7$.

autonomous growth and differentiation. It may also react in a complex fashion to hormones or exogenous materials that do not occur in the course of normal development. As far as these reactions are concerned, and also with regard to pathological malformations, isolation in culture has made it possible to distinguish the role of the factors intrinsic to the rudiment itself and the role of the humoral influences that affect the rudiment in the intact organism.

B. Effects of Hormones on the Structure and Function of the Mammary Gland *in Vitro*

Using organ culture techniques and experimental animals (mice), many workers have tried to elucidate the hormonal factors necessary for structural differentiation and functional activity of the mammary gland [Lasfargues (1959–1962), Elias *et al.* (1959–1963) and Prop (1960–1961)].

It has been possible to show that many hormones have an effect on the mammary gland *in vivo*, but a clear-cut picture of the mechanisms of their action has remained elusive. When the ovarian hormones estradiol and progesterone are given to mice in a ratio of 1/1000, development of the ducts and alveoli is induced. These hormones do not stimulate mammary growth in hypophysectomized animals, and synergically only with pituitary hormone (prolactin). Other experiments have shown the effect of the adreno-cortical hormones. Mammary tissue regresses rapidly in the adrenalectomized animal and the administration of cortisone induced enlargement of the ducts without normal growth or differentiation. Growth of the mammary gland can be obtained in the hypophysectomized, ovariectomized animal by daily injections of insulin retard together with an appropriate combination of estradiol and progesterone. Thus, this growth occurs in the absence of pituitary hormones. Lastly, prolactin or somatotrophin together with cortisol is the minimal combination capable of inducing lactation in hypophysectomized, ovariectomized, adrenalectomized mice. Thus the mammary gland is susceptible to the effects of estradiol, progesterone, pituitary hormones, corticosteroids, and insulin. However, studies on the intact animal present a confused picture, where it is difficult to determine the true role of each hormone, since different hormonal combinations can induce growth of the gland. Ablation of all of the endocrine glands results in a complete physiological upset, incompatible with life, and induces secondary reactions that may mask the phenomena under investigation. Organ culture is thus the ideal technique for studying the separate or combined effects of hormones on an organ where the anatomical and physiological integrity are maintained.

The experiments discussed have all made use of similar culture techniques, derived either from Chen's method, Trowell's method, or Wolff and Haffen's method. Morgan's synthetic medium 199 with a known composition was used most commonly. The atmosphere in contact with the explants was either air (for embryonic organs) or $95\% \, O_2 + 5\% \, CO_2$ (for adult organs). The slight variations in techniques are certainly not responsible for the observed differences between the results.

The experiments on explantation were carried out at different stages of maturation of the mammary gland:

1. Undifferentiated embryonic rudiment.

2. Immature adult gland, or adult gland in the physiological resting stage between periods of gestation.

3. Prelactating gland at the beginning of gestation.

4. Prelactating gland at the end of gestation.

1. THE EMBRYONIC RUDIMENT

The influences of several hormones on the differentiation and growth of the embryonic mammary rudiment have been studied (61). Pieces of abdominal skin were taken from 10–15 day embryos of the C 57 B strain, and were cultured for 10–12 days. The sex of the embryos was not determined. This strain was chosen because it never shows the "milk factor" that may modify the cellular responses. The hormones tested were 17β-estradiol and progesterone (dissolved in alcohol and diluted in the culture medium), growth hormone, prolactin, and cortisol (in aqueous solution). The concentrations used for the first two were determined from the literature, and for the other two by direct trial. Several types of control media were used: "normal" medium 199, medium 199 with alcohol (the same amount was added as used for the solvent for the ovarian hormones), and medium 199 enriched with crystalline bovine albumin to reproduce the possible nutrient effect of the protein hormones. These controls showed that alcohol at the concentrations used was not toxic and that albumin had a slightly favorable effect, though for smaller than the specific effects of the hormones.

The primitive ducts in the rudiment are formed by a tubular invagination of the germinal layer of the epidermis. This invagination extends and ramifies in the underlying adipose and connective tissues. All the canalicular tissue can be formed in culture from undifferentiated epidermis (44). Lasfargues and Murray found that most of the glands differentiated from buds that were already present at the time of explantation. The newly formed tubules showed an empty lumen lined by two layers of cubical cells and a basement membrane. Similar differentiation occurred in 60% of the explants on a biological medium (based on embryo extract) and in 40% of the explants on synthetic medium 199. The walls of the tubules were irregular and often thicker on the synthetic than on the biological medium. The adipose and

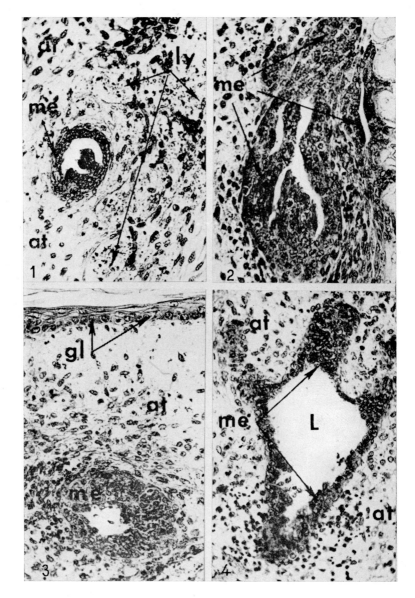

Plate II. Development of embryonic mammary gland cultured on medium 199 in the presence of various hormones. × 224. After Lasfargues and Murray (1959).

Fig. 1. Estradiol + progesterone in the ratio of 1/1000. Epithelium (me) poorly developed, adipose tissue (at) prominent. Zones of necrosis (ly) in the connective tissue.

Fig. 2. Growth hormone. Marked epithelial hyperplasia (me).

connective tissues showed well-developed active zones close to necrotic areas. The germinal layer of the skin was often discontinuous with compact hair follicles.

Differentiation of the mammary epithelium ceased completely in the presence of estradiol. The connective tissue was degenerate or absent, and the hair follicles were stunted. In contrast, the adipose tissue was stimulated.

Progesterone induced general necrosis of the explants.

The combination of estradiol and progesterone in the ratio of 1/1000 partially restored the normal appearance of the explants. There was a slight inhibition of the growth of the mammary epithelium. The adipose tissue was well developed and active (Plate II, Fig. 1).

Apart from their specific effects, which will be analyzed later, the pituitary hormones improved the general development of the explants. In their presence the percentage of explants that differentiated rose to 60 and 80%.

Prolactin increased the degree of differentiation of the mammary epithelium. The ducts were lined by 3–4 layers of large epithelial cells (Plate II, Fig. 3). Adipose tissue invaded large areas of connective tissue, which nevertheless was healthy. This last effect, which seems specific to prolactin, may be a preparatory phase before secretion occurs.

Growth hormone produced the most spectacular results. The mammary epithelium and the different epithelial structures of the skin (germinal layer, hair follicles) showed extremely active growth. Many mammary ducts were often grouped together in a single epithelial mass with many mitoses (Plate II, Fig. 2). The cells were large, almost turgid, but they did not show the cytoplasmic vacuoles indicative of secretion. In direct contrast to the effect of prolactin, the connective tissue was well-developed with many collagen fibers, while the adipose tissue was limited to small areas.

The combination of growth hormone and prolactin induced a similar morphology of the epithelium. However, the connective and adipose tissues were more regularly distributed and the adipose tissue was active. It is evident that the effects of the two hormones on the epithelium overlap. In contrast, their effects on the glandular stroma were different and complementary. Prolactin stimulated the development of the adipose tissue, while the growth hormone induced development of the connective tissue and an overproduction of collagen.

The combination of the two ovarian hormones with each of the pituitary hormones and then of the two pituitary hormones with each of the ovarian

---

Fig. 3.   Prolactin. Epithelial hyperplasia less marked (gl = germinal layer of the skin).

Fig. 4.   Cortisol. Exfoliation of the epithelial cells into the lumen (L), the adipose tissue very prominent (at), walls of the lumen distended.

hormones showed that the specific effect of the pituitary hormones was always dominant. The only exception occurred with the pituitary hormones plus progesterone, where complete necrosis took place (progesterone effect).

When the four hormones were associated, a balance was reestablished. The cultures showed large epithelial masses, and the connective and adipose tissues were almost equally distributed.

The last experiment was on the effect of cortisol on the embryonic rudiments. It was shown that the mammary epithelium differentiated, but presented a structure that was typical of secretion. The lumen of the tubes was distended and they were lined by a flattened epithelium whose cells showed large cytoplasmic vacuoles. Well-developed adipose tissue replaced the connective tissue almost completely (Plate II, Fig. 4). When it was associated with the other hormones, cortisol imposed its own effect. Associated with prolactin, cortisol seemed to stimulate secretion even more strongly than when it was alone. The cytoplasm of the epithelial cells was filled with secretory products and the lumen of the ducts contained abundant cellular debris.

These experiments establish certain properties of the embryonic rudiment:

1. Differentiation occurs on a synthetic medium in the absence of hormones.

2. The primary structures are very sensitive to specific hormonal stimulation and some of the reactions of the adult gland *in vivo* are manifested by the embryonic gland *in vitro*:

      a. There is a critical ratio between the concentrations of estradiol and progesterone (1/1000).

      b. Pituitary hormones induce epithelial development.

      c. Cortisol evokes a secretory response.

In fact, a single hormone, that is, the growth hormone, seems to be implicated in the growth of primitive mammary epithelium.

The results of this work are summarized in Table I.

2. THE IMMATURE ADULT GLAND

Lasfargues (58) used the same experimental conditions to study the effect of the ovarian hormones on cultures of completely differentiated mammary gland during the physiological resting stage. The glands were taken from 3-month-old virgin mice. At the time of explantation, the tissues showed a system of ducts with secondary and some tertiary branching, but no lobule formation. The ducts were narrow and were surrounded by connective tissue. The adipose tissue showed closely packed fat globules. When they were cultured for 10–14 days on medium 199, the explants

TABLE I

RESPONSE OF THE EMBRYONIC MAMMARY RUDIMENT TO DIFFERENT COMBINATIONS
OF HORMONES (61)[a]

Hormones	Epithelium	Connective tissue	Adipose tissue
No hormones	+	+	+
Estradiol	0	−	+ +
Progesterone	−	−	−
Estr. + Progest.	+ to ±	+	+ +
Prolactin	+ +	+ to ±	+ +
Growth hormone (STH)	+ + +	+ +	±
Prolact. + STH	+ + +	+	+ +
Estr. + Progest. + Prolact.	+ +	+	+ +
Estr. + Progest. + STH	+ + +	+ +	±
Estr. + Prolact. + STH	+ + +	+	+ +
Prolact. + Progest. + STH	−	−	−
Cortisol	Secretion	−	+ +
Cort. + Estr. + Prog.	Secretion	−	+ +
Cortisol + STH	Secretion	−	+ +
Cortisol + Prol.	Secretion	−	+ +

[a]Key:

+	normal differentiation	0	no differentiation
+ +	slight stimulation	−	necrosis
+ + +	marked stimulation	±	inhibition

retained almost the same appearance. A few necrotic areas appeared but these were considered to be due to the relative poverty of the medium.

In the presence of estradiol, the epithelium seemed to be stimulated, judging by its excellent morphological appearance and by the numerous mitoses present. The adipose tissue was entirely necrotic and the collagen very abundant. The influence of estradiol on the adult gland was thus very different from its effect in the embryonic rudiment, where it inhibited epithelial differentiation.

As in the embryonic organ, progesterone induced generalized necrosis.

Normal appearance was restored when both hormones were added to the culture medium in appropriate proportions.

Meanwhile, Prop (73) and Rivera (79) had obtained significantly different results using analogous materials. In both cases the mammary glands were taken from 3–6 week old mice. There was regression of the primary ducts after 5–12 days of culture on medium 199 (Rivera) or on a medium based on a hydrolysate of lactalbumin with human serum. The canals became progressively thinner and the terminal buds disappeared (Plate III, Fig. 2). According to these two authors, insulin can prevent this regression.

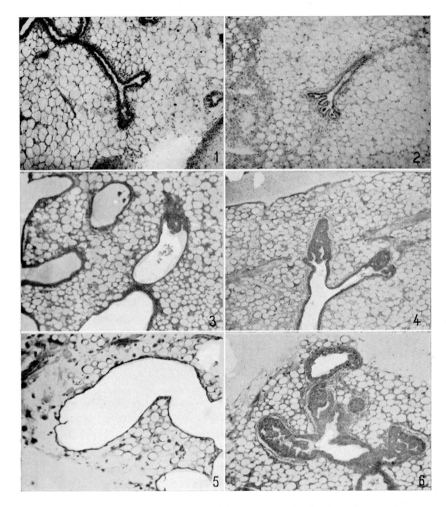

Plate III. Development of the immature adult mammary gland cultured on medium 199. After Prop (1961).

FIG. 1.   Six-week-old gland before culture.

FIG. 2.   After 5 days of culture without hormones. Regression.

FIG. 3.   Cultured in the presence of insulin. Proliferation of blind epithelial channels, ducts a little enlarged.

FIG. 4.   Insulin + progesterone. Proliferation a little more marked than in the preceding example.

FIG. 5.   Insulin + hydrocortisone. Proliferation arrested, the epithelium flattened, ducts distended.

FIG. 6.   Insulin + prolactin + progesterone. Intraluminal papillomatous growth.

Trowell (85) defined a culture medium for adult organs, in which insulin improved survival of the explants. Prop (72) obtained development of secretory alveoli in immature mammary glands from 6-week mice by a modification of this technique. The medium contained insulin, prolactin, progesterone, and hydrocortisone. It was shown (1961) that of all these hormones, only insulin could prevent regression of the ducts in culture (Plate III, Fig. 3). In addition, the other three hormones could only affect the gland in the presence of insulin. The different combinations of hormones gave the following results:

insulin + progesterone → stimulated proliferation and induced edema of the ducts (Plate III, Fig. 4).

insulin + prolactin → maintenance of the ducts (same effect as insulin alone).

insulin + hydrocortisone → extreme edema of the ducts; flattened epithelium (Plate III, Fig. 5).

insulin + progesterone + hydrocortisone → ditto

insulin + prolactin + progesterone → swollen ducts; papillomatous intraluminal growth (Plate III, Fig. 6).

insulin + prolactin + hydrocortisone → thinning of the ducts and appearances of secretion.

Rivera and Bern (80) also attributed a fundamental role to insulin in the survival of the mammary gland from a nonpregnant animal. They worked with multiparous mice and the glands were taken 2 weeks after weaning. At the time of explantation, the tissue was composed of alveoli in the course of regression and duct elements. On medium 199, the mammary tissue became necrotic. The addition of insulin maintained the structure and insulin together with cortisol induced some reorganization of the alveoli.

These different experiments show that as the isolated mammary gland differentiates further, its hormonal requirements become more complex. The situation complicates itself further when the gland is studied during the period of physiological activity during pregnancy.

3. The Mammary Gland of Pregnancy

Two phases may be distinguished in the preparation of the mammary gland for gestation. The first phase lasts until the 12th–14th days: This is the phase of development or reorganization of the alveoli. During the second phase, that is, at the end of gestation, signs of secretory activity begin to appear in the alveolar cells—intracytoplasmic vacuoles and accumulation of secretions in the lumen of the alveoli. These two phases will be called early and late prelactation.

Rivera and Bern (80) and Lasfargues (60) have studied the mammary gland during early prelactation and agree that rapid necrosis of the explants

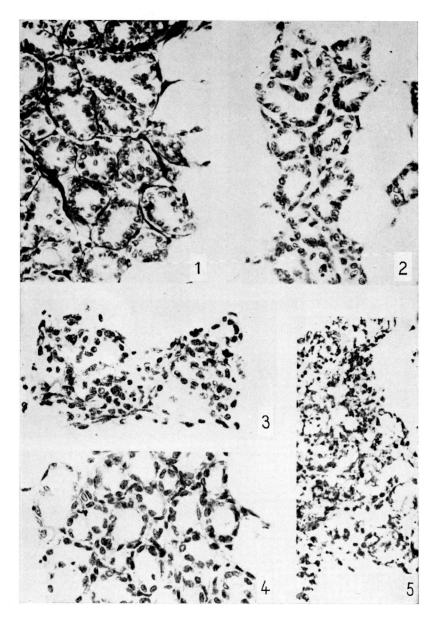

Plates IV and V. Culture of the mammary gland at various stages during and after gestation using medium 199 with various added hormones. × 380. After Rivera and Bern (1961).

Plate IV. Different functional stages on a medium containing insulin and cortisone (I + C).
  FIG. 1. Late prelactation (end of gestation).
  FIG. 2. Early prelactation.
  FIG. 3. Nonpregnant (I = 50 μg/ml + C = 5 μg/ml).
  FIG. 4. Nonpregnant (I = 25 μg/ml + C = 8 μg/ml).
  FIG. 5. Late prelactation without hormones. Necrosis.

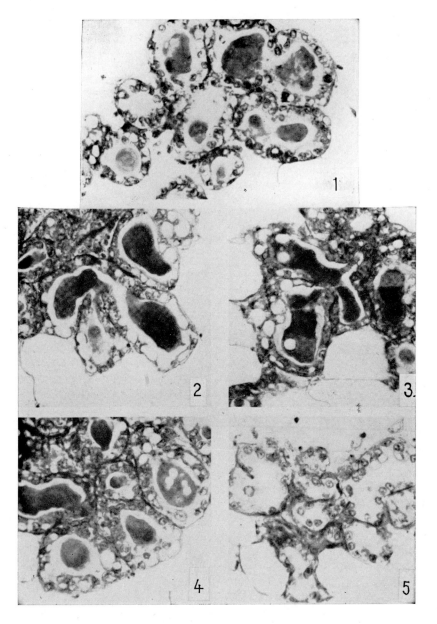

Plate V. Medium containing insulin + cortisone + various pituitary hormones (MH = prolactin, STH = somatotrophic hormone). After Rivera and Bern (1961).

FIG. 1. Late prelactation; I + C + MH + STH.
FIG. 2. Early prelactation; I + C + MH; advanced secretory activity.
FIG. 3. Early prelactation; I + C + MH + STH; as above.
FIG. 4. Early prelactation; I + C + MH + STH; as above.
FIG. 5. Nonpregnant; I + C + MH + STH; some secretory activity.

occurred on medium 199 without addition of hormones. They disagree on the hormonal combinations necessary or sufficient for maintenance of the alveolar structure or for stimulation of the secretion. Rivera and Bern found that insulin on its own permitted survival of explants taken between the 10th and 12th days of gestation. After 5 days of culture the explants retained their alveolar structure, although it had regressed a little and there were some areas of necrosis. When insulin and cortisol were combined, the explants retained the structure that they had at the time of explantation (Plate IV, Figs. 2, 3, and 4). With cortisol alone, the explants became necrotic. Lastly, addition of either prolactin, growth hormone, or the two pituitary hormones to the insulin-cortisol combination induced the appearance of secretion, as seen in the phase of late prelactation. If insulin or cortisol was omitted from these combinations, degeneration of the explants occurred.

Lasfargues (60) attempted to show that insulin played neither a fundamental role in structural maintenance, nor a permissive role in the action of other hormones as had been suggested by other workers. According to Lasfargues, cultures in the presence of insulin alone died by the end of 8 days, with only the adipose tissue retaining an almost normal appearance. It must be noted that there is no fundamental incompatibility between this result and that reported by Rivera and Bern. The latter authors found only an indifferent maintenance of structure for 5 days with evidence of necrosis at that time. In contrast, Lasfargues obtained survival of the glandular epithelium in the presence of the ovarian hormones (estradiol and progesterone) in combination with prolactin. However, the connective tissue stroma and the adipose tissue became necrotic under these conditions. The addition of insulin to this combination not only assured survival of all of the tissues, but also a true growth of the acini. Lastly, the combination insulin-cortisol-prolactin arrested development but induced a secretory appearance, while causing pyknosis of some epithelial cells. The explants were taken very early, before the 10th day of gestation. Pyknosis did not appear in explants that were taken at a later stage. Lasfargues concluded from these results that insulin has no specific effect on the mammary epithelial cells, though it may reinforce the action of specific hormones, perhaps by favoring their entry into the cell.

A last group of experiments (13, 14, 80) is concerned with the survival and maintenance of secretion in the mammary gland during the last stages of gestation. Summarizing these experiments, it seems that insulin alone can only support an indifferent type of survival, whilst insulin and cortisol maintain the alveoli (Plate IV, Fig. 1). The secretory level reached at the time of explantation is maintained in culture if the medium contains insulin, cortisol, prolactin, and somatotrophin (Plate V, Fig. 1). The tissues in the last stages of gestation require doses of the last two hormones four times weaker than the doses required by the tissues in the early stage. Either the sensitivity of the tissues increases or a stronger dose is needed to bring about the secretory phase than is needed to maintain it. There is only one possible discrepancy in the observations on the gland at the end of gestation. Elias and Rivera (14) noted that cortisol and prolactin were sufficient to ensure maintenance of the secretory state. It is possible that the prolactin used was contaminated by insulin activity (80).

Certain conclusions can be drawn from the group of experiments on the mammary gland that are summarized in Table II.

1. The hormonal requirements increase with increasing degree of differentiation. The embryonic rudiment will differentiate on a hormone-free medium. The immature adult gland survives but regresses in the absence of hormones. Lastly, once preparation for lactation has commenced, the gland dies if relatively complex combinations of hormones are not available.

2. Whatever divergencies occur in the interpretation of the results, the following hormones act on the isolated mammary gland at different stages in its maturation:

Insulin	Prolactin
Estradiol	Growth hormone
Progesterone	Cortisol

The action of some of these hormones has been firmly established. Cortisol induces secretion; prolactin and growth hormone induce growth of the mammary epithelium. Different combinations of hormones can act in an analogous fashion on the different stages of the gland. It is reasonable to think that complex interactions, and occasionally substitutions, occur *in vivo*. It is certain that there is a predetermined sequence of hormonal actions and that the gland cannot react to a hormone or certain combination of hormones until it has reached a given stage of development, which itself is controlled by other hormones. The role of organ culture is obvious in such a complex subject and this technique has already furnished new precise information.

III. GENERAL CONCLUSIONS

A general principle emerging from the discussed experiments is that embryonic organs are relatively independent as far as hormones are concerned, even though the hormonal requirements of differentiated organs increase as their development progresses. Organ culture allows the organs

TABLE II

ANALYTICAL SUMMARY OF THE HORMONAL REQUIREMENTS OF THE MAMMARY GLAND AT DIFFERENT FUNCTIONAL STAGES, AS DETERMINED BY VARIOUS AUTHORS[a]

Stage at explantation of the mammary gland	Differentiation achieved in culture	Maintenance of the structure present at explantation	Secretory activity	Reference
Embryonic rudiment	Without hormones Prol → ++ STH → +++		C	(61)
Immature adult		Without hormone, slight necrosis		(58)
		E + Prog		
		Prog + Prol + I	Prog + Prol + I + C	(72)
		I		(73)
		I		(79)
Adult during the physiological resting stage		I or I + C		(80)
Prelactating gland				
(1) Early stage of gestation		I + C	I + C + Prol or	(80)
		Prog + Prol + E or	I + C + STH	
		I + Prog + Prol + E	I + C + Prol	(60)
		I + C		
(2) Late stage of gestation			C + Prol	(13)
				(14)
		I + C	I + C + Prol + STH	(80)

[a] Key:

C = corticoids   E = estradiol   Prol = prolactin
I = insulin   Prog = progesterone   STH = somatotrophic hormone

to survive in a very simplified environment and as a result it has been possible to analyze not only the hormonal requirements but also the mechanism by which many substances act, divorced from the interference of the secondary effects that occur in the intact organism.

BIBLIOGRAPHY

1. Ancel P. "La chimiotératogénèse. Réalisation des monstruosités par des substances chimiques chez les Vertébrés", 1950, G. Doin, Paris, pp. 324–340.
2. Bazin S., Girard H. and Delaunay A. Effets biochimiques exercés par la papaïne sur des ébauches cartilagineuses d'embryons de Poulet. *Ann. Inst. Pasteur*, 1962, **102**, 346–352.
3. Bern H. A. and Rivera E. M. Effect of hormones on organ cultures of mouse mammary tissues. *Proc. Am. Ass. Cancer Res.*, 1960, **3**, 94.
4. Chen J. M. The effect of insulin on embryonic limb-bones cultivated *in vitro*. *J. Physiol.* (U.S.A.), 1954, **125**, 148–162.
5. De Voogd van der Straaten W. A. The influence of parathyroid extract on the glycine binding capacity of the cultivated radius of the 15 day-old mouse embryo. *Proc. Akad. Amst. Ser. C.*, 1962, **65**, 231–239.
6. De Voogd van der Straaten W. A. A further radiometrical analysis of the influence of parathyroid extract on the glycine binding capacity of the cultivated mouse radius rudiment. The effect of a lowered glucose content on the medium. *Proc. Kon. Ned. Akad. Wet. Ser. C.*, 1962, **65**, 506–521.
7. De Voogd van der Straaten W. A. Some data concerning the mode of action of parathyroid hormone on bone tissue. *Seconde Réunion Européenne d'Endocrinologie comparée*, 1963. Bruxelles, 16–19 sept. 1963. Abstract.
8. Dieterlen-Lièvre F. Influence du pancréas embryonnaire sur la formation du glycogène hépatique chez le Poulet étudiée par la méthode des parabioses *in vitro*. *C. R. Acad. Sc.*, 1960, **250**, 1349–1351.
9. Dieterlen-Lièvre F. Démonstration de l'activité précoce des cellules A du pancréas chez l'embryon de Poulet. *C. R. Acad. Sc.*, 1963, **256**, 1597–1599.
10. Dingle J. T. Studies on the mode of action excess vitamin A. 3: Release of a bound protease by the action of vitamin A. *Biochem. J.*, 1961, **79**, 509–512.
11. Dingle J. T. Penetration and stabilization of biological membranes by vitamin A. *Biochem. J.*, 1964, **90**, 36 p.
12. Elias J. J. Cultivation of adult mouse mammary gland in hormone-enriched synthetic medium. *Science*, 1957, **126**, 842–844.
13. Elias J. J. Effect of insulin and cortisol on organ cultures of adult mouse mammary glands. *Proc. Soc. exp. Biol. Med.*, 1959, **101**, 500.
14. Elias J. J. and Rivera E. M. Comparison of the responses of normal, precancerous and neoplastic mouse mammary tissues to hormones *in vitro*. *Cancer Res.*, 1959, **19**, 505–511.
15. Fell H. B. Experiments on the action of vitamin A on the ground substance of cartilage and bone. *Coll. intern. C.N.R.S., Nogent-sur-Marne*, 1961, 85–94.
16. Fell H. B. Some effects of hypervitaminosis A on cells and their organelles. *Biochem. J.*, 1964, **90**, 35 p.
17. Fell, Dingle J. T. and Webb M. Studies on the mode of action of excess of vitamin A. 4: The specificity of the effect on embryonic chick-limb cartilage in culture and on isolated rat liver lysosomes. *Biochem. J.*, 1962, **83**, 63–69.

18. Fell H. B., Lucy J. A. and Dingle J. T. Studies on the mode of action of excess vitamin A. 1: The metabolism, composition and degradation of chick-limb cartilage *in vitro*. *Biochem. J.*, 1961, **78**, 11 p.

19. Fell H. B. and Mellanby E. Effects of hypervitaminosis on foetal mouse bones cultivated *in vitro*. *Brit. Med. J.*, 1950, **2**, 535–539.

20. Fell H. B. and Mellanby E. The effect of hypervitaminosis A on embryonic limb-bones cultivated *in vitro*. *J. Physiol.*, 1952, **116**, 320–349.

21. Fell H. B. and Mellanby E. Biological action of thyroxine embryonic bones grown in tissue culture. *J. Physiol.*, 1955, **127**, 427–447.

22. Fell H. B. and Mellanby E. The effect of 1-tri-iodothyronine on the growth and development of embryonic chick limb-bones in tissue culture. *J. Physiol.*, 1956, **133**, 89–100.

23. Fell H. B., Mellanby E. and Pelc S. R. Influence of excess vitamin A on the sulfate metabolism of bone rudiments grown *in vitro*. *J. Physiol.*, 1956, **134**, 179–188.

24. Fell H. B. and Robison R. The growth, development and phosphatase activity of embryonic avian femora and limb-buds cultivated *in vitro*. *Biochem. J.*, 1929, **23**, 767–784.

25. Fell H. B. and Thomas L. Comparison of the effects of papain and vitamin A on cartilage. II: The effects on organ culture of embryonic skeletal tissue. *J. Exp. Med.*, 1960, **11**, 719–744.

26. Gaillard P. J. Parathyroid gland tissue and bone *in vitro*. *Exp. Cell. Res.* 1955, suppl. 3, 154–159.

27. Gaillard P. J. Parathyroid gland tissue and bone *in vitro*. *Koninkl. Ned. Akad. Wetenschap.*, 1955, Proc. C **58**, 279–293.

28. Gaillard P. J. Parathyroid gland and bone *in vitro*. *Schweiz. med. Wochsch.*, 1957, suppl. **14**, 447–450.

29. Gaillard P. J. Parathyroid gland and bone *in vitro*. *Acta Physiol. et Pharmacol. Neerl.*, 1958, **7**, 142–143.

30. Gaillard P. J. Parathyroid gland and bone *in vitro*. *Dev. Biol.*, 1959, **1**, 152–181.

31. Gaillard P. J. The influence of parathyroid hormone on osseous tissue in culture. *Verb. Vlaam. Akad. Geneesk. Belg.*, 1960, **22**, 24–35.

32. Gaillard P. J. Over het mechanisme van de werking van het bijschildklierhormoon. *Versl. kon. Akad.*, 1960, **69**, 147–149.

33. Gaillard P. J. Bone primordia and parathyroid secretions *in vitro*. *Coll. Intern. C.N.R.S.*, *Nogent-sur-Marne*, 1961, 15–32.

34. Gaillard P. J. The influence of parathyroid extract on the explanted radius of albino mouse embryos. *Proc. Konink. Ned. Akad. Wetensch. Ser. C*, 1961, **64**, 119–128.

35. Gaillard P. J. Parathyroid and bone in tissue culture. *In R. O. Greep and R. V. Talmage*. "The parathyroids", Thomas, Springfield, édit., 1961, 19–48.

36. Gaillard P. J. A comparative study on the influence of thyroxine and of parathyroid extract on the histological structure of the embryonic explanted embryonic radius rudiment. *Acta morph. Neerl. Scand.*, 1962, **5**, 21–36.

37. Gaillard P. J. Parathyroid hormone and bone *in vitro*. *Voeding*, 1962, **23**, 283–301.

38. Gaillard P. J. Observations on the effect of thyroid and parathyroid secretions on explanted mouse radius rudiments. *Dev. Biol.*, 1963, **7**, 103–116.

39. Gaillard P. J. The influence of parathyroid and thyroid secretions on explants of long bones of mouse embryos. *Seconde Réunion Européenne d'Endocrinologie comparée*. Bruxelles, 16–19 sept. 1963. Abst.

40. Girard H. Les conditions de réapparition de la substance fondamentale du cartilage embryonnaire de Poulet détruite par la papaïne. *C. R. Acad. Sc.*, 1961, 253, 2407–2409.

41. Girard H.   Influence de la papaïne sur le tibia embryonnaire de Poulet cultivé *in vitro. J. Embryol. exp. Morph.*, 1962, **10**, 231–247.
42. Guillemin R. and Rosenberg B.   Humoral hypothalamic control of anterior pituitary: a study with combined tissue cultures. *Endocrinol.*, 1955, **57**, 599–607.
43. Hancox N. M.   Effect of commercial parathyroid extract on embryonic avian bone *in vitro. J. Anat.*, 1961, **95**, 411–415.
44. Hardy M.   The development *in vitro* of the mammary glands of the mouse. *J. Anat.*, 1950, **84**, 455–458.
45. Hay M. F.   The effect of growth hormone and insulin on limb-bone rudiments of the embryonic chick cultivated *in vitro. J. Physiol.*, 1958, **144**, 490–504.
46. Hekkelman J. W.   Bone metabolism and the effect on parathyroid extract. *Gen. Comp. Endoc.*, 1962, 2, 607 (abstract).
47. Herbertson M. A.   The reversibility of the effect of hypervitaminosis A on embryonic limb-bones cultivated *in vitro. J. Embryol. exp. Morph.*, 1955, **3**, 355–365.
48. Hermann-Erlee M. P. M.   A histochemical investigation of embryonic long bones: the effect of parathyroid hormone on the activity of a number of enzymes. *Proc. Akad. Amst. Ser. C*, 1962, **65**, 22–40.
49. Ito Y., Takamura K. and Endo H.   The effect of growth hormone on the incorporation of labeled sulfate into the chick embryo femur in tissue culture. *Endoc. Japon*, 1960, **7**, 327–335.
50. Ito Y. and Endo H.   Direct action of growth hormone on skeletal tissue, with special reference to S 35 sulfate uptake of chick-embryo femur growing *in vitro. Endocr. Japon.*, 1962, **38**, 340.
51. Kieny M.   Contribution à l'étude des besoins nutritifs des tibias embryonnaires d'Oiseau cultivés en milieux naturels et synthétiques. *Arch. Anat. micr. Morph. exp.*, 1958, **47**, 85–169.
52. Kieny M.   Action de diverses fractions de jus d'embryons "Creeper" sur la croissance de tibiotarses normaux cultivés *in vitro. C. R. Acad. Sc.*, 1962, **254**, 360–462.
53. Kieny M.   Action de diverses fractions de l'extrait d'embryon Creeper sur la croissance de tibiotarses normaux en culture *in vitro. Arch. Anat. micr. Morphol. exp.*, 1962, **51**, 577–586.
54. Kieny M. and Abbott U. K.   L'extrait d'embryon diplopode-4 inhibe la croissance des ébauches cartilagineuses normales cultivées *in vitro. C. R. Acad. Sc.*, 1962, **254**, 1520–1522.
55. Kieny M. and Abbott U. K.   Contribution à l'étude de la diplopodie liée au sexe et de l'achondroplasie Creeper chez l'embryon de Poulet: culture *in vitro* des ébauches cartilagineuses du tibiotarse et du péroné. *Dev. Biol.*, 1962, **4**, 473–488.
56. Landauer W.   Induced rumplesness of chicken. V: The effect of insulin on the axial skeleton of chicks and adult fowl. *J. exp. Zool.*, 1947, **105**, 317–328.
57. Lasfargues E. Y.   Cultivation and behavior *in vitro* of the normal mammary epithelium of the adult mouse. *Exp. Cell Res.*, 1957, **13**, 553–562.
58. Lasfargues E. Y.   Action de l'œstradiol et de la progestérone sur des cultures del glandes mammaires de jeunes Souris. *C. R. Soc. Biol.*, 1960, **154**, 1720–1722.
59. Lasfargues E. Y.   Influences hormonales sur le développement structural et fonctionnel d'organes en culture. *Path. Biol.*, 1961, **9**, 633–637.
60. Lasfargues E. Y.   Concerning the role of insulin in the differentiation and functional activity of mouse mammary tissues. *Exp. Cell Res.*, 1962, **28**, 531–542.
61. Lasfargues E. Y. and Murray M. R.   Hormonal influences on the differentiation and growth of embryonic mammary glands in organ culture. *Dev. Biol.*, 1959, **1**, 413–435.
62. Lasfargues E. Y. and Murray M. R.   Comparative hormonal responses *in vitro* of

mouse mammary glands from agent-carrying and agent-free strains. Formation of hyperplasic nodules. *VIII Intern. Cancer Congr.*, 1962, Abstr., p. 196.

63. Lawson K. The differential growth-response of embryonic chick limb-bone rudiments to tri-iodothyronine *in vitro*. I: Stage of development and organ size. *J. Embryol. exp. Morph.*, 1961, **9**, 42–51.

64. Lawson K. The differential growth-response of embryonic chick limb-bone rudiments to tri-iodothyronine *in vitro*. II: Growth rate. *J. Embryol. exp. Morph.*, 1961, **9**, 534–555.

65. Lawson K. The differential growth-response of embryonic chick limb-bone rudiments to tri-iodothyronine *in vitro*. III: Hormone concentration. *J. Embryol. exp. Morph.*, 1963, **11**, 383–398.

66. Lucy J. A., Dingle J. T. and Fell H. B. Studies on the mode of action of excess vitamin A. 2: A possible role of intracellular proteases in the degradation of cartilage matrix. *Biochem. J.*, 1961, **79**, 500–508.

67. McCluskey R. T. and Thomas L. The removal and cartilage matrix, *in vivo*, by papain. Identification of crystalline papain protease as the cause of the phenomenon *J. exp. Med.*, 1958, **108**, 371.

68. Miahle P. Glucagon, insuline et régulation endocrine de la glycémie chez le Canard. *Acta endocr.*, 1958, Suppl., **36**, 1–134.

69. Moszkowska A. L'antagonisme épiphyso-hypophysaire. Étude *in vivo* et *in vitro* chez l'embryon de Poulet Sussex. *Ann. Endoc.*, 1958, **19**, 69–79.

70. Moszkowska A. L'antagonisme épiphyso-hypophysaire. *Ann. Endoc.*, 1962, **24**, 215–226.

71. Petrovic A. Recherches sur la préhypophyse en culture organotypique; évolution structurale et action sur les organes effecteurs associés *in vitro*. Un vol. Imprimerie Alsatia, Colmar, 1961, 179 p.

72. Prop F. J. A. Development of alveoli in organ cultures of total mammary glands of six weeks old virgin mice. *Exp. Cell Res.*, 1960, **20**, 256–258.

73. Prop F. J. A. Effects of hormones on mouse mammary glands *in vitro*. Analysis of the factors that cause lobulo-alveolar development. *Path. Biol.*, 1961, **9**, 640–645.

74. Raisz L. G. Stimulation of bone resorption by parathyroid hormone in tissue culture. *Nature*, 1963, **197**, 1015–1016.

75. Schaberg A. The influence of A.C.T.H. and the anterior lobe of the hypophysis on the adrenal cortex *in vitro*. *Proc. Koninkl. Ned. Akad. v. Wetensch.*, 1957, **60**, 464–470.

76. Schaberg A. Adrenal cortex and anterior hypophysis *in vitro*. *Coll. intern. C.N.R.S.*, Nogent-sur-Marne, 1961, 33–44.

77. Schaberg A. and De Groot C. A. The influence of the anterior hypophysis on the morphology and function of the adrenal cortex *in vitro*. *Exp. Cell. Res.*, 1958, **15**, 475–483.

78. Schaberg A., De Groot C. A. and Sollewijn Gelpke A. Corticotrophic activity of the fœtal and neonatal anterior hypophysis *in vitro*. *Acta Physiol. pharmacol. Neerl.*, 1960, **8**, 447–456.

79. Rivera E. M. Hormonal requirements for survival and growth of mouse primary mammary ducts in organ culture. *Proc. Soc. exp. Biol. Med.*, 1963, **114**, 735.

80. Rivera E. M. and Bern H. A. Influence of insulin on maintenance and secretory stimulation of mouse mammary tissues by hormones in organ-culture. *Endocrin.*, 1961, **69**, 340–353.

81. Thomas L. Reversible collapse of rabbit ears after intravenous papain and prevention of recovery by cortisone. *J. exp. Med.*, 1956, **104**, 245.

82. Thomas L., McCluskey R., Potter J. L. and Weissmann G. Comparison of the effects of papain and vitamin A on cartilage. I: The effects in rabbit. *J. exp. Med.*, 1960, **111**, 705–718.

83. Tixier-Vidal A. Étude chronologique *in vivo* et *in vitro* des corrélations hypophyse-thyroïde chez l'embryon de Poulet. *Arch. Anat. micr. Morph. exp.*, 1956, **45**, 236–253.

84. Tixier-Vidal A. Étude histophysiologique des relations hypophyse et thyroïde chez l'embryon de Poulet. *Arch. Anat. micr. Morph.*, 1958, **47**, 236–340.

85. Trowell O. A. The culture of mature organs in a synthetic medium. *Exp. Cell Res.*, 1959, **16**, 118–147.

86. Vuylsteke C. A. and De Duve C. Le contenu en glucagon du pancréas aviaire. *Arch. Int. Physiol.*, 1953, **61**, 273.

87. Wolff Em. Le stockage d'hormones sexuelles par un organe embryonnaire du Canard. *C. R. Soc. Biol.*, 1960, **154**, 2184–2186.

88. Wolff Em. Sécrétion et stockage d'hormones sexuelles par les organes de l'embryon d'Oiseau associés *in vitro* à des organes effecteurs. *Coll. intern. C.N.R.S.*, 1961, 61–72.

89. Wolff Et., Haffen K. and Dieterlen F. Influence des états nutritionnels sur la différenciation et le fonctionnement des glandes endocrines embryonnaires. *Ann. Nutr. Aliment.*, 1960, **14** (6), B 11-B 29.

90. Wolff Et. and Kieny M. Mise en évidence d'une action inhibitrice de l'extrait d'embryons de la race de Poules "Courtes-pattes" Creeper sur la croissance des tibias cultivés *in vitro*. *C. R. Acad. Sc.*, 1957, **244**, 1089–1091.

91. Wolff Et. and Kieny M. Recherches sur la nature d'un facteur inhibiteur de la croissance des os longs dans la race de Poule Creeper. *Dev. Biol.*, 1963, **7**, 324–341.

92. Zwilling E. Association of hypoglycemia with insulin micromelia in chick embryos. *J. exp. Zool.*, 1948, **109**, 197–214.

93. Zwilling E. Micromelia as a direct effect of insulin. Evidence from in vitro and in vivo experiments. *J. Morph.*, 1959, **104**, 159–179.

ADDENDUM

At the time it was written, the main chapter was planned to illustrate the possibilities of organ culture in enlightening developmental problems in regard to hormones and inhibiting sustances; it did not pretend to be an exhaustive review on the subject. The reader is therefore referred to the article by Lasnitzki (42) for earlier studies that were not included in the main chapter.

This addendum will be restricted to organ culture studies in the field of endocrinology. Some recent work has been dedicated to the effect of inhibitors incorporated into synthetic culture media; such studies are analyzed in Chapter III.

On the other hand, research on hormonal actions in organ culture has thrived, and numerous studies have appeared since 1964, investigating either the conditions for *in vitro* activity of endocrine glands—usually involving incorporation of hormones into the medium—or the response of a target organ to a hormone or a hormone combination incorporated into the culture medium. All studies concerning sex hormones are excluded from this analysis as they are dealt with in Chapter IV.

I. HYPOTHALAMO–HYPOPHYSIS INTERRELATIONSHIPS

Most studies on the liberation of pituitary hormones under the influence of hypothalamic releasing factors have used short incubation techniques. However some authors, using organ culture experiments, have tried to prevent the functional rest which usually happens when the anterior pituitary is explanted *in vitro*. The cultivated hypophysis loses its cell-type variety (61), the only remaining cell types being the prolactin cell (11) and another cell type which might be either MSH or LH type (91, 92).

Deuben and Meites (18) showed that the addition of a hypothalamic extract to rat anterior pituitaries precultivated for 6 days reinitiates the release of growth hormone into the medium, even though this release had ceased for 3 days. Mittler, Redding, and Schally (49) investigated further the mechanism and extent of action of hypothalamic releasing factors, to find whether the thyrotropin-releasing factor (TRF) stimulates synthesis as well as release of thyrotropin (TSH). They found that TRF added to the culture medium causes an increase in TSH activity of both media and pituitary tissue.

Birge, Peake, Mariz, and Daugmaday (6) investigated *in vitro* the more

215

complex influences of cortisol and diethylstilbestrol on rat pituitary. Both hormones depress *in vivo* release of growth hormone. Organ culture experiments show that the amount of growth hormone in the medium is decreased in the presence of cortisol; however, the amount of GH in the cultivated pituitary is the same after control or cortisol culture; thus cortisol has affected synthesis as well as release of growth hormone, and the result suggests that the effect is a direct one. On the other hand diethylstilbestrol has no influence *in vitro* on GH secretion; *in vivo* effects of this hormone are probably mediated by the hypothalamus.

II. THYROID GLAND DIFFERENTIATION *IN VITRO* UNDER THE INFLUENCE OF HORMONES

Numerous reports have shown that embryonic thyroid glands of chick (2, 8, 9, 29, 32, 64, 90, 109), rat (10), and mice (13) continue some development and differentiation in organ culture either on natural or synthetic media.

More recently one group of workers has studied the hormonal factors capable of initiating and stimulating thyroid function *in vitro* (56–58, 83, 84). Thyroid function, as judged from iodine uptake and incorporation into organic compounds, is initiated in young explants or stimulated in older ones, if the medium is supplemented with TSH. Studies of labeled leucine and iodine incorporation as well as experiments with inhibitors of protein synthesis show that TSH stimulates the iodide-concentrating ability of the explants and, moreover, accelerates the conversion of monoiodotyrosine to diiodotyrosine and the formation of thyroxine.

The same authors demonstrated insulin also has a powerful effect on embryonic thyroid metabolism in organ culture. This is the first evidence of this effect of insulin hitherto unsuspected. Alone or with TSH, insulin enhances significantly ^{131}I incorporation into organic compounds. The formation of diiodothyronine and thyroxine is especially stimulated. No morphogenetic effect was detected. Incorporation studies indicate that insulin enhances the formation of both protein and ribonucleic acid by the fetal thyroid gland in culture.

III. EFFECTS OF THYROID HORMONE IN THE MEDIUM ON DIFFERENTIATION PROCESSES

A. Tadpole Tail Resorption in Tissue Culture

It is well-known that the anuran tadpole tail regresses in response to thyroid hormone during metamorphosis. The fine biochemical mechanism of this event has been extensively studied *in vitro* since Weber (103) and

Schaffer (79) showed that *Xenopus* tadpole tails could be maintained in culture and that their regression was induced by thyroid hormone incorporated into the medium. There is a direct relationship between concentration of the hormone and the extent of shrinkage in an isolated tail fragment (16); the tissue sensitivity increasing with progressive stages of metamorphosis. Anterior pituitary hormones (prolactin or growth hormone) have an antagonistic effect on this action. (17). What is the mechanism of action of thyroxine Weber (104) has detected a rise in cathepsin activity during thyroxine-induced regression and concluded that it was more likely due to new enzyme formation than to activation of latent enzymes. Tata (89) found from incorporation studies that cultured tails synthesize RNA and proteins. Furthermore, during hormone-induced regression, synthesis of both RNA and proteins is accelerated. Actinomycin D, puromycin, or cycloheximide abolish the regression and the increase in hydrolase activity mediated by thyroxine. This result demonstrates that hormone-induced regression of the isolated tadpole tail is an active process involving a continuous generation of RNA and protein and supports the hypothesis of new hydrolytic enzyme synthesis.

B. Maturation of Embryonic or Young Organs in Culture

Thyroid dependency of an embryonic organ for differentiation was demonstrated by Wessells (108): 8- and 10-day chick embryo skin does not continue differentiation when explanted onto a synthetic medium; epidermal differentiation will proceed if thyroxine is present.

Another example is the maturation of the nervous system: the role of thyroid hormone for this maturation in higher vertebrates is well-known, mostly from pathological findings. However, the approach to this problem is difficult in the whole animal. Hamburgh (33, and earlier work) has studied the evolution of cultivated cerebella from newborn rats and mice. Thyroxine in the medium accelerates myelogenesis and this process is preceded by considerable resorption of the excess cell population of the explant. This result argues in favor of a direct action of thyroid hormone on nervous system development.

IV. PARATHYROID HORMONE AND CALCITONIN

Roth and Raisz (78) have studied in organ culture the ultrastructural features of the chief cells in the parathyroid gland of the rat in relationship to their functional state: these features change in response to variations of the calcium concentration in the medium.

Vaes (see 99 for review of earlier work) studied the fine biochemical mechanisms of bone resorption in organ culture when parathyroid hormone is incorporated into the medium. The hormone induces synthesis and release of acid hydrolases by the lysosomes.

The hypocalcemic hormone, calcitonin, was isolated from the thyroid gland in 1963; its effects were presumed to be primarily on bone; this has been proved since in a number of organ culture studies (1, 27, 28, 48, 67–69, 88). The experiments were designed to unravel the mechanisms of bone resorption under the influence of parathormone and calcitonin, working either alone or together. Effects were measured by the release of previously incorporated ^{45}Ca. The results demonstrate that calcitonin is a potent inhibitor of bone resorption; this inhibition is best shown when resorption is stimulated by parathormone or by vitamin A, but it can occur independently. After prolonged administration of calcitonin in organ culture the bone becomes insensitive to its antiresoptive action. This "escape" phenomenon fits the hypothesis that calcitonin is an emergency hormone secreted intermittently in response to hypercalcemic stress.

The time course and points of impact of the two hormones were also investigated by following RNA synthesis and Ca release in different experimental conditions such as the presence of actinomycin D. The results suggest that parathyroid hormone acts on different processes: (1) it stimulates the translocation of calcium from bone to the medium by already present osteoclasts; (2) it inhibits bone formation by osteoblasts; (3) it stimulates the differentiation of new osteoblasts. Calcitonin would have a direct, separate action on bone-resorbing cells, possibly at a step preceding the parathormone-sensitive step.

Recent studies by Reynolds and Dingle (74) indicate species differences in activity of calcitonin from different sources. Reynolds (73) also investigated further the interactions on bone of vitamin A and calcitonin. Vitamin A causes bone resorption with a concomitant loss of weight and mineral. Calcitonin prevents bone resorption and loss of mineral but only partially prevents the loss of weight. This loss of weight can be correlated with an increased release of lysosomal proteolytic enzyme, which is evolved by vitamin A and not inhibited by calcitonin. The author concluded that there is a lack of correlation between bone resorption and release of lysosomal enzymes. This is confirmed at the histological level, since calcitonin suppresses the appearance of multinucleate osteoclasts but does not prevent loss of osteocytes or transformation of osteoblasts into fibroblasts, all changes evoked by vitamin A or parathormone. Calcitonin action would thus appear to be primarily on osteoclasts.

V. ENDOCRINE PANCREAS DIFFERENTIATION AND FUNCTION

Endocrine differentiation proceeds in mammalian fetal pancreas explanted in organ culture at a precocious stage (81, 105); granulation of the B cells, indicating elaboration and storage of insulin, is acquired *in vitro;* elevated concentrations of glucose in the medium provoke degranulation of the B cells (23, 34, 106, 107); similar findings are noted when the explants come from fetuses of diabetic mothers. Insulin in the medium results in an increase in the number of granulated B cells (24). All these studies indicate parallel differentiation *in vitro* as compared to *in vivo*, secretion or storage resulting analogously from similar stimuli.

On the basis of former observations by Fautrez, Vakaet, and Van Strijthem (25) and by Zagury (110), Murrell (53), Murrell, Morgan, and Lazarow (54) found that the presence of hydrocortisone in the medium favors a selective endocrine differentiation of cultured fetal pancreas. The explants in these conditions develop no acini and contain more aldehyde–fuchsin-positive (B) cells than normal pancreatic tissue of comparable age, and more insulin can be recovered from the culture and medium than from corresponding normal organs.

On the other hand, cultivating adult guinea pig isolated islets of Langerhans or pancreatic fragments from young rabbits, Moskalewski (52) and Takaki and Okada (87) observed that degranulation of endocrine cells occurs and increases with time of culture.

The effects of the pancreatic hormones, insulin and glucagon, in culture media have been studied by a number of workers. Earlier work has demonstrated a potent anabolic influence of insulin in culture conditions; more recent experiments are analyzed in different sections of this addendum, since insulin is found to be active on any organ when it is tried. We shall further mention Lostroh's studies (46, 47) evidencing such an influence on mouse accessory sex organs explanted onto a synthetic medium; insulin promotes protein synthesis in them and potentiates the effects of sex hormones.

The action of glucagon on liver cells has been extensively studied by Verne and Hébert (101), but the experiments were done with monolayer cultures and as such are beyond the scope of this review. Vecchio, Luyckx, Zahnd, and Renold (100) investigated the mechanism of release of insulin by cultured fetal rat pancreas; glucagon induces in such explants a clear-cut dose-dependent release of insulin and is even more effective than glucose in this respect. This observation confirms *in vivo* results and suggests that stimulation of insulin secretion by oral glucose is mediated by glucagon release.

VI. ERYTHROPOIETIN

Krantz, Gallien-Lartigue, and Goldwasser (41) have shown that this hormonal factor, elaborated by the kidney, stimulates heme synthesis by marrow cells *in vitro*. Gallien-Lartigue (30, 31) demonstrated that erythropoietin restores erythropoiesis in mouse fetal liver grown in organ culture.

Cole and Paul (12) found that this response of fetal mouse liver cells *in vitro* is restricted to certain stages of development, and heme synthesis in the explanted mouse yolk sac is insensitive to erythropoietin.

VII. ADRENAL DIFFERENTIATION AND FUNCTION *IN VITRO*

Chick embryo adrenals 6- to 10-days-old elaborate lipids in organ culture only if ACTH is present in the medium (60). Coupland, MacDougall, and Biswas (15), Biswas, MacDougall, and Coupland (7) found a marked improvement in adult rat adrenal histology when they are cultured under hyperbaric oxygen. However, the steroid output of the explants is stimulated in these conditions only during the first 24 hours of culture. The subsequent fall in the secretion rate is prevented by addition of progesterone and of a NADPH–regenerating system; ACTH addition results in a further increase in steroid secretion (14).

VIII. EFFECTS OF CORTICOSTEROIDS ON CULTIVATED ORGANS

A. Embryonic Bone

Schryver (80) and Reynolds (72) showed that hydrocortisone added to the medium in low concentrations exerts a beneficial effect on cultivated chick bone rudiments by preventing the excessive uptake of water usual *in vitro;* however, increasing doses of the hormone cause a progressive inhibition of growth.

In an attempt to clarify the problems involved in the pathogenesis of rheumatoid arthritis, H. B. Fell and her collaborators studied the influence and interactions on cultivated fetal bone of antiserum and hydrocortisone. The hormone protects the terminal cartilage against the extensive degradation provoked by antiserum (20, 26). It also exerts a protective influence against the release of lysosomal enzymes that occurs when limb-bone rudiments are cultivated in the presence of poorly metabolized sugars (21); but hydrocortisone does not inhibit the changes induced in bone by excess vitamin A (22). It is concluded from these different studies that hydrocortisone presumably exerts its protective influence by stabilizing the lysosomal membranes.

B. Embryonic Thymus

Various steroid hormones are known to influence thymus morphogenesis *in vivo*. Sidky (82) tested a number of steroid hormones on embryonic mouse thymus in organ culture. Cortisone, hydrocortisone, and, especially, corticosterone inhibit lymphoid development.

C. Embryonic Retina

Glutamine synthetase activity, characteristic of the neural retina, increases markedly toward the end of embryonic development in the chick embryo. Moscona and co-workers have shown that this activity appears several days earlier if the retina is explanted in organ culture on a medium containing adult serum. Piddington (62) could demonstrate that hydrocortisone or cortisone was capable of eliciting *in vitro* this precocious rise in enzymatic activity. Other corticoids are active in this respect, steroid structure playing a role in the capacity of induction (71). Moscona, Moscona, and Saenz (50) investigated the influence of the hormone on transcription and translation during the process of enzymatic induction. Some characteristics of the system had been defined by Kirk (38) with a serum-containing medium. The system is especially interesting from the point of view of study of the fine events of differentiation in eukaryotic cells, because it provides a specific, measurable response characteristic of differentiation, elicited by a chemically defined inducer. In the absence of the steroid there is only a slight increase in glutamine synthetase (GS) activity. No measurable increase in cell number or overall protein synthesis occurs either in induced or control cultures.

1. REQUIREMENT FOR PROTEIN SYNTHESIS

The induction of retinal GS activity is blocked by inhibiting protein synthesis either by cycloheximide or puromycin. If the inhibitor is added to the culture medium some time after the beginning of induction, further increase in GS is blocked. Incorporation of ^{3}H-uridine into RNA is not decreased by these inhibitors. Therefore, it is protein synthesis that is essential for initial and continued increase in GS activity. These results suggest that the induced increase in GS activity is due to synthesis of enzyme protein; however, other possibilities, such as synthesis of proteins which regulate GS synthesis of activity, should not be excluded.

2. RNA SYNTHESIS AND GS INDUCTION

Actinomycin D blocks ^{3}H-uridine incorporation into RNA and completely prevents GS induction. Therefore, RNA synthesis is essential for the enzyme induction. However, if actinomycin D is added at various times between 0 and 6 hours of incubation, it is evident that GS induction becomes progressively less dependent on new RNA synthesis. When actinomycin D is added after 4 hours GS activity rises to values close to those of controls. This suggests that relatively stable RNA accumulates in cells during the first 4 hours of induction. This stable RNA serves either directly as a template for enzyme synthesis or controls the rate of transcriptional processes.

3. Transcription-Independent Increase of GS Activity Requires
Protein Synthesis

If cycloheximide is added, together with actinomycin D, after 4 hours of
incubation with the steroid inducer there is no increase in GS activity. Thus,
at the time when transcription is no longer required, protein continues to be
essential.

4. During the Transcription Period No Protein Synthesis Is Required

If cycloheximide is added to the medium during the first 4 hours of incubation at the time when RNA synthesis is essential and if the tissues are then
washed and transferred to a medium containing actinomycin D and, in some
cases, the inducer, GS activity increases in all experiments, whether the
inducer is present or not. Therefore, continuous protein synthesis is not
essential during the first 4 hours. The independence from further transcription is due to accumulation of stable RNA, after which the inducer action
becomes unnecessary.

IX. INFLUENCE OF MULTIPLE HORMONE COMBINATIONS ON DIFFERENTIATION OF MAMMARY GLANDS *IN VITRO*

A. Morphological Differentiation

New information has been acquired which is in line with the data analyzed
in the main chapter.

1. The influence of the age and physiological state of the mammary gland
on its reactivity *in vitro* have been further investigated. Ichinose and Nandi
(35) emphasized the incapacity of adult immature mouse glands to undergo
lobuloalveolar development *in vitro*, even on a hormone-supplemented
medium. Development comparable to that of late pregnancy could be
attained in culture only if the glands had been prepared by administration of
mammogenic hormones to the animal prior to cultivation. The necessity of
such priming was confirmed by Voytovich and Topper (102). Prop (65)
investigated the effect of different hormonal combinations on young virgin
mouse mammary glands; he found that the pattern of reactivity of *in vitro*
reactions depends on the donor's age and progresses parallel to *in vivo*
differentiation.

2. Different workers have tried to define the hormonal requirements of the
cultivated glands. The basic necessity for insulin has been confirmed. Prop
and Hendrix (66) demonstrated that the mitotic rate increases in the epithelial
cells with the dose of insulin. Insulin alone ensures survival of the explanted

glands (36). Parenchymal proliferation and some morphogenesis in glands from untreated mice can be obtained on complex media containing serum, insulin, and ovarian, adrenocortical, and anterior pituitary hormones (39, 40, 70, 75). But true lobuloalveolar development occurs only in glands from hormone-primed animals or from pregnant animals on media containing steroid hormones, anterior pituitary hormones (prolactin and growth hormone), and insulin (36). Rivera (76) demonstrated that cortisol, corticosterone, or aldosterone are interchangeable, any of them meeting the minimal steroid requirement in hormone combinations capable of inducing secretion in mammary glands from 10-day pregnant mice.

Studies by Rivera (77) and Barnawell (3, 4) extended to *in vitro* conditions some *in vivo* observations concerning the differential responsiveness to anterior pituitary hormones in various species or even strains of mammals.

These experiments are concerned with the response of prepared, prelactating glands to prolactin and growth hormone introduced into a synthetic medium of culture. The importance of these two hormones in lactogenesis is well known from *in vivo* as well as *in vitro* results (see main chapter). That these two hormones were not interchangeable in all species was indicated by some experiments *in vivo*. Rivera (77) confirmed in organ culture the results of Nandi (55), concerning a differential responsiveness of mouse strains C3H and A; whereas the C3H-strain mammary gland is induced to secretion by a growth hormone–corticoid combination as well as by a prolactin–corticoid combination; prolactin is an absolute requirement for secretion in the A strain. Barnawell (3, 4) extended such comparative studies to five mammalian species: two strains of laboratory rats, golden hamster, guinea pig, rabbit, and dog. Mammary tissues from the dog, guinea pig, and rabbit showed some ability to survive in unsupplemented "199" medium. Supplementation of the medium with insulin resulted in improvement in survival of mammary tissue from all species. The further addition of a corticosteroid led to an augmentation of survival in tissues of the five species, with some indication that the glucocorticoid principally characteristic of the concerned species is more effective than the others. Prolactin (MH) and growth hormone (STH) were assayed separately or together in media containing insulin and a corticoid. MH stimulated secretion in all species studied with the exception of the guinea pig. In all species, secretory response to STH was quite low compared to response to MH at equivalent levels. Any of these apparent secretory effects of STH could be accounted for by contamination with MH. Consequently this study indicates an absolute requirement for MH in four of the species. There is a species difference in sensitivity to MH: dog and rabbit are most sensitive, hamster and rat are less; no difference could be detected between the two strains of rats. The lack of responsiveness of the guinea pig gland is unexplained.

B. Biochemical Differentiation of the Mammary Gland *in Vitro*

1. BIOCHEMICAL CHARACTERISTICS OF THE SYSTEM

Since 1965 a group of workers has been actively engaged in unraveling the complex mechanism of action of hormones on the mammary gland *in vitro* on a biochemical and molecular level. They confirmed that the minimal hormonal requirement for biochemical differentiation of mammary glands from mice in midpregnancy includes insulin, hydrocortisone, and prolactin (37). Biochemical differentiation is judged by the stimulation of "casein-like" phosphoprotein synthesis. A maximal histological response coincides with the maximal stimulation of synthesis. Starch-gel electrophoresis demonstrates that the phosphoproteins elaborated *in vitro* are identical with those formed *in vivo* by lactating mice (96). The biosynthetic response to the three-hormone combination is specific; casein synthesis alone is stimulated, while the synthesis of other phosphoproteins is only slightly stimulated (85). Whey protein synthesis is also stimulated in a parallel way. On the other hand, synthesis of nonmilk protein is stimulated maximally by insulin alone and is unaffected by hydrocortisone and prolactin; therefore, it is believed to reflect proliferation of the epithelial cells rather than differentiation (44).

2. DISSOCIATION OF THE STEPS OF HORMONAL ACTIONS

The authors next tried to determine the sequence of action of the hormones. The differentiative processes themselves can be divided into two phases: in the first phase multiplication of the epithelial cells occurs, thus giving rise to the lobuloalveolar architecture; the second phase is cytological and functional development of the epithelial cells. The two processes are necessarily coupled and the second one cannot occur if the first has not taken place.

In order to determine the sequence of action of the hormones, the culture was divided into periods during which the explants were grown on media containing different hormone combinations. Synthesis of DNA and mitosis occur extensively during the first 48 hours of culture. Both processes virtually cease by the third day. Insulin is the only hormone required during this period. The next question is whether hydrocortisone and prolactin need to be present during proliferation, to ensure subsequent differentiation, or whether they can act after mitosis. To answer this question, the explants received during a first period either insulin alone, or insulin plus hydrocortisone, or insulin plus prolactin; insulin being present in all systems, an identical degree of proliferation was ensured in the three cases. In the second period all three hormones were present in the medium (43). If the second period is initiated after 1 day (cells still being engaged in DNA synthesis and mitosis), the level of casein synthesis reached at the end is independent of the initial hormone composition. But, if the first period lasts 3 days, the rate of casein synthesis increases only in the system which contained hydrocortisone during proliferation. These results demonstrate that hydrocortisone acts during the proliferative period, while prolactin can act after mitosis. Another experiment confirmed this last point: a mitotic inhibitor, colchicine, does not prevent prolactin action if the tissue has been previously incubated for 3 days in a medium containing insulin and hydrocortisone (97).

Moreover, if hydrocortisone is removed during the second period, the increase in casein synthesis is still manifest. On the other hand, if insulin is removed during the second period, no increase occurs.

In summary, insulin is the hormone involved in the stimulation of cell proliferation, but its presence remains necessary after mitosis. Hydrocortisone, though not necessary for proliferation, has to be present during this phase for any subsequent differentiation to be possible. On the contrary, prolactin is necessary only after mitosis and ensures overt differentiation.

All these reactions concerned mammary glands from midpregnancy. The effects of hormones could be further dissociated by testing the reactions of mammary glands from immature animals. These glands undergo DNA synthesis and mitosis *in vitro* independent of exogenous insulin (102). In the presence of the full three-hormone complement, these tissues after 24 hours in culture, make only whey proteins and one of the four casein components. The ability to make all the major caseins is acquired only after several days in culture with all hormones. Despite this active secretory function, no alveolar structures appear in these immature glands. In this case development of histological structure and development of casein-synthetic capacity are dissociated.

Since in these explants mitosis occurs independently of insulin, explants were cultured for 96 hours on media containing hydrocortisone and prolactin, then 24 hours with the three hormones. No casein synthesis occurred. This paradoxical result suggests that actions of insulin other than initiation of DNA synthesis and postmitotic synergism with prolactin must occur for functional differentiation to be expressed.

3. Effects of Hormones on Intracellular Processes

Lockwood, Stockdale, and Topper (43) and Turkington (94) investigated the role of insulin in initiation of DNA synthesis, either in glands from postpubertal virgin mice or in glands from midpregnancy animals. In the presence of insulin DNA polymerase activity appears after 20 hours of culture, reaches a maximum between 48 and 72 hours, and remains high for 5 days; glucose is not required for this effect; actinomycin D and puromycin prevent it, indicating that concurrent protein synthesis is necessary for the initiation of DNA synthesis and for completion of DNA replication in these cells.

To investigate the role of the three hormones in modifying transcriptional events, Turkington and Ward (98) examined the RNA polymerase activity of isolated nuclei from cultivated mammary glands. Insulin causes an important rise in RNA polymerase activity after 8 hours of incubation. The effect is DNA-dependent and represents an early effect of insulin on nuclear transcription, since the insulin effect on DNA synthesis does not appear until 12 hours of incubation. Prolactin stimulates RNA synthesis and RNA polymerase activity only in epithelial cells that are "covertly" differentiated after proliferation in the presence of hydrocortisone. Cycloheximide and puromycin decrease the rate of RNA synthesis in the explants and completely inhibit the prolactin stimulatory effect, thus demonstrating the dependence of this effect on the continued synthesis of protein. Since the stimulation of RNA polymerase activity and RNA synthesis by prolactin occurs prior to the induction of specific milk proteins, the early effect of prolactin also appears to be on nuclear transcription. Neither insulin nor prolactin exerts a stimulatory effect upon isolated nuclei under the conditions of RNA polymerase assay; this result is consistent with the concept that these hormones may require an intact cell for their action upon RNA synthesis. Hydrocortisone does not detectably alter the activity of RNA polymerase in these assays, either in the presence or absence of insulin, despite the fact that it exerts a profound alteration in the state of differentiation of the mammary epithelial cells.

X. EFFECT OF MULTIPLE HORMONE COMBINATIONS ON SALIVARY GLANDS OF THE CHIMNEY SWIFT

The salivary glands of this bird undergo pronounced development at the time of reproduction. The endocrine control of this development was unknown until Barnawell (5) investigated its nature by organ culture experiments. Contrary to expectation, prolactin, testosterone, and anterior pituitary hormones did not induce secretion; insulin, glucagon, or corticosterone promoted survival; a combination of insulin plus corticosterone or insulin plus glucagon induced secretion. Thus, it seems that hormones of carbohydrate metabolism play a leading part in the functional differentiation of this organ. The possibility should not be excluded that the salivary gland is already primed by the hormones present *in vivo* and that this priming may be essential for *in vitro* secretion, as is the case for the mammary gland.

XI. CONCLUSIONS

Recent literature demonstrates that organ culture offers unique opportunitites to the field of endocrinology. By providing an autonomous living system which retains inter- and intracellular reactions of organs it bridges the gap between biochemical reactions on one hand and the more complex intracellular machinery on the other. It allows the investigation of stepwise reactions and adaptations of cells. The mechanisms of hormone-dependent embryological differentiation or of functional differentiation of adult tissues may be studied in detail by this technique.

All data show that adult organs enter a state of functional inertia when cultivated on synthetic media and resume activity through new enzyme synthesis only if the medium is hormone-supplemented. Insulin and corticoids seem to play general and fundamental roles in this respect, their presence appearing as a prerequisite for function of many organs. In several instances such a role was unsuspected and has been shown for the first time by the use of organ culture. Another interesting recent contribution of organ culture studies has been the breaking up of the sequence of intracellular events evolved by hormonal action and including DNA-dependent protein synthesis, as exemplified by mammary gland and embryonic retina. It is clear from the number and quality of the results obtained in organ culture that this technique will continue to yield important information concerning hormonal action at the intracellular level. In particular, mediation of hormonal action by the "second messenger," cyclic AMP, now being studied extensively by short incubation techniques, would seem to offer a promising field for investigation by organ culture techniques.

BIBLIOGRAPHY

1. Aliapoulos M. A., Goldhaber P. and Munson P. L.   Thyrocalcitonin inhibition of bone resorption by parathyroid hormone in tissue culture. *Science*, 1966, **151**, 330.
2. Bakker-Sauer E. K.   Some effects of thyrotropic hormone on thyroid tissue *in vitro*. *Koninkl. Ned. Akad. Wetenschap.*, *Proc.*, *Ser. C*, 1961, **64**, 86–95.
3. Barnawell E. B.   Comparative interchangeability of mammotropin and somatotropin in the induction of secretory activity in organ cultures of mammary tissues from several mammalian species. *Amer. Zool.*, 1964, **4**, Abstr. 117.
4. Barnawell E. B.   A comparative study of the responses of mammary tissues from several mammalian species to hormones *in vitro*. *J. exp. Zool.*, 1965, **160**, 189–206.
5. Barnawell E. B.   Hormonal influence on salivary glands of chimney-swift (Chaetura pelagica) in organ culture. *J. exp. Zool.*, 1968, **169**, 161–172.
6. Birge C. A., Peake G. T., Mariz I. K. and Daugmaday W. M.   Effects of cortisol and diethylstilbestrol on growth hormone release by rat pituitary *in vitro*. *Proc. Soc. exp. Biol. Med.*, 1967, **126**, 342–345.
7. Biswas S., MacDougall J. B. and Coupland R. E.   Effect of hyperbaric oxygen on corticosteroid secretion and morphology of organ cultures of adult rat adrenal glands. *J. Endocr.*, 1967, **39**, 233–249.
8. Carpenter E.   Differentiation of chick embryo thyroids in tissue culture. *J. exp. Zool.*, 1942, **89**, 407–431.
9. Carpenter E., Beattie J. and Chambers R. D.   The uptake of ^{131}I by embryonic chick thyroid glands *in vivo* and *in vitro*. *J. exp. Zool.*, 1954, **127**, 249–269.

10. Carpenter E. and Rondon-Tarchetti T. Differentiation of embryonic rat thyroid *in vivo* and *in vitro*. *J. exp. Zool.*, 1957, **136**, 394–417.

11. Cohere G., Bousquet J. and Meunier J. M. Ultrastructure d'explants de glande pituitaire de Ratte adulte cultivés sur milieux artificiels: action de variations hormonales. *C. R. Soc. Biol.*, 1964, **158**, 1056–1058.

12. Cole R. J. and Paul J. The effects of erythropoietin on haem synthesis in mouse yolk-sac and cultured fetal cells. *J. Embryol. exp. Morph.*, 1966, **15**, 245–266.

13. Colle-Vandevelde A. Étude de la thyroïde embryonnaire de Souris cultivée *in vitro* en présence de fragments préhypophysaires. *C. R. Soc. Biol.*, 1968, **162**, 1245–1247.

14. Coupland R. E., Biswas S. and MacDougall J. D. B. The effect of progesterone, glucose-6-phosphate dehydrogenase, adrenocorticotrophic hormone and metyrapone on adrenocortical secretion of rat adrenal glands cultured under hyperbaric oxygen. *J. Endocr.*, 1969, **43**, 265–270.

15. Coupland R. E., MacDougall J. D. B. and Biswas S. Survival of the rat adrenal cortex in organ cultures under conditions of hyperbaric oxygen. *J. Endocr.*, 1966, **34**, XVI.

16. Derby A. An *in vitro* analysis of the response of tadpole tissue to thyroxine. *J. exp. Zool.*, 1968, **168**, 147–156.

17. Derby A. and Etkin W. Thyroxine induced tail resorption *in vitro* as affected by anterior pituitary hormones. *J. exp. Zool.*, 1968, **169**, 1–8.

18. Deuben R. and Meites J. *In vitro* reinitiation of pituitary somatotropin release by an acid extract of hypothalamus. *Proc. Soc. exp. Biol. Med.*, 1965, **118**, 409–412.

19. Dilley W. G. and Nandi S. Rat mammary gland differentiation *in vitro* in the absence of steroids. *Science*, 1968, **161**, 59–60.

20. Dingle J. T., Fell H. B. and Coombs R. R. A. The breakdown of embryonic (chick) cartilage and bone cultivated in the presence of complement-sufficient antiserum. 2. Biochemical changes and the role of the lysosomal system. *Int. Arch. Allergy*, 1967, **31**, 283–303.

21. Dingle J. T., Fell H. B. and Glauert A. M. Endocytosis of sugars. IV. Lysosomal and other biochemical effects. General discussion. *J. Cell Sc.*, 1969, **4**, 139–154.

22. Dingle J. T., Fell H. B. and Lucy J. A. Synthesis of connective tissue components. The effect of retinol and hydrocortisone on cultured limb-bone rudiments. *Biochem. J.*, 1966, **98**, 173–181.

23. Erlandsen S. L. Effects of glucose on organ cultures of fetal pancreases from normal and diabetic rats: granulations of the islets of Langerhans and the insulin content of the media (abstr.). *Anat. Rec.*, 1968, **160**, 345.

24. Erlandsen S. L., Wells L. J. and Lazarow A. Effects of beef insulin upon the granulations of beta cells in cultures of pancreases of fetal rats from diabetic mothers. *Anat. Rec.*, 1967, **157**, 415–424.

25. Fautrez J., Vakaet L and Van Strijthem, N. L'action antimitotique des stéroïdes cortico-surrénaliens sur le pancréas en culture organotypique. *Rev. Fr. Et. Clin. Biol.*, 1960, **5**, 608–609.

26. Fell H. B. and Weiss L. The effect of antiserum, alone and with hydrocortisone on foetal mouse bones in culture. *J. exp. Med.*, 1965, **121**, 551–560.

27. Friedman J., Au W. Y. W. and Raisz L. G. Response of fetal rat bone to thyrocalcitonin in tissue culture. *Endocrin.*, 1968, **82**, 149–156.

28. Friedman J. and Raisz L. G. Thyrocalcitonin: inhibitor of bone resorption in tissue culture. *Science*, 1965, **150**, 1465.

29. Gaillard P. J. Differentiation phenomena in explants of the embryonic chick thyroid gland. *Acta Physiol. pharmacol. Neerl.*, 1954, **3**, 432–448.

30. Gallien-Lartigue O. Action du facteur erythropoïétique du plasma sur l'hémopoïèse *in vitro* du foie de Souris embryonnaire. *Exp. Cell Res.*, 1966, **41**, 109–116.

31. Gallien-Lartigue, O. Arrêt et reprise de l'érythropoïèse dans le foie foetal de Souris *in vitro* sous l'action de l'érythropoïètine. *C. R. Acad. Sc.*, 1967, **264**, 1066–-1068.

32. Gonzales F. Evidence of functional differentiation of the embryonic chick thyroid in tissue culture. *Texas Rep. Biol. Med.*, 1954, **12**, 828–832.

33. Hamburgh M. An analysis of the action of thyroid hormone on development based on *in vivo* and *in vitro* studies. *Gen. Comp. Endocr.*, 1968, **10**, 198–213.

34. Hegre O. D. and Wells L. J. Response of beta cells to different levels of glucose: fetal pancreases grown in organ culture and subsequently grafted into maternal hosts. *Anat. Rec.*, 1968, **160**, 364 (abstr.).

35. Ichinose R. R. and Nandi S. Lobulo-alveolar differentiation in mouse mammary tissues *in vitro*. *Science*, 1964, **145**, 496–497.

36. Ichinose R. R. and Nandi S. Influence of hormones on lobuloalveolar differentiation of mouse mammary glands *in vitro*. *J. Endocr.*, 1966, **35**, 331–340.

37. Juergens W. G., Stockdale F. E., Topper Y. J. and Elias J. J. Hormone dependent differentiation of mammary gland *in vitro*. *Proc. Nat. Acad. Sci.*, 1965, **54**, 629–634.

38. Kirk D. L. The role of RNA synthesis in the production of glutamine synthetase by developing chick neural retina. *Proc. Nat. Acad. Sci.*, 1965, **54**, 1345–1353.

39. Koziorowska J. Influence of hormones on mouse mammary glands cultured *in vitro*. *Acta, Unio Int. contra Cancrum*, 1962, **18**, 211–214.

40. Koziorowska J. The influence of ovarian hormones and insulin on the mouse mammary glands *in vitro*. *Acta med. Polona*, 1962, **3**, 237–245.

41. Krantz S. B., Gallien-Lartigue O. and Goldwasser E. The effect of erythropoietin upon heme synthesis by marrow cells *in vitro*. *J. biol. Chem.*, 1963, **238**, 4085–4090.

42. Lasnitzki I. The action of hormones on cell and organ cultures. *In* "Cells and Tissues in Culture" (E. N. Willmer, ed.), Vol. 1, pp. 591–658. Academic Press, New York, 1965.

43. Lockwood D. H., Stockdale F. E. and Topper Y. J. Hormone dependent differentiation of mammary gland: sequence of action of hormones in relation to cell cycle. *Science*, 1967, **156**, 945–946.

44. Lockwood D. H., Turkington R. W. and Topper Y. J. Hormone dependent development of milk protein synthesis in mammary gland *in vitro*. *Biochim. biophys. Acta*, 1966, **130**, 493–501.

45. Lockwood D. H., Voytovich A. E. and Topper Y. J. Insulin dependent DNA polymerase and DNA synthesis in mammary epithelial cells *in vitro*. *Proc. Nat. Acad. Sc.*, 1967, **58**, 658–664.

46. Lostroh A. J. Synthetic activity in mouse organs maintained on chemically-defined media. *Acta endocr.*, 1964, **47**, 331–337.

47. Lostroh A. J. Regulation by testosterone and insulin of citrate secretion and protein synthesis in explanted mouse prostates. *Proc. Nat. Acad. Sc.*, 1968, **60**, 1312–1318.

48. Mecca C. E., Martin G. R. and Goldhaber P. Alteration of bone metabolism in tissue culture in response to parathyroid extract. *Proc. Soc. exp. Biol. Med.*, 1963, **113**, 538–540.

49. Mittler J. C., Redding T. W. and Schally A. V. Stimulation of thyrotropin secretion by TSH-releasing factor in organ cultures of anterior pituitary. *Proc. Soc. exp. biol. Med.*, 1969, **130**, 406.

50. Moscona A. A., Moscona N. H. and Saenz N. Enzyme induction in embryonic retina: the role of transcription and translation. *Proc. Nat. Acad. Sc.*, 1968, **61**, 160–167.

51. Moscona A. A. and Piddington R.   Stimulation by hydrocortisone of premature changes in the developmental pattern of glutamine-synthetase in embryonic retina. *Biochim. biophys. Acta*, 1966, **121**, 409–411.
52. Moskalewski S.   Isolation and culture of the islets of Langerhans of the guinea-pig. *Gen. Comp. Endocr.*, 1965, **5**, 342–353.
53. Murrell L. R.   Mammalian pancreatic islet tissue in organ culture. I. Methods of culture and *in vitro* histogenesis. *Exp. Cell Res.*, 1966, **41**, 350–364.
54. Murrell L. R., Morgan C. R. and Lazarow A.   Mammalian pancreatic islet tissue in organ culture. II. Insulin content of tissues and culture medium. *Exp. Cell Res.*, 1966, **41**, 365–375.
55. Nandi S.   Differential responsiveness of A and C3H mouse mammary tissues to somatotropin-containing hormone combinations. *Proc. Soc. exp. Biol. Med.*, 1961, **108**, 1–3.
56. Nataf B. M.   Fetal rat thyroid gland in organ culture. *Gen. Comp. Endocr.*, 1968, **10**, 159–173.
57. Nataf B. M. and Chaikoff I. L.   The effect of insulin on iodine metabolism of fetal rat thyroid glands in organ culture. *Life Sc.*, 1964, **3**, 895–898.
58. Nataf B. M. and Chaikoff I. L.   The effect of insulin on iodine metabolism of fetal thyroid glands in organ culture. *Biochim. biophys. Acta*, 1965, **111**, 422–428.
59. Nataf B. M., Rivera E. M. and Chaikoff I. L.   Role of thyrotropic hormone in iodine metabolism of embryonic thyroid glands in organ culture. *Endocrin.*, 1965, **76**, 35–42.
60. Pedernera E. A.   Differentiation *in vitro* of chick embryo adrenal glands. *Experientia*, 1968, **24**, 938–939.
61. Petrovic A.   Cytophysiologie de l'adénohypophyse des Mammifères en culture organotypique: fonctions gonadotrope, thyréotrope et corticotrope. *In* "Cytologie de l'adénohypophyse" (Benoît and Da Lage, eds.), pp. 121–135. C.N.R.S., Paris, 1963.
62. Piddington R.   Hormonal effects on the development of glutamine-synthetase in the embryonic chick retina. *Dev. Biol.*, 1967, **16**, 168–188.
63. Piddington R. and Moscona A. A.   Precocious induction of retinal glutamine synthetase by hydrocortisone in the embryo and in culture. Age-dependent differences in tissue response. *Biochim. biophys. Acta*, 1967, **141**, 429–432.
64. Porte A. and Petrovic A.   Sur les caractères ultrastructuraux de la thyroïde d'embryons de Poulet en culture organotypique et leur signification fonctionnelle. *C. R. Soc. Biol.*, 1961, **155**, 1701–1705.
65. Prop F. J. A.   Effect of donor age on hormone reactivity of mouse mammary gland organ cultures. *Exp. Cell Res.*, 1966, **42**, 386–388.
66. Prop F. J. A. and Hendrix S. E. A. M.   Effect of insulin on mitotic rate in organ cultures of total mammary glands of the mouse. *Exp. Cell Res.*, 1965, **40**, 277–281.
67. Raisz L. G.   Bone resorption in tissue culture: factors influencing the response to parathyroid hormone. *J. clin. Invest.*, 1965, **44**, 103.
68. Raisz L. G., Au W. Y. W., Friedman Y. and Niemann I.   Thyrocalcitonin and bone resorption (studies employing a tissue culture bioassay). *Amer. J. Med.*, 1967, **43**, 684.
69. Raisz L. G. and Niemann I.   I Early effects of parathyroid hormone and thyrocalcitonin on bone in organ culture. *Nature*, 1967, **214**, 486–487.
70. Ranadive K. J. and Chapekar W. T.   *In vitro* studies on mouse mammary gland response to hormonal treatment. *Brit. J. Cancer*, 1964, **18**, 308–311.

71. Reif-Lehrer L.   Induction of glutamine-synthetase in chick embryo retina: effects of serum and steroid structure. *Biochim. biophys. Acta*, 1968, **170**, 263–270.
72. Reynolds J. J.   The effect of hydrocortisone on the growth of chick bone rudiments in chemically define medium. *Exp. Cell Res.*, 1966, **41**, 174–189.
73. Reynolds J. J.   Inhibition by calcitonin of bone resorption induced *in vitro* by vitamin A. *Proc. Roy. Soc. London, B*, 1968, **170**, 61–69.
74. Reynolds J. J. and Dingle J. T.   Time course of action of calcitonin on resorbing mouse bones *in vitro*. *Nature*, 1968, **218**, 1178–1179.
75. Rivera E. M.   Maintenance and development of whole mammary glands of mice in organ culture. *J. Endocr.*, 1964, **30**, 33–39.
76. Rivera E. M.   Interchangeability of adrenocortical hormones in initiating mammary secretion *in vitro*. *Proc. Soc. exp. Biol. Med.*, 1964, **116**, 568–572.
77. Rivera E. M.   Differential responsiveness to hormones of C3H and A mouse mammary tissues in organ culture. *Endocrin.*, 1964, **74**, 853–864.
78. Roth S. I. and Raisz L. G.   The course and reversibility of the calcium effect on the ultrastructure of the rat parathyroid gland in organ culture. *Lab. Invest.*, 1966, **15**, 1187–1211.
79. Schaffer B. M.   The isolated Xenopus laevis tail: a preparation for studying the central nervous system and metamorphosis in culture. *J. Embryol. exp. Morph.*, 1963, **11**, 77–90.
80. Schryver H. F.   The influence of hydrocortisone on the water uptake of embryonic chick tibiotarsi in organ culture. *Exp. Cell Res.*, 1965, **37**, 327–337.
81. Schweisthal M. R., Wells L. J. and Céas M. P.   Development of islets and acini from the explanted primordium of the pancreas of the rat embryo. *Anat. Rec.*, 1965, **151**, 93–105.
82. Sidky Y. A.   Effect of steroids on thymus lymphoid development *in vitro*. *Anat. Rec.*, 1968, **161**, 187–196.
83. Singh V. N. and Chaikoff I. L.   Effect of 1-methyl-2-mercaptoimidazole and perchlorate on the insulin-mediated enhancement of ^{131}I incorporation into iodoaminoacids by fetal thyroid glands in organ culture. *Endocrin.*, 1966, **78**, 339–342.
84. Singh V. N., Nataf B. M. and Chaikoff I. L.   The effect of insulin on the formation of protein and ribonucleic acid by fetal thyroid glands in organ culture. *Life Sc.*, 1965, **4**, 1603–1616.
85. Stockdale F. E., Juergens W. G. and Topper Y. J.   A histochemical and biochemical study of hormone dependent differentiation of mammary gland tissue *in vitro*. *Dev. Biol.*, 1966, **13**, 266–281.
86. Stockdale F. E. and Topper Y. J.   The role of DNA synthesis and mitosis in hormone-dependent differentiation. *Proc. Nat. Acad. Sc.*, 1966, **56**, 1283–1289.
87. Takaki R. and Okada N.   Pancreatic alpha cells in organ culture. Bright field and immunofluorescent studies. *Proc. Japan Acad.*, 1967, **43**, 556–561.
88. Talmage R. V., Cooper C. W. and Neuenschwander J.   The effect of actinomycin D on parathyroid induced changes in bone and kidney. *Gen. Comp. Endocr.*, 1965, **5**, 475–483.
89. Tata R.   Requirement for RNA and protein synthesis for induced regression of the tadpole tail in organ culture. *Dev. Biol.*, 1966, **13**, 77–94.
90. Tixier-Vidal A.   Étude histophysiologique des relations hypophyse et thyroïde chez l'embryon de Poulet. *Arch. Anat. micr. Morph. exp.*, 1958, **47**, 235–240.
91. Tixier-Vidal A. and Gourdji D.   Évolution cytologique ultrastructurale de l'hypophyse du Canard en culture organotypique. Élaboration autonome de prolactine par les explants. *C. R. Acad. Sc.*, 1965, **261**, 805–808.

92. Tixier-Vidal A. and Picart R. Étude quantitative par radioautographie au microscope électronique de l'utilisation de la DL-leucine-^{3}H par les cellules de l'hypophyse du Canard en culture organotypique. *J. Cell Biol.*, 1967, **35**, 501–519.

93. Topper Y. J. Multiple hormone interactions related to growth and differentiation of mammary gland *in vitro*. *Trans. N. Y. Acad. Sc.*, 1968, **30**, 869–974.

94. Turkington R. W. Hormone-induced synthesis of DNA by mammary gland *in vitro*. *Endocrin.*, 1968, **82**, 540.

95. Turkington R. W. Induction of milk protein synthesis by placental lactogen and prolactin *in vitro*. *Endocrin.*, 1968, **82**, 575–583.

96. Turkington R. W., Juergens W. G. and Topper Y. J. Hormone dependent synthesis of casein *in vitro*. *Biochim. biophys. Acta*, 1965, **111**, 573–576.

97. Turkington R. W., Lockwood D. H. and Topper Y. J. The induction of milk protein synthesis in post mitotic mammary epithelial cells exposed to prolactin. *Biochim. biophys. Acta*, 1967, **148**, 475–480.

98. Turkington R. W. and Ward O. T. Hormonal stimulation of RNA polymerase in mammary gland *in vitro*. *Biochim. biophys. Acta*, 1969, **174**, 291–301.

99. Vaes G. On the mechanisms of bone resorption. *J. Cell Biol.*, 1968, **39**, 676–697.

100. Vecchio D., Luyckx A., Zahnd G. R. and Renold A. E. Insulin release induced by glucagon in organ cultures of fetal rat pancreas. *Metab.*, 1966, **15**, 577–581.

101. Verne J. and Hébert S. Action du glucagon sur les hépatocytes en culture. *C. R. Soc. Biol.*, 1963, **157**, 984–986.

102. Voytovich A. E. and Topper Y. J. Hormone dependent differentiation of immature mouse mammary gland *in vitro*. *Science*, 1967, **158**, 1326–1327.

103. Weber R. Induced metamorphosis in isolated tails of xenopus laevis. *Experientia*, 1962, **18**, 84–85.

104. Weber R. Behavioral properties of acid hydrolases in regressing tails of tadpoles during spontaneous and induced metamorphosis *in vitro*. *Ciba Found. Symp. Lysosomes*, 1963, p. 282.

105. Wells L. J., Erlandsen L. and Eguchi Y. Development of pancreases and adrenals of rat embryos in organ culture. *Anat. Rec.*, 1968, **160**, 201–206.

106. Wells L. J. and Lazarow A. Organ cultures of pancreases of fetuses from diabetic rats. *Diabetes*, 1967, **16**, 846–851.

107. Wells L. J., Schweisthal M. R., Nunamaker-Marx R., McKay M., Saccoman F. and Lazarow A. Effects of different levels of glucose upon the development of granulated beta cells in cultures of pancreatic primordia from normal rat embryos. *Diabetes*, 1967, **16**, 839–845.

108. Wessells N. K. Thyroxine initiation of epidermal differentiation as studied *in vitro* in chemically defined medium. *Exp. Cell Res.*, 1961, **24**, 131–142.

109. Wolff E., Haffen K. and Dieterlen F. Influence des états nutritionnels sur la différenciation et le fonctionnement des glandes endocrines embryonnaires. *Ann. Nutr. Aliment.*, 1960, **14**, 11–29.

110. Zagury D. Contribution à l'étude morphologique des sécrétions pancréatiques chez le Rat. *Ann. Sc. Nat.*, 1961, **3**, 196–296.

CHAPTER VI

CULTURE AND PARABIOSIS
OF BLASTODERMS

Berthe Salzgeber

INSTITUT D'EMBRYOLOGIE ET DE TÉRATOLOGIE EXPÉRIMENTALE DU C.N.R.S.
PARIS, FRANCE

I. INTRODUCTION

The culture of embryos has been carried out in different species of oviparous and viviparous vertebrates, particularly mammals and birds, which will be referred to in this chapter.

The technique of organ culture is useful in studying viviparous species where the egg or embryo is difficult to reach. The early stages of morphogenesis can be studied and operations can be carried out directly on the egg or the embryo.

Among the oviparous species, experiments carried out on the blastoderm *in vitro* have confirmed, defined, or developed experiments already carried out *in ovo*. The bird embryo, which is more accessible than the mammalian embryo, lends itself to many experiments that have already yielded many fruitful results. For example:

1. Experiments in polyembryony, carried out by splitting the blastoderm of nonincubated duck embryos (Lutz, 1949; Lutz *et al.*, 1963).

2. Localization and displacement of rudiments during embryonic development (Pasteels, 1937).

3. Experiments on the circulatory system of the embryo (Stephan, 1952).

4. Many experiments in teratogenesis (Ancel, 1950).

Culture *in vitro* makes operations easier, since:

a. When the young blastoderm is isolated from its vitelline support it is easier to see on a transparent medium than in the egg.

b. Some experiments carried out *in vivo* have been developed *in vitro*, since excisions, surgical removals, and grafts can be carried out without danger to the embryo.

233

Finally, organ culture techniques have enabled some new experiments to be performed. These relate to problems concerning the nutritional and metabolic requirements of embryos.

II. THE CULTURE OF AVIAN BLASTODERMS

A. Methods of Culture

The simplest method consists of pouring the contents of the egg, that is, the blastoderm, yolk, and albumin, into a sterilized glass container to prevent desiccation and bacterial infection (see Assheton, 1896; Vollmar, 1935; Romanoff, 1943).

The embryos survive for about 48 hours, but experimentation on these blastoderms is haɪdly possible because of the presence of the yolk.

The first experiments in which the blastoderm was explanted onto a culture medium were carried out by Waddington (1932). Waddington used Fell and Robinson's (1929) technique for tissue culture. Whole chick or duck blastoderms were transplanted onto a coagulum composed of adult bird blood and chick embryo extract. This semisolid medium was contained in a watch glass inside a Petri dish containing moist cotton wool. The blastoderms survived, but their development was limited and blood circulation rarely developed. The technique did, however, clarify some of the problems of experimental embryology.

Spratt (1947) and Et. Wolff and Simon (1955) used a medium based on agar and containing nutrient materials. Spratt used a mixture of yolk and albumin diluted with physiological saline (Ringer's solution), whilst Wolff and Simon (1955) used chick embryo extract. Wolff and Haffen's method of organ culture (1951) was adapted by Wolff and Simon for chick embryo blastoderm. The medium, composed of agar (12 parts), Tyrode's solution (4 parts), and 7–9 day chick embryo extract (4 parts), is poured between two watch glasses to produce a medium with a curved surface like an egg yolk (see Fig. 1).

The explanted embryos survived and developed for 2–3 days and their circulation was active. In order to encourage the extension of the blastoderm and to improve the survival of the embryo, fragments of additional blastoderm from other embryos were grafted into the extraembryonic region of the explanted blastoderm.

In all the experiments to be considered, the blastoderm was removed from the vitelline membrane and was spread out with the ventral surface on the medium.

New (1955) cultured blastoderms with the vitelline membrane closely adjoining the blastoderm. The dorsal surface was in contact with the medium (Fig. 2). A glass ring (internal diameter 28 mm, external diameter 33 mm) was placed on the vitelline membrane. Peripheral extension of the blastoderm occurred, the outer cells of the blastoderm proliferated, and the whole blastoderm stretched out on the vitelline membrane. Under these conditions, embryos taken during the first 48 hours of incubation developed, grew, and established a circulation. Sometimes the embryos reached the 20-somite stage. The nutrient medium was simply composed of fluid albumin placed in a watch glass. The vitelline membrane was in contact with the albumin.

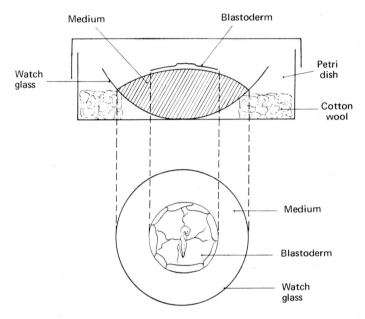

FIG. 1. Wolff and Simon's technique for culturing the blastoderm. The blastoderm is spread out on a curved medium. Pieces of supplementary blastoderm from other embryos are grafted around the extraembryonic region. After Wolff and Simon.

Nicolet and Gallera (1961–1963) modified New's technique and were able to grow the blastoderm with the ventral surface on the medium. The vitelline membrane was wedged between two glass rings. Direct intervention on the dorsal surface of the blastoderm thus became possible.

The study of early and late embryonic morphogenesis has been carried out using these techniques. Nutritional requirements, metabolic and enzymic activity, and teratogenesis of embryos have also been studied.

B. Problems of Morphogenesis

Research into morphogenesis was among the first problems to be studied by the method of culture of whole blastoderms. Operations that are too injurious to the blastoderm when carried out *in ovo* can be performed using this method.

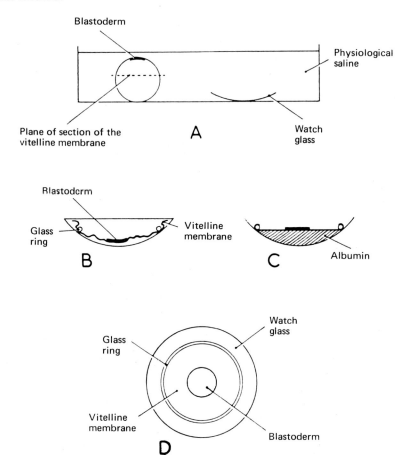

FIG. 2.   The technique for explanting the blastoderm (A) and the mode of culture on an albumin medium (B, C) (New's method). A glass ring is placed on the vitelline membrane (D). After New (1955).

All of these experiments on the development of the early stages of chick embryos were carried out on blastoderm cultured *in vitro*. The following problems of morphogenesis have been tackled:

1. Localization of rudiments and study of the organizing center.

2. Morphogenetic movements.

3. The potential for regulation possessed by pieces or regions of the blastoderm.

4. Experimental study of the embryonic circulatory system.

5. Transport of the primary gonocytes in avian blastoderms cultured *in vitro*.

1. EARLY MORPHOGENESIS BEFORE THE ESTABLISHMENT OF THE CIRCULATORY SYSTEM

a. Localization of Rudiments and Study of the Organizing Center. Spratt (1942–1946) studied the localization and development of different rudiments by placing markers (particles of carbon) on the blastoderm cultured *in vitro*. He also sectioned and removed certain regions. The experiments confirmed or defined more precisely the previous work that had been carried out *in ovo* using colored markers (Wetzel, 1929; Gräper, 1929); Pasteels, 1937).

According to Spratt, the chordamesoblastic region occupies the posterior half of the area pellucida of the nonincubated blastoderm. However, Pasteels found this zone to be less extensive and localized more in the posterior region. During development, this region is displaced and progressively invaginated into primitive streak.

Spratt (1952) studied the localization of the presumptive neural plate and its relations with other embryonic structures, in particular with the primitive streak. A map of this rudiment was prepared at the stage of the definitive primitive streak and at the head process stage (Fig. 3). According to Spratt, the neural plate has a horseshoe shape and its oblique posterior edges are bordered by a narrow zone of epiblastic material which becomes incorporated in the tail bud to form the spinal medulla. Between this zone and the primitive streak could be seen a small amount of noninvaginated mesoderm.

Experiments on the organizing center, carried out by Waddington (1932–1935), Spratt (1955–1958), and Hara (1961), showed that Hensen's node and the anterior end of the primitive streak have the same organizing properties as the lip of the blastopore in amphibians.

Waddington (1932–1935) carried out the first investigations on the organizing center in chick embryos using both whole and fragmented blastoderms. The primitive streak induced the formation of neural tissue in ectoderm placed above it. The area of Hensen's node was especially active. As in the amphibians, the organizer showed no specificity. Waddington and Schmidt (1933) grafted pieces of the primitive streak of chick embryos into the area pellucida of duck embryos. The graft induced the formation of an embryonic axis with the neural plate, notochord, and somites.

Waddington showed also that the endoderm is capable of inducing a supplementary primitive streak oriented according to the axis of the graft. These experiments were confirmed by Lutz (1953) following his experiments involving the splitting of embryos and by Lutz and Lutz-Ostertag (1955).

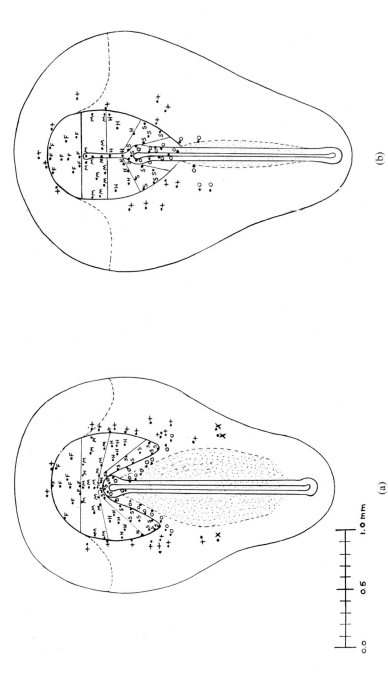

(a)

(b)

Fig. 3. Area pellucida of a blastoderm at the primitive streak stage. Mapping of regions: (a) at the stage of the definitive streak; (b) at the head process stage. The points represent the localization of carbon markers. The letters and symbols indicate the movement of cells after 20 hours of development *in vitro*, that is, after formation of the brain and the spinal cord. After Spratt (1952).

Key: Dotted area: noninvaginated mesoderm; F = Forebrain = prosencephalon; M = Midbrain = mesencephalon; H = Hindbrain = rhombencephalon; S = Spinal cord; O = Posterior part of the spinal cord; + = Skin of the head and trunk; x = Skin of the trunk at the region of the 20th somite.

These workers showed that an endodermal graft could induce embryo formation in the nonincubated blastoderm of the duck egg. The embryo had the same orientation as the graft. The culture was carried out on a semisolid medium.

Grabowski (1957) obtained the same results as Waddington. The development of a secondary embryo could be induced if the region of Hensen's node was grafted between the endoderm and the mesoderm of another blastoderm. The graft was placed away from the axial region of the blastoderm.

Hara (1961) repeated and extended Waddington's experiments, and has carried out explants of pure ectoderm and mesodermal inductor.

The ectodermal explants were taken from the anterior and lateral regions of the blastoderm (primitive streak stage before development of the head process).

The mesodermal inductor (notochordal rudiment) was taken at different stages of the primitive streak and head process.

The ectodermal and mesodermal explants were associated and cultured on gelatin beneath a vitelline membrane. The association was maintained for 30 minutes at 38°C *in vitro*, in Locke's solution (lacking calcium). It was then grafted into the coelom of a $2\frac{1}{2}$-day chick embryo, in order to obtain adequate differentiation. The host embryos were killed at 14 days of incubation. In order to eliminate the effects of the host embryos, the following control tests were carried out.

1. With explants of pure ectoderm from the anterolateral region; neural differentiation never occurred, although epidermis and feathers did differentiate.

2. With explants overlying the axial mesoderm, with previous induction; neural differentiation identical to that in the combined explants was always observed.

3. Associations of ectoderm and mesoderm; clear regional structures were obtained.

This series of experiments produced the following results (Fig. 4).

At the stage of the primitive streak, differentiation of the prosencephalon was predominant.

At an early stage of the head process, the prechordal region induced differentiation of the prosencephalon; the chordal region gave rise to the mesencephalon, rhombencephalon, and some parts of the spinal cord.

During the head process stage the prechordal part induced differentiation of the prosencephalon; the anterior rudiment of the notochord induced the mesencephalon and the rhombencephalon; the posterior rudiment of the notochord induced the rhombencephalon and parts of the spinal cord.

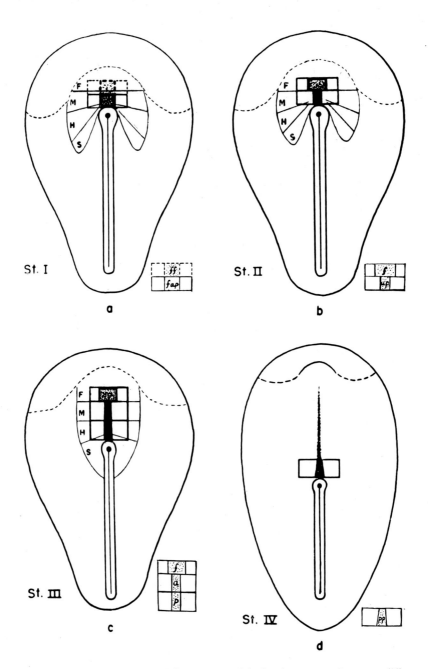

Fig. 4. Regional induction of different parts of the head process acting on undifferentiated ectoderm. F, Prosencephalon; M, mesencephalon; H, rhombencephalon; S, spinal cord. The different regions taken are indicated by the dotted areas. f, Prechordal mesoderm; a, p, anterior and posterior parts of the head process. After Hara (1961).

Summarizing:

1. The prechordal mesoderm induces prosencephalic formations.

2. The anterior part of the notochordal rudiment induces mesencephalic and rhombencephalic differentiation.

3. The posterior part of the notochordal rudiment induces rhomben-cephalic and spinal differentiation.

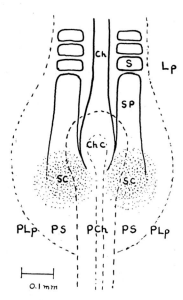

Fig. 5. Mesodermal organizing centers. The region of Hensen's node in a 4–5 somite blastoderm. The ectodermal structures (neutral plate, node, furrow of the primitive streak) are represented by dotted lines. The mesodermal structures (notochord, dorsal swelling, somites) are represented by continuous lines. Ch, Differentiated notochord; Chc, noto-chordal center; Sc, somatic center; Pch, presumptive notochord; Ps, presumptive somites; PLp, presumptive lateral plate; SP, segmentation plate; S, somites. After Spratt (1955).

Hara concluded that there was a regional differentiation of the organizing center, and stressed the remarkable parallels between amphibians and birds.

Spratt (1955, 1957, 1958) showed the presence of an organizing center for the notochord and two organizing centers for the somites in the region of Hensen's node (Fig. 5). Excision of the supposed organizing center from the notochord, which appeared as a bulbous swelling both at the head process stage and at the early stages in somite formation, prevented differentiation of the notochord.

Excision of the two somatic centers which lay on either side of the posterior half of the node suppressed the development of other somites posterior to the center. Spratt concluded that the continued formation of the notochord and the somites depended on the presence of these centers, which were precisely localized groups of specialized cells.

Spratt (1957) then analyzed the regulating and inducing properties of the centers for the notochord and the somites. The notochordal or somatic organizing centers were placed in contact with presumptive tissues that would normally form notochord, somites, or lateral plates. The following results were obtained:

$$\text{notochordal center} \Bigg\langle \begin{array}{l} \text{— + presumptive cells for notochord} \;\rightarrow \text{notochord} \\ \text{— + presumptive cells for somites} \;\;\;\;\;\rightarrow \text{notochord} \\ \text{— + presumptive cells for lateral plate} \rightarrow \text{notochord} \end{array}$$

$$\text{somatic center} \Bigg\langle \begin{array}{l} \text{— + presumptive cells for notochord} \;\rightarrow \text{somites} \\ \text{— + presumptive cells for somites} \;\;\;\;\;\rightarrow \text{somites} \\ \text{— + presumptive cells for lateral plate} \rightarrow \text{somites} \end{array}$$

Thus, the notochordal and somatic centers act as more than organizers, since they induce mesodermal cells situated behind the node to form either notochord or somites.

Fraser (1960) used the same culture techniques as Spratt and found that the somatic organizing centers were not sufficient to induce the development of somites from undifferentiated mesoderm. Contact with the neural rudiment was necessary to determine the morphogenesis of the somites. The following are some of Fraser's observations.

1. To deduce the importance of Hensen's node in the differentiation of the somites the region of the node was grafted into another blastoderm, away from the axial organs: somites were formed.

2. In certain cases in culture, when there was no contact between the nervous system and the unsegmented somatic region, the somites did not form.

3. Explanted *in vitro*, Hensen's node consisting of notochord and neural rudiments gave only notochord and no somites.

4. When explanted *in vitro*, the paraxial mesoderm gave rise to a nervous system and somites but no notochord.

Meanwhile, some further experiments have not given the expected precise results. Thus, grafts of the nervous system into the paraxial region or grafts of parts of the nervous system superimposed on Hensen's node have not formed true somites. Only a mesenchymal condensation appeared around the graft.

b. Study of Morphogenetic Movements.   These movements were studied *in ovo* by Pasteels (1937) and Lutz (1953–1955). The latter author showed that the movements contributed to the positioning of the endoderm. Spratt and Haas (1960) studied these processes *in vitro*. Blastoderms were explanted *in vitro* onto a medium composed of agar, albumin, and yolk. The blastoderms were taken both from nonincubated eggs and from eggs that had been incubated for several hours and had reached the blastula or primitive streak stage. Normal development up to 10 somites was achieved. During culture the ectodermal or the superficial layer was placed against the medium, since adherence of the endoderm to the substrate restrained the morphogenetic movements.

The movements were studied by marking the internal and the external layers with carbon particles or carmine powder.

In the deeper layer of the blastoderm, the movements are considerable (Fig. 6). They begin from a region localized posteriorly, at the junction between the area pellucida and the area opaca. From this point, the movements occur in all directions. They are particularly marked toward the anterior region, and then diminish progressively toward the lateral zones and the posterior region. The movements occur during the formation of the primitive streak and continue until the definitive streak is formed. Then the anterior movements stop and the lateral and posterior movements predominate. The importance and the role of these morphogenetic movements in the deep layer of the nonincubated blastoderm have been demonstrated by Spratt and Haas (1960). They inhibited the movements, either by explanting the nonincubated blastoderm with the inner layer next to the medium, or by putting large amounts of carmine powder on the inner layer of the blastoderm which had been explanted with its outer surface applied to the culture medium

Not only did the morphogenetic movements not occur, but the embryo did not form. It was suggested that the whole series of cellular movements was necessary to produce a complete axial embryonic system.

Movements also occur in the superficial layer (ectoderm), but here they are less marked (Fig. 6). These movements of cellular material are very small during the formation of the primitive streak.

In a recent paper, Gallera (1963) considered that Spratt and Haas had minimized the importance of morphogenetic movements in the ectoderm. Gallera considered that the ectoderm adheres strongly to the substrate when the blastoderm is cultured with the outer layer against the agar, thus preventing the extension of movements in this layer.

Spratt and Haas (1962) concluded that the primitive streak does not correspond to the blastopore of the amphibia, but that it represents an elongated center of cellular proliferation. These conclusions were based on their observations on the morphogenetic movements and their experiments in grafting the primitive streak into the anterior and posterior regions of nonincubated blastoderms.

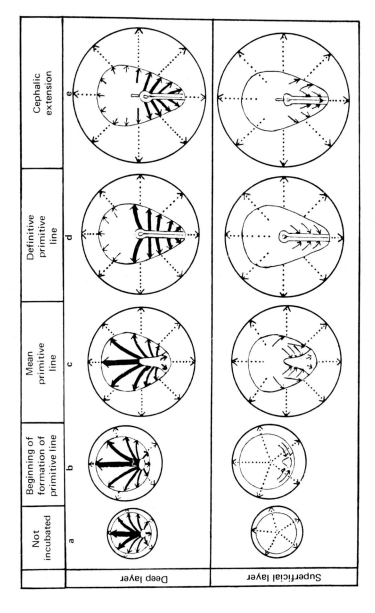

Fig. 6. Morphogenetic movements in the deep endodermal layer and the superficial layer at different stages. (a) Nonincubated; (b) early formation of the primitive streak; (c) medium-length primitive streak; (d) definitive primitive streak; (e) head process. After Spratt and Haas (1960).

c. The Potentialities for Regulation in the Blastoderm. Experiments carried out by Lutz (1949) on the nonincubated duck egg, showed the capacity for regulation possessed by the germ cell (Fig. 7). The nonincubated blastoderm was split using fine glass needles. Each part could give rise to a complete embryo, even if the blastoderm was split into several strips. Partial splits induced monsters in the form of Y or χ. These experiments, which were carried out *in vivo*, were repeated *in vitro* by Spratt and Haas (1960). These authors used the same method of splitting the blastoderm and confirmed the

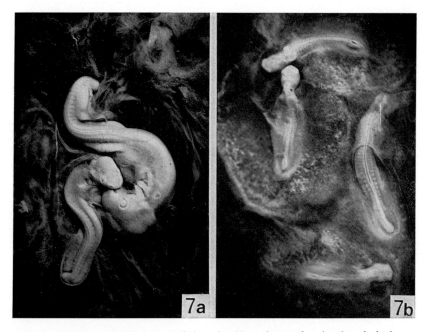

FIG. 7. Embryos obtained by splitting the blastoderm of unincubated duck eggs (experiments carried out *in ovo*).   (7a) Twin embryos obtained after splitting the blastoderm perpendicular to the presumptive embryonic axis.   (b) 4 embryos derived from small pieces: anterior, posterior, and lateral. The whole central region of the blastoderm was submerged in the yolk. After Lutz (1949) and Lutz, Departout Hubert, and Pieau (1963).

previous results, that is, that the nonincubated blastoderm is capable of regulation. The blastoderms were cultured in an inverted position, with the ventral surface uppermost. The medium was composed of agar, physiological saline, and egg extract.

The nonincubated blastoderm of the hen's egg showed the same capacity for regulation as the duck blastoderm developing in the egg (Fig. 8). Each part of the nonincubated embryonic area could organize a complete embryonic axis. However, according to the experiments of Spratt and Haas, only the area pellucida possessed this property, with the fragmented area opaca being unable to form an embryo. Also, the posterior region always gave a higher proportion of embryonic axes than did the anterior region.

In contrast, experiments carried out *in ovo* by Lutz (1949) and by Lutz *et al.* (1963) showed that the nonincubated blastoderm of the duck eggs is totipotent. "If any part is physiologically isolated, it can give rise to a complete embryo." After splitting the blastoderm and eliminating part of it by sinking it in the yolk, embryos were always obtained from the remaining fragments (Fig. 7b). No region of the blastoderm had any preferential capacity for development. Each segment, anterior, posterior, or lateral, showed the same potentialities for regulation.

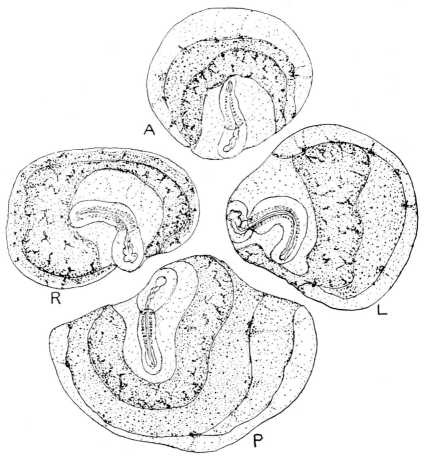

FIG. 8. Splitting the blastoderm of hen's eggs. Experiments carried out *in vitro*. The blastoderm was split into 4 pieces and each piece produced an embryo. After Spratt and Haas (1960).

Experiments carried out on blastoderms incubated for $9\frac{1}{2}$–11 hours before the appearance of the primitive streak, and just at the time of its appearance, have shown that older blastoderms have a reduced capacity for regulation (Fig. 9).

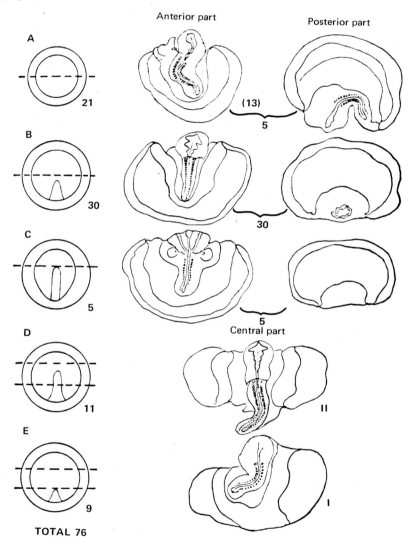

FIG. 9. Regulation of incubated blastoderm (after $9\frac{1}{2}$ hours of incubation) (A). Blastoderm split at different stages of differentiation; the development of anterior, posterior, and central parts is illustrated. Results obtained 24 hours after explantation. After Spratt and Haas (1960).

In the course of such experiments, the potentialities for both growth and regulation were analyzed in whole embryos and in united fragments. Lutz (1962) combined *in ovo* parts of nonincubated duck blastoderms. Spratt and Haas (1961) carried out similar experiments with chick blastoderms *in vitro* and produced similar results. Each isolated part of a blastoderm was capable of producing a whole embryo. When they were joined together, the different parts only gave rise to partial formations. When the fragments fused together, only one embryo was formed.

The results of this work show the potentialities for regulation possessed by avian blastoderms (Lutz, 1962). Deficiencies can be regulated, with each piece of blastoderm giving rise to a complete embryo. Excesses too can be regulated, with the fragments fusing to form a single embryo with normal organization.

According to Spratt, there is a gradient of capacity for embryonic formation that corresponds to a gradient of cellular density (Fig. 10). This gradient is at

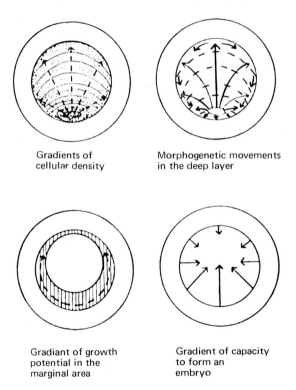

Gradients of
cellular density

Morphogenetic movements
in the deep layer

Gradiant of growth
potential in the
marginal area

Gradient of capacity
to form an
embryo

FIG. 10.   Diagram illustrating the properties of nonincubated blastoderm. Comparison of the different gradients and morphogenetic movements (gradients of cellular density, gradient of growth potential in the marginal area, and gradient of capacity to form an embryo. After Spratt and Haas (1960).

a maximum in the presumptive posteromedian zone. In the anterior region the potential for regulation is weak. The morphogenetic movements correspond to this gradient, which is dominant in the median and posterior regions. In these areas morphogenetic movements are equally very marked.

The existence of such gradients had already been established by Wolff (1948). According to this author, "... the embryonic area is subjected to a double gradient, a postero-anterior gradient and a medio-lateral gradient. The dominant region is situated in the postero-median sector of the entire embryonic area; it corresponds to the presumptive rudiment of the organizing center; it inhibits the organization of regions both anterior and lateral to it. If there is a relaxation in the bond between these areas and the dominant region they recover their autonomy and become embryogenic."

2. Late Morphogenesis. Appearance of the Circulatory System

a. Study of the Circulation in Embryos Explanted in Vitro. Removal of extraembryonic regions and parabiosis between blastoderms were carried out by Simon (1956), who showed the adaptability of the extraembryonic circulation and its potentialities of regulation (Fig. 11). After a region has been excised, for example, the region extending between the 15th and 30th pairs of somites, the circulation was reestablished. In the surviving zone vitelline

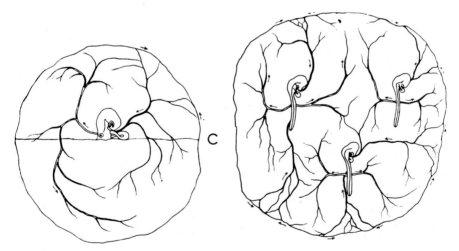

Fig. 11. The results of operations on chick embryo blastoderm cultured *in vitro* by Wolff and Simon's technique. *Left:* Embryo sectioned at the level of the first pair of somites and rejoined to the posterior part of the extraembryonic area. Despite the extent of the ablation, circulation has been established *in vitro.* C = scar. *Right:* Circulatory parabiosis between three embryos. There is a vascular anastomosis at the center of the explant. The anterior embryos communicate directly with the anterior vitelline vein of the posterior embryo. After Simon (1960).

arteries developed in the vascular area posterior to the embryo (Fig. 12c). Widespread resections that deprived the embryo of its posterior region did not prevent survival and the establishment of a circulatory network. Another series of experiments consisted of associating 2 or 3 whole blastoderms. These parabiotic embryos developed a communal circulatory network (Figs. 12d and 12e). Lastly, combinations of pieces of different embryos resulted in monsters that were deficient or had accessory parts (Fig. 12b).

Embryos explanted *in vitro* before the development of the circulation developed blood islets in the area vasculosa. These were the forerunners of the vascular network.

Under normal conditions of culture, the circulation was established in the majority of cases. Accidental circulatory anomalies did nevertheless appear, including arteriovenous anastomoses and anomalies of the venous network.

While carrying out resections or grafting regions of the blastoderm, Simon (1960) observed malformations in the circulatory system.

These experiments show that the chick embryo blastoderm can be subjected to various experimental procedures. The embryos survive considerable amputation. When associated in the region of the area vasculosa they establish a communal circulation, even if they belong to different species of bird, for example, chicken and duck (Fig. 12d).

These experiments confirm the results of work carried out *in ovo* by Stephan (1952). The destruction of one part of the extraembryonic area or the ligation of a vessel resulted in modifications of the whole extraembryonic circulation.

The two series of experiments, one carried out *in ovo*, the other on the blastoderm *in vitro*, reached the same results. They demonstrated the extraordinary plasticity of the embryonic circulatory system and its possibilities of regulation.

b. Experiments on the Transport of Germinal Cells in the Chick Embryo. It is generally accepted that the germinal cells are localized in the extraembryonic "germinal crescent," between the 1st and 2nd days of incubation. This is the stage when the primitive streak and the first somites appear (Swift, 1914). Some authors (Matsumoto, 1932; Essenberg, 1939) deny the existence of the germinal crescent. Simon's experiments (1960) proved the presence of gonocytes in the germinal crescent and their migration from the crescent toward the gonadial region of the embryo. The experiments were carried out in culture on a watch glass, using Wolff and Simon's technique (1955).

In a first series of experiments, the germinal crescent was excised from embryos at both the primitive streak and the 10-somite stage. Embryos operated upon were sterile.

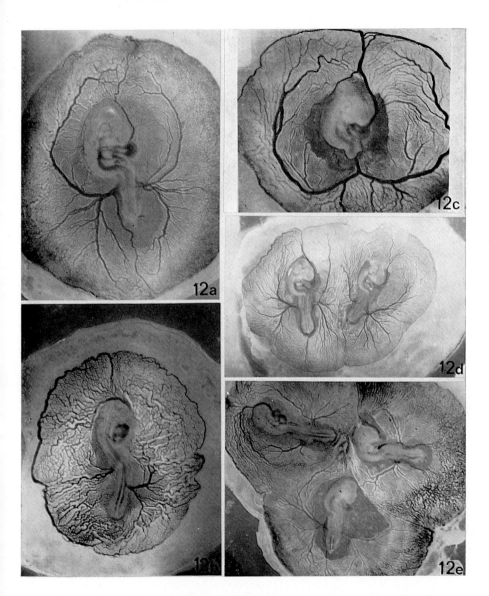

FIG. 12.   The results of operations on chick embryo blastoderms.   (a) Chick embryo cultured for 48 hours *in vitro*.   (b) Association between the anterior part of one embryo and the posterior part of a second embryo.   (c) Embryo deprived of its posterior part below the level of the 15th pair of somites. The vitelline arteries originate from the vascular area behind the embryo.   (d) Heterogeneous parabiosis between a chick embryo on the left and a duck embryo on the right. The photograph shows the communal circulation of the two explants.   (e) Parabiosis between three embryos.   After Simon (1956, 1959).

In a second series of experiments, Simon induced parabiosis between two blastoderms, one of which had had the germinal crescent removed. The gonads of both embryos were colonized by gonocytes from the remaining germinal crescent. Owing to the common circulation established between the two embryos, the germinal cells were distributed between them. These experiments show that the gonocytes of the extraembryonic area migrate toward the genital region by way of the circulatory system. A similar combination carried out between chick and duck embryos before the migration of the germinal cells showed that the genital region of one species could be colonized by the gonocytes of the other species.

When the gonadial region of an embryo was excised at the 12-somite stage (the posterior part of the embryo behind the 20th pair of somites was removed), there was an accumulation of germinal cells in the blood vessels. The gonocytes were unable to colonize any other region of the embryo.

As a result of these experiments, Simon concluded that the germinal crescent represented the source of the gonocytes in the chick embryo, and that the germinal cells were carried from the germinal crescent to the gonads by means of the circulatory system.

Present experiments by Dubois (1964) have provided more precise information on the migration of the primordial germ cells and the colonization of the gonads by these cells.

A genital region that had been previously sterilized by X-rays was associated *in vitro* with fragments of fertile germinal crescent on Wolff and Haffen's culture medium. Dubois showed that in the absence of a circulatory system the primordial germ cells from the crescent could colonize the gonadial rudiments. He considered that the germinal epithelium of the gonads produced a specific substance that attracted the gonocytes toward the gonads. To prove this hypothesis, Dubois studied the ability of an immature germinal epithelium in undifferentiated gonads to attract the germinal elements. He carried out two series of experiments.

1. A previously sterilized gonadial region of a 30–somite blastoderm was associated with a small strip from the left gonad of a 5–7$\frac{1}{2}$ day embryo.

2. An opening was made into the coelomic cavity of a previously sterilized 30-somite blastoderm. A piece of undissociated left gonad was placed in the cavity, which was then closed. The whole object was then transferred to a culture medium. The contralateral germinal epithelium served as a control. In both cases the culture was carried out for 12 to 40 hours.

These experiments showed that the primary gonocytes left the left gonad and migrated toward the younger germinal epithelium of the gonadial rudiment of the sterilized embryo (Figs. 13a,b,c). The germinal cells retained this ability to migrate even after several days of development in the gonad.

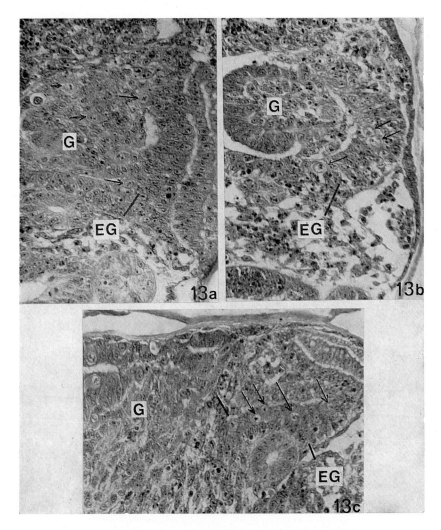

Fig. 13. The results of the *in vitro* experiments of R. Dubois (1964) on the attraction of gonocytes from undifferentiated chick embryo gonads, by young germinal epithelium. After Dubois (1964). (a) 30-somite embryo with 5½-day gonad. A migrating gonocyte escapes from its normal environment in the gonad and penetrates the germinal epithelium of the host. Two germinal cells have already settled in a corner of the coelom. 20 hours' culture. (b) 24-somite embryo with a 5½-day gonad. Three germ cells have migrated and colonized the germinal epithelium of the host. 14 hours' culture. (c) 26-somite embryo with 6-day gonad. Many exogenous germ cells are already established in the germinal epithelium of the host. A migrating gonocyte penetrates the mesenchyme in the region of the germinal epithelium. Other germinal elements are seen in the piece of gonad. 24 hours' culture. G, Piece of left gonad; EG, germinal epithelium. The short arrows indicate the gonocytes. A line outlines the junction between the host tissues and the piece of associated gonad.

253

Dubois concluded from these experiments that the germinal epithelium exerts an attraction, probably chemotactic, on the primordial germinal cells.

C. Nutritional Requirements

1. NUTRITIONAL REQUIREMENTS OF THE WHOLE BLASTODERM

One of the most important problems posed by the *in vitro* culture of blastoderms is that of the nutrition of the organisms. Culture in a synthetic medium makes it possible to study the nutrient substances that are needed for the survival, growth, and differentiation of the explants.

The first experiments with synthetic media were carried out by Spratt (1948), who explanted blastoderms onto many types of synthetic media. These media were composed of an agar substrate to which were added various nutrient materials, vitamins, and physiological solutions. The explanted blastoderms were taken between the primitive streak and 10-somite stages.

A simple medium composed of agar and physiological saline allowed cells and organs to survive for 48 hours but it was not suitable for the culture of blastoderms, which degenerated within an hour of explantation.

A synthetic medium described by White (1946) was found to be satisfactory. This medium contains:

physiological saline with phosphate buffer, bicarbonate, and agar
10 essential amino acids (Rose)
vitamins A, B, and C
glucose

The pH of the medium was maintained between 7.5 and 8.0
65 embryos were explanted at the primitive streak stage, and developed for 24 hours; 44 reached the head process; 9 reached the first stages of somite development.

Development obtained in this way was not equivalent to that obtained on natural media. Growth on this synthetic medium was limited.

Some constituents were eliminated from the complete synthetic medium:

a. All amino acids were removed.

b. All amino acids and the vitamins were removed.

c. Glucose was removed.

According to these experiments, only glucose was found to be absolutely indispensable. In the absence of this substance the blastoderms degenerated within 10 hours of explanation.

Glucose thus plays an essential role. It is an energy source that is absolutely indispensable to the culture of blastoderms, their morphogenesis, their differentiation, and their growth. The importance of glucose as more than an oxygen-using energy source was confirmed by other experiments. A very simple medium of buffered Ringer's solution and glucose was found to be adequate for the survival and development of blastoderms.

Can glucose be replaced by other sugars in the culture medium? Spratt (1949, 1958) substituted other sugars for glucose (Fig. 14) and showed that

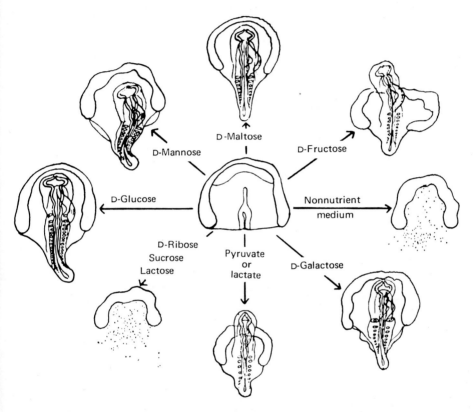

FIG. 14. The development of blastoderms on a Ringer medium containing various carbohydrates and metabolites as a source of nutrients. After Spratt (1958).

D-mannose, D-fructose, D-galactose, and D-maltose were used by the embryo. Lactose and sucrose were scarcely adequate for the survival and development of blastoderms.

These sugars were active at different concentrations: 20 mg/100 ml for glucose and mannose; 50 mg/100 ml for fructose; 200 mg/100 ml for galactose; 400 mg/100 ml for maltose.

For a similar molar concentration, the relative activities of the sugars were as follows: Glucose = mannose > fructose > galactose = maltose.

2. The Different Nutritional Requirements of Certain Organs (Heart and Brain)

Spratt's experiments (1950) have shown the nutritional requirements of certain organs during the processes of morphogenesis and differentiation. The embryos were explanted on a nonnutrient buffered medium with Ringer's solution and containing different nutrients, that is, glucose, mannose, fructose, galactose, sodium pyruvate, and sodium lactate. Some embryos were also cultured anaerobically or on a medium with a pH below 7.3. The nervous system was particularly sensitive to external factors, such as changing pH, and to anaerobic conditions. The heart was affected less than the brain by a reduction in the glucose or fructose concentration of the medium. Spratt concluded that there was a differential sensitivity of the organs as regards exogenous factors, and that the morphogenetic processes (folding of the primitive streak, formation of the notochord and the cephalic folds, formation and closure of the neural gutter, and flexion of the head) require fewer energy-yielding nutrients than processes of differentiation (histogenesis of the brain, the optic vesicles, the heart, the otocysts, and the somites). There was a certain gradation in the nutritional requirements which increased as the embryo differentiated and grew:

Survival → morphogenetic movements → differentiation → growth

3. The Nutritional Requirements of Certain Regions of the Blastoderm (Hensen's Node and Somites)

Different regions of the young blastoderm also show different nutritional requirements and metabolic activities in the course of their morphogenesis. Spratt (1955, 1958) studied the region of Hensen's node, and Fraser (1957) investigated differentiation of the somites.

a. The Region of Hensen's Node. Spratt (1955-1958) cultured the region of Hensen's node from blastoderms (primitive streak stage to the 10-somite stage) on various media.

The explants developed on a medium composed of albumin, glucose, or physiological saline (Fig. 15). The medium with albumin was better than the one with glucose, and favored the differentiation of the node, which increased in length, grew, and formed somites. It must be noted that an explant cultured for 12 hours on a medium based on physiological saline, which does not favor development, differentiated when it was transplanted onto a medium based on albumin.

The effects of different sugars and metabolites, alone or in combination, on the differentiation of the node have been tested.

If the culture medium containing glucose was combined with galactose, succinate, or pyruvate the development was not modified. It was the same as with glucose alone. On the other hand, when fructose was combined in the culture medium with glucose or galactose, extensive degeneration and cellular dispersion of the explants was induced. Even minimal concentrations of fructose (2×10^{-2} mole) could inhibit the utilization of exogenous galactose, or of exogenous and endogenous glucose.

b. Differentiation of the Somites.   Fraser (1957) explanted chick embryo blastoderms at the primitive streak stage (21 hours of incubation) onto Spratt's medium, consisting of agar and Ringer's solution. Many substances or fractions derived from albumin were added to this basic medium, and their

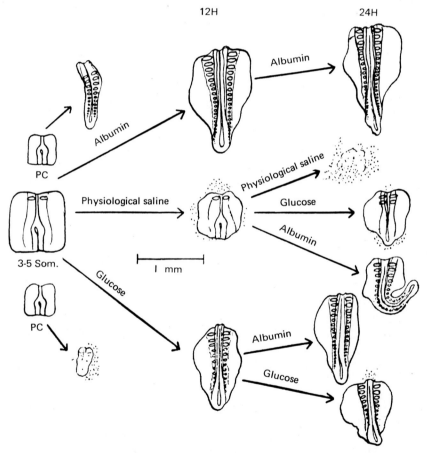

FIG. 15.   Development of the nodal region cultured on media based on albumin, glucose, and physiological saline. Duration of culture: 12 hours and 24 hours. After Spratt (1958).

effect on the formation of the somites was tested. The culture was carried out for 22–23 hours, and the following results were obtained:

On an nonnutrient agar medium, the somites did not form and the region of the node degenerated;

On a medium containing albumin or the dialyzable fraction of albumin, the mean number of pairs of somites was respectively 5.6 and 4.7. The non-dialyzable fraction or crystalline ovalbumin never induced formation of the somites. These facts suggest that small molecules are more active in this process than are larger molecules.

Fraser analyzed the effect of the free amino acids that existed in the albumin (leucine, valine, alanine, lysine, glutamic acid, and aspartic acid) and found a differentiation of around 1.9 somites. Glutamic acid, known to be of considerable importance in intermediary metabolism, was inactive, as was its analog glutamine. The other amino acids with the exception of alanine, which was utilized in the presence of glucose, were found to be inactive or poorly active.

From these experiments it was concluded that several factors present in the albumin were responsible for its activity during the development of the somites. These factors include glucose, alanine, some substances of low molecular weight, and a fraction of large molecules containing a sulfhydryl group. Fraser (1960) had studied the effect of substances containing sulfhydryl groups on the development of the somites. Blastoderms at the primitive streak stage were explanted into a moist chamber on an agar gel containing various substances:

1. Media containing cysteine, cystine, and glucose. Cysteine alone (10 mg/ 100 ml) favored the development of the somites (6.4 pairs of somites were formed). The results obtained with a higher concentration of cysteine (25 mg/ 100 ml) were not as good (3.5 pairs of somites):

If part of the cysteine (8 mg/100 ml) was replaced by cystine (2 mg/100 ml) 6.5 pairs of somites were obtained. This result was identical with that obtained for cysteine alone.

2. Media containing other sulfhydryl components. Certain sulfhydryl-containing substances (DL-methionine, taurine, glutamic acid, and glycine) were inactive. Others had a weak activity (thiamine, DL-homocysteine, and glutathione (20 mg/100 ml). From these results, Fraser concluded that the stimulating effect of cysteine was not due solely to its reducing capacity.

Later, seeking to define the role of cysteine in the cell, Fraser (1960) concluded that most of its activity was due to its incorporation into the nonspecific cellular proteins. In these, the active sulfur is probably in the disulfide form (S–S) and not in the sulfhydryl form (S–H). Two experiments demonstrate this point:

1. The explants were treated with mercuric chloride ($HgCl_2$) at a concentration of 4×10^{-5} mole for 10 minutes. This blocked the sulfhydryl groups by the formation of mercaptides, Hg being substituted for the H of the SH group.

The development of the somites was inhibited. Not only did cysteine (with its SH group) increase this inhibition but so did the dialyzate of albumin (without the SH group).

2. Pretreatment of the blastoderms with hydrogen peroxide (1.5×10^{-2} mole for 10 minutes) resulted in selective inhibition of somite development. Culture of the blastoderms on a medium containing either cysteine or albumin dialyzate protected the somites against the inhibiting effect of hydrogen peroxide.

D. Study of Metabolic and Enzymic Activities

Several methods are available for the study of these activities.

1. The technique of colored indicators for reducing enzymes was used by Spratt (1952). With the aid of neotetrazolium chloride, methylene blue, and potassium tellurite, Spratt was able to show strong enzymic activity in certain regions of the embryo, that is, in Hensen's node, the anterior part of the brain, the notochord, the somites, and the neural tube.

The reducing activity of these regions differed according to the sugar supplied.

Under aerobic conditions and in the presence of glucose, mannose, pyruvate, or lactate, only the node was able to reduce neotetrazolium. The brain and the notochord were unable to do so. In the presence of galactose, fructose, maltose, and succinate the node, the brain, and the notochord showed reducing activity.

Under anaerobic conditions, the node, the brain, and the notochord were active in the presence of glucose, mannose, and fructose, but only the node showed activity on a medium containing galactose, succinate, malate, pyruvate, lactate, and α-ketoglutarate. Hensen's node is thus one of the principal centers of enzymic activity and alone is able to reduce tetrazolium in the presence of all of the substrates used under both aerobic and anaerobic conditions.

2. The use of labeled substances. The intensity of certain metabolic processes has been analyzed by the use of labels. Labeled amino acids are administered to the embryo and the formation of proteins and the incorporation of the tracers can then be measured quantitatively under varying experimental conditions during the early stages of development.

Herrmann and Schultz (1958) studied the incorporation of ^{14}C-labeled glycine into the proteins of chick embryos explanted *in vitro*. The embryos were explanted at the 4–7 somite or 11–13 somite stage, and were cultured for 4–8 hours on Spratt's culture medium containing labeled amino acids.

The total quantity of proteins in the embryo did not vary during the 8 hours of culture. Over the same period *in situ* the protein content would have doubled. This shows that during the first 8 hours of culture the growth was almost completely stopped.

The cultured embryos incorporated the labeled glycine. In embryos explanted at the 4–7 somite stage the amount of labeled glycine rose from $51.71 \times 10^3 \, \mu g$ at the beginning of culture to $314.93 \times 10^3 \, \mu g$ after 8 hours. Meanwhile, the total quantity of glycine incorporated into protein in the embryo was not increased ($4 \, \mu g$).

The labeled glycine was not liberated from the proteins in the explant, since when embryos that had been cultured for 2 hours on a medium containing labeled glycine were transferred to a medium containing unlabeled glycine for 6 hours, the amount of labeled glycine in the proteins did not vary in a significant fashion.

During previous experiments Schultz and Herrmann (1958) had shown that the embryonic rudiments incorporated variable amounts of labeled glycine. The highest activity was found at the level of Hensen's node and the neural tube. There was less activity in the region of the notochord. These experiments corroborate those of Spratt on the enzymic activity of different regions of the blastoderm.

Hayashi and Hermann (1959) reexamined the problem of glycine incorporation by embryonic explants, but they altered the conditions of culture.

According to Britt and Herrmann (1959), the concentration of proteins in the embryo increased when the embryo together with a significant amount of the extraembryonic area, was explanted onto a medium containing a concentrated egg homogenate. Embryos were taken at the 11–13 somite stage and were cut out close to the marginal sinus (narrow border) or well away from the marginal sinus (wide border) (Hayashi and Herrmann).

Culture was carried out on various natural and synthetic media, and was continued for 8–24 hours. The growth was well marked where the blastoderm was associated with a large amount of extraembryonic material and when it was cultured on a natural medium.

An explant undergoing rapid growth incorporated little ^{14}C-labeled glycine into its protein. An explant undergoing little growth but actively differentiating showed a high incorporation of ^{14}C-glycine. These experiments show that the nutritional requirements for growth and differentiation are not the same. Growth requires complex molecules that can be obtained from the natural medium; differentiation, which is possible on a synthetic medium, can make use of peptides, such as glycine.

Using labeled amino acids, Herrmann and Marchok (1962) showed that there was only a significant degradation of proteins in explanted chick embryos that were undergoing little growth.

E. Teratogenic Effects Induced by Chemical Substances

Many factors that disturb metabolism have been studied and have been found to be the cause of more or less specific malformations.

1. EFFECT OF METABOLIC ANALOGS

The analogs studied have chemical structures that closely resemble those of certain vitamins, intermediate metabolites, and other cell constituents. They act by the mechanism of competitive inhibition and induce malformations.

The substances that have been tested include the following:

1. The analogs of leucine, DL-ω-bromoallylglycine (Herrmann, 1953; Rothfels, 1954; Herrmann et al., 1955; Hahn and Herrmann, 1962).

2. The analogs of valine (Herrman, 1953).

3. The analogs of methionine (Hermann et al., 1955).

4. The analogs of folic acid (O'Dell and McKenzie, 1963).

The results of these experiments show that the analogs of phenylalanine induce general inhibition of growth and several more or less specific malformations, occurring mainly in the nervous system. The analogs of leucine induce selective inhibition of somatic segmentation. The addition of specific or other amino acids protects the embryo against the teratogenic effects of amino acid analogs.

The action of one analog of leucine (ω-bromoallylglycine) has been studied and was found to prevent segmentation of the somites (Herrmann, 1953; Rothfels, 1954; Herrmann et al., 1955).

While the role of ATPase in the segmentation of the somites was being studied (Deucher, 1960) a diminution in the ATPase activity of the somatic mesoderm after addition of bromoallylglycine to the culture medium was observed. When leucine was added at the same time, the ATPase activity was reestablished.

Schultz and Herrmann (1958) analyzed the effects of bromoallylglycine on the incorporation of glycine into the proteins of embryos explanted at the 11–13 somite stage. A decrease in the amount of glycine contained in the protein was observed for both Hensen's node and the somites. There was also a decrease in the incorporation of labeled glycine in the region of Hensen's node, but not in the region of the somites. Is there a decrease in synthesis of proteins, or are the proteins degraded by proteolysis? In the latter case, the results would agree with those of Jensen, Lehmann, and Weber (1956), who noted an increase in the cathepsin activity (that is, an increase in proteolysis) in the tissues of amphibians that had been grown in the presence of leucine analogs.

In order to analyze this problem, Deuchar (1960) and Hahn and Herrmann (1963) investigated the activity of cathepsins (proteolytic enzymes) in different regions of chick embryo blastoderm.

Deuchar (1960) studied the activity of the cathepsins in somatic mesoderm from 45-hour embryos (stage 11 of Hamburger and Hamilton). The activity of cathepsins was considered to be higher in unsegmented somatic mesoderm than in the region undergoing segmentation. The activities, expressed in micrograms of soluble casein per microgram of total nitrogen, are: 0.292 for segmented mesoderm and 0.481 for unsegmented mesoderm.

Embryonic somatic mesoderm that had been cultured for 10 hours on an agar-glucose medium containing 0.15 mg/ml of the leucine analog ω-bromoallylglycine (BAG) showed a marked increase in the cathepsin activity, when compared with somatic mesoderm from control embryos cultured without this substance. The value for the cathepsin activity in the control tissues was 0.139, rising to 0.375 after treatment with BAG.

According to Deuchar, these results confirm the experiments of Schultz and Herrmann (1958), who investigated the amount of radioactive glycine incorporated into the tissues. The small amount of glycine in the protein of the treated tissues was a result of the abnormally high level of protein degradation.

Meanwhile, Hahn and Herrmann (1962) studied the effects of two analogs of leucine, aminoketone F and γ-bromoallylglycine, on both cathepsin activity and nitrogen content of proteins in the brain, neural tube, and axial mesoderm of explanted chick embryo (11–13 somite stage).

The amount of nitrogen contained in the protein did not increase in the same proportion in the treated organs as it did in the controls. The increase in treated organs was never more than 20% of the increase shown by the controls. However, the overall activity of cathepsins was unchanged in these organs. The decrease in the content of protein nitrogen was not linked to an increase in proteolytic activity. In contrast, fluorophenylalanine, which is not an analog of leucine, inhibited both the activity of cathepsin and the increase in the protein nitrogen content of the organs studied.

2. The Action of Metabolic Inhibitors

Using metabolic inhibitors, that is, substances that block or interfere with enzymic activity, Spratt (1950) showed that some organs possessed a differential sensitivity toward inhibitors, for example, sodium monoiodo-acetate, sodium fluoride, sodium citrate, sodium malonate, sodium cyanide, and sodium cyanide and sodium azide (Fig. 16). Embryos explanted onto a medium containing glucose and monoiodoacetate (10^{-4} to 5×10^{-5} M) or glucose and sodium fluoride (10^{-2} M) underwent complete degeneration.

At lower concentrations of monoiodoacetate (2×10^{-5} M) the central nervous system degenerated, or did not form, but the heart developed and started beating. Sodium fluoride had the opposite specific effect to monoiodoacetate. Used at a concentration of 5×10^{-3} M, sodium fluoride affected the development of the heart, but had no effect on the central nervous system. The addition of sodium lactate or sodium pyruvate to the culture medium protected the embryo from the toxic effects of monoiodoacetate and sodium fluoride.

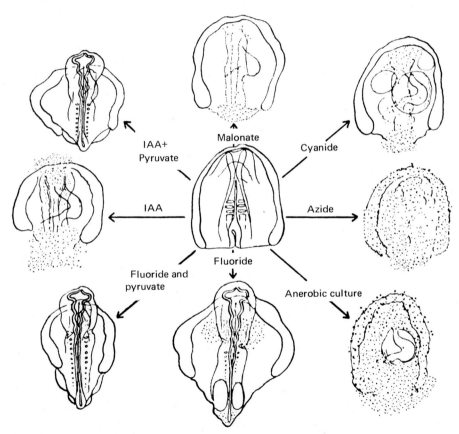

FIG. 16. The effects of different metabolic inhibitors on the development of the explants. In most cases the inhibitors were added to a Ringer-glucose medium. When pyruvates are substituted for glucose, they protect the explant against the toxic effects of iodoacetic acid. After Spratt (1958).

The effects obtained and the ability to protect against these effects suggest that certain enzyme systems, such as triose-phosphate dehydrogenase and enolase, can be inhibited by sodium monoiodoacetate or sodium fluoride. Finally these experiments show that organs such as heart and nervous system possess varying levels of metabolic activity.

3. THE EFFECT OF TOXIC SUBSTANCES ON THE CHICK EMBRYO CULTURED *IN VITRO*

It has been shown (Ancel, 1950) that various chemicals exert a teratogenic effect on certain regions of the chick embryo when they are placed on the embryo at an early stage of its development. Few experiments have been carried out *in vitro*, since the survival of the embryos is limited, but some work has recently been done by Jurand (1958–1963). Chick embryo blastoderms were subjected to the action of various cytotoxic, antitumoral agents. The embryos were explanted after 22–23 hours of incubation and cultured on a watch glass using New's technique. The toxic substance was added in solution to the liquid albumin, and explanted embryos were cultured for 24 hours. The following results were obtained.

1. Triethylenemelamine (TEM) used at a concentration of 2–$5 \times 10^{-6} M$ (Jurand, 1958) slowed the growth of the embryo. Six to nine somites were formed, whereas the controls formed 12–16 somites; when used in higher doses, TEM exerted a selective action on the somites, which degenerated.

2. *N-p*-Aminophenyl-2,2′-dichlorodiethylamine and its acetyl derivative (Jurand, 1960) induced degeneration of the neural tube and the somatic cells. Endodermal structures, the notochord, the heart, and the lateral mesoderm were not affected.

At low concentrations, the fluoroacetyl derivative (Jurand, 1961), which is rapidly destroyed by hydrolyzing enzymes, prevented closure of the neural tube. At high concentrations it destroyed the medullary plate.

3. When used at a concentration of 50–$100 \, \mu g/ml$, *p-(N,N*-di-2-chloroethylamino)phenyl-*N′*-(*p*-carboxyphenyl)carbamate, a derivative of mustard gas, inhibited segmentation of the somatic mesoderm (Fig. 17).

These experiments demonstrate the teratogenic and selective action of certain compounds derived from mustard gas. The somatic region is particularly sensitive and the inhibition of somatic segmentation produced recalls that obtained with analogs of amino acids (Rothfels, 1954; Herrmann *et al.*, 1955). It can be asked whether these teratogenic agents act on the same metabolic pathways.

Barron and McKenzie (1962) gave insulin to 24-hour chick embryos that had been explanted using New's technique. Insulin had a teratogenic effect, especially on the development of the neural tube and the brain. The somites

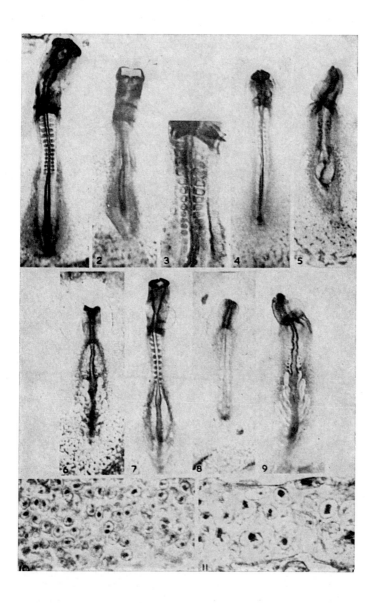

FIG. 17. Embryos treated with mustard gas derivatives. (1) Control embryo at the 15-somite stage. (2–9) Embryos treated with the toxic agent which affects the somatic region. Partial or complete degeneration of the somites. (10) Cells of the neural tube in a control 15-somite embryo. (11) Cells of the neural tube in an embryo treated with a mustard gas derivative (10^{-4} M). After Jurand (1960).

and the heart were only affected by high doses. When oxidized nicotinamide-adenine dinucleotide was given with the insulin there was no teratogenic effect. The reduced form of NAD had no such action.

Emanuelson (1961), Nicolet (1961), and Rogers (1963) have studied the effect of lithium chloride on young chicken blastoderms, cultured *in vitro*.

Nicolet (1961) explanted blastoderms at the early primitive streak stage and up to the appearance of the first somites on a medium containing lithium chloride. The treatment was never administered for more than 8 hours, and the explants were fixed after 36–48 hours of incubation. Lithium chloride was found to affect the morphogenetic movements and at the early stages it prevented the formation of the axial components. The neural rudiment was particularly affected and showed many malformations.

Rogers (1963) obtained one-eyed embryos after culturing blastoderms in the presence of lithium chloride (11.8 and 15.7 millimoles).

These experiments demonstrate the selective effect of chemical substances on the development of certain regions of the blastoderm.

III. *IN VITRO* CULTURE OF MAMMALIAN OVA

Experiments on mammalian ova are more difficult than those on birds, since the ovum soon becomes attached to the uterine mucosa and further development is maintained through the placenta. Many attempts have been made to culture ova away from the maternal tissues.

Initially, these experiments were concerned with fertilization of ova *in vitro*. The ova were taken from the ovaries or oviducts of several mammalian species, particularly the rabbit. In most cases only parthenogenetic development of the ova was obtained (Pincus, 1939; Thibault, 1947, 1948). To avoid parthenogenetic activation of the ovum, work was carried out at a temperature of 38°–39°C (Dauzier *et al.*, 1954). It was also shown that the spermatozoa had to mature in the genital tract of the female before fertilization could occur. This confirmed the *in vivo* experiments of Chang (1951) and Austin (1961). A detailed cytological study confirmed that actual fertilization had occurred. Of 88 oocytes treated in this way 33 were fertilized.

A second type of experiment was devoted to the culture of ova or embryos at different stages: segmenting eggs taken from the oviducts, and blastocysts from the uterus.

Mammalian fetuses (of sheep and cattle, for example) have been maintained outside the uterus using a technique of aseptic perfusion (Thomas, 1948; Thomas *et al.*, 1948).

The ovum developed much better, and for longer when it was taken at a relatively late stage (8-blastomere stage or later). However, survival was limited, and did not exceed 72 hours.

To overcome this difficulty, the embryos were reimplanted in the uterus of the female in which pregnancy had been induced.

Lastly, the technique of culture not only allows study of nutritional requirements, but also direct intervention on the mammalian ovum. Such experiments have yielded interesting results.

A. Culture and Nutritional Requirements

1. CULTURE OF THE TUBAL OVUM

The first experiments with tubal ova were carried out using rabbits, guinea pigs, rats, and mice. Lewis and Gregory (1929) and Gregory (1930) studied the development of naturally fertilized rabbit ova, and obtained the blastocyst stage from ova that had been cultured after fertilization. Pincus and Werthessen (1938) placed the ova in Carrel flasks with 6–8 ml of serum. Hammond (1949), working with mouse ova, used a medium based on yolk extract. After 2 days of culture, ova taken at the 2-blastomere stage showed no development, but ova cultured from the 4-blastomere stage were able to develop and 5 out of the 9 cultured reached the blastocyst stage. Ova cultured at the 8-blastomere stage all developed into blastocysts. Hammond thought that there was a critical stage associated with physiological differences between the 2-blastomere and the 8-blastomere stages.

Washburn (1951) cultured rat embryos on a medium based on physiological saline. Ringer's, Tyrode's, or Gey's solutions were used with other substances such as fluid from the anterior chamber of the eye, rat plasma (10–15%), bone marrow, or hen's egg yolk with or without albumin. Several cellular divisions were obtained.

Wintemberger, Dauzier, and Thibault (1963) studied the *in vitro* development of sheep and goat ova. The ova were taken at 38°–39°C by perfusion with homologous serum and were cultured in glass tubes with the homologous serum and streptomycin. Nonsegmented ova could divide *in vitro*, but none developed past the 9-blastomere stage. The best results were obtained with ova containing 15–20 blastomeres, which developed to the blastocyst stage.

Whitten (1956–1957), Brinster (1963), and Purshottan and Pincus (1961) studied the nutritional needs of ova from different mammalian species, from the time of fertilization until implantation had occurred (blastocyst stage).

Whitten (1956) used mouse ova at the 8-blastomere stage and cultured them on a medium containing bicarbonate-buffered Krebs-Ringer solution (pH 7.4), glucose, and crystalline bovine albumin (Armour) at a concentration of 0.03–6%. Of 148 ova used, 145 developed into blastulas. The latter were normal and continued to grow when grafted under the renal capsule of adult mice.

Later, Whitten (1957) defined the culture conditions. Growth did not occur when the ova were cultured on the Krebs-Ringer solution alone.

Beef albumin could be replaced by egg albumin or even by glycine (0.003 M) or other simple amino acids and by peptides.

The energy-producing nutrients were provided by glucose or mannose, but not by fructose, galactose, maltose, or lactose. Lactates, pyruvates, and malates also allowed gtowth of the blastulas but development was most rapid in the presence of lactates.

Purshottan and Pincus (1961) cultured rabbit and mouse ova on a synthetic medium to which they had added small amounts of serum. Several media were tested:

1. Bicarbonate-buffered Krebs-Ringer solution with 1% glucose and 2% albumin.

2. Medium based on Eagle's medium

    a. without added serum,
    b. with 10% horse serum,
    c. with 10% human serum,
    d. with 10% rabbit serum.

3. 100% rabbit serum.

4. Waymouth's synthetic medium lacking proteins.

Early ova, taken at the 2-blastomere or the morula stage, developed on Eagle's synthetic medium without added serum. This medium was more favorable for the development of mouse ova than it was for the development of rabbit ova.

The bicarbonate-buffered Krebs-Ringer medium with added glucose and albumin was also more suitable for mouse ova.

The conditions for development were nevertheless improved by the addition of 10% of horse serum to the culture medium. Serum had to be present for morulas to develop into blastocysts.

From these experiments, it has been concluded that ova have different nutritional requirements, according to their developmental stage at the time of explantation. The blastocyst stage at the time of formation and implantation is at a critical stage, requiring more complex and more specific factors than do young ova in the course of segmentation.

2. Culture of Uterine Ova

It is during the uterine stage that the ovum develops the germinal disk and the primitive streak. The first attempts at culture were made by Brachet (1913), who used a medium containing coagulated rabbit plasma. Blastodermal vesicles were collected from the uterus at the 7th day of gestation and were placed in tubes containing plasma. After 24–48 hours, development had begun. There was an embryonic axis, with a primitive streak, head process, and mesodermal rings. Trophoblastic villi also appeared. Maximow (1925) and Waddington and Waterman (1933) cultured rabbit ova, and da Costa and Pires Soares cultured guinea pig ova on media based on coagulated plasma.

The results were not constant and survival was limited.

Other workers have tested homologous plasma. This had been made incoagulable at 39°C by the addition of heparin (Nicholas and Rudnick, 1934, 1938) or by removing part of the fibrin content (Jolly and Lieure, 1938). Nicholas and Rudnick specified for the culture of rat embryos a medium composed of heparinized rat plasma and rat embryo extract prepared from 14–15 day embryos.

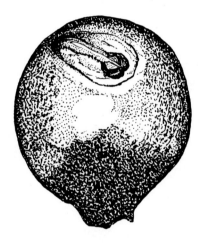

Fig. 18. Development of a guinea pig ovum cultured from the beginning of the 14th day. Duration of culture 25 hours. The embryonic axis, brain, medulla, 5–6 pairs of somites, and double cardiac rudiment have developed. After Jolly and Lieure (1938).

Embryos taken from the uterus with the decidua intact developed for 24–36 hours. In the more successful experiments, there was a development of an embryonic axis with the nervous system, the formation of blood islets, and the appearance of 2–16 somites.

Jolly and Lieure (1938) cultured young rat and guinea pig embryos taken at the primitive streak stage. A liquid medium was used, composed of homologous plasma with the addition of a few drops of decidual extract.

The temperature at which the culture took place was critical; 38°C for the rat and 39°C for the guinea pig. In this way, starting with the germinal disk and the primitive streak, the authors obtained the appearance of the embryonic axis, the neural tube, some somites, the heart, main vessels, and hemoglobin. In the rat, the heart began to beat. The period of culture varied from 30 to 36 hours, and exceptionally from 48 to 60 hours (Figs. 18 and 19). Culture of older ova resulted in differentiation of the optic and otic vesicles, the formation of the liver rudiments, and the appearance of limb buds.

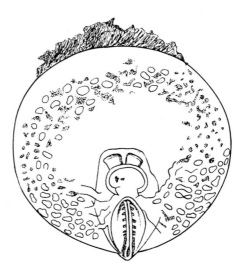

Fɪɢ. 19. Guinea pig ovum cultured from the beginning of the 14th day. Culture continued for 30 hours. The ovum has developed a complete embryonic axis, the area vasculosa has developed, and the blood islets are separating. After Jolly and Lieure (1938).

New and Stein (1963, 1964) recently carried out experiments on mouse and rat embryos using a medium composed of a coagulum of 15 drops of chicken plasma and 5 drops of chick or mouse embryo extract. The embryos, which were explanted after 7–10 days in the case of mice, and after 9–10½ days in the case of rats, were cultured on this substrate in the presence of air, where the carbon dioxide concentration had been raised to 4–5%.

Of embryos taken at the 1–7 somite stage, 72% developed a blood circulation, and 33% reached the limb bud stage.

Of 19 embryos taken at the 8–12 somite stage, 17 developed a blood circulation and 13 developed 24 to 32 somites and limb buds.

In the case of the rats, 22 embryos cultured at the 6–12 somite stage developed anterior limbs.

The development observed in culture corresponded to 26 hours of development *in situ*. The heart could beat for longer than 72 hours.

B. Reimplantation of Ova or Embryos into the Female after Culture *in Vitro*

In order to prolong the survival of cultured embryos beyond 72 hours, many workers have tried to reimplant them into a female prepared by a fertilizing coitus. The duration of culture prior to reimplantation varied. In some instances, the embryo was reimplanted into the uterus immediately after treatment. Other embryos were cultured for several hours or days before reimplantation.

Working with the 2-blastomere rat ovum, Nicholas and Hall (1936–1942) used the combination of two techniques. After having been removed from the oviducts the ova were immersed in acidified Ringer's solution (0.0002 M) for 3 hours in order to remove the zona pellucida. Normal embryos developed until the 9th day.

This useful technique was also used by other workers. Pincus (1939) implanted rabbit ova that had been artifically activated *in vitro*. Of 19 rabbits, 3 gave birth to young. Older ova (16-blastomere stage) (Adams, 1956) were incubated for $21\frac{1}{2}$ hours in a bicarbonate-buffered Krebs-Ringer solution containing 2 mg/ml of beef albumin (fraction V, Armour). Segmentation continued normally. The ova were then transferred into the uterus of a receptive female, prepared by mating with a male 3 days previously. Normal embryos developed.

Working with mouse embryos and using Whitten's synthetic medium, McLaren and Biggers (1958) cultured embryos for 2 days after they had been taken at the 8–16 blastomere stage. On this culture medium, 216 out of 249 embryos (87%) developed into blastocysts. A comparable degree of development could be observed *in vivo* in 24 hours. The cultured and non-cultured control blastocysts were then implanted into the uteruses of receptive females, $2\frac{1}{2}$ days after mating. The females were killed on the 16th and 19th days of gestation.

Differences in eye color permitted differentiation between the implanted embryos and those that had developed *in situ*.

The results are summarized in Table I.

The proportion of living embryos obtained after culture (20.4%) is close to that observed after implantation on noncultured embryos (21.7%).

These experiments demonstrate the possibilities for the survival and development of ova and embryos from rabbits, rats, and mice that have been cultured *in vitro*, and then reimplanted into the uteruses of female hosts.

Some workers have followed the development of ova that had been previously cultured. Others have used these techniques to carry out experiments that would be impossible under normal conditions. The most recent of these experiments were carried out by Tarkowski (1959). Interesting results were obtained on Whitten's medium concerning the early morphogenesis of the mouse embryo.

TABLE I

Mice with implanted cultured blastocysts		Mice with implanted noncultured control blastocysts	
No. of mouse	(Number of living embryos obtained) (number of blastocysts introduced into the uterus)	No. of mouse	(Number of living embryos obtained) (number of blastocysts introduced into the uterus)
1	5/9	9	0/9
2	4/11	10	0/11
3	1/9	11	3/12
4	2/11	12	7/17
5	2/16	13	5/20
6	1/12		
7	0/10		
8	4/15		
Total	19/93	Total	15/69

C. Experimental Work on Mammalian Ova

The topics studied in this field are the same as those that have been studied in birds. However, since experiments on mammalian ova are difficult to carry out *in situ*, the development of culture techniques was necessary before the experiments could be performed. The ability of isolated blastomeres or fused ova to regulate their development could only be studied once these techniques had been developed. The first experiments to be carried out were reported by Nicholas and Hall (1942). Later, Seidel (1952, 1960) and Tarkowski (1959, 1961) and Jolly and Lieure (1936–1938) studied the problem of the formation of the embryonic vascular system and the regulatory capacities of the cardiac rudiments.

1. EXPERIMENTS ON THE REGULATORY CAPACITY OF THE CARDIAC RUDIMENTS AND ON THE FORMATION OF THE VASCULAR SYSTEM OF THE EMBRYO

It is known that the heart of the higher vertebrates develops from two separate rudiments situated symmetrically on either side of the median line. Later, the two rudiments come together and fuse. If the two rudiments fail to unite, monsters with two hearts may develop.

Jolly and Lieure (1938) worked with guinea pig and rat embryos and destroyed one of the two cardiac rudiments before this fusion could occur. After 24 hours of culture, a small lateral heart had formed and had begun to beat rhythmically. These experiments show that in mammals one of the cardiac rudiments is able to regulate itself and develop into a functional heart.

In addition, if the region that separated the two rudiments was destroyed at an early stage, so that they could not unite, two lateral hearts beating independently of each other were developed. Complete destruction of the two rudiments resulted in an embryo with no heart.

These operations on the egg and on the embryo were carried out either by surgical destruction or by localized electrolysis.

In a second series of experiments, Jolly and Lieure studied the appearance of the primary blood islets in guinea pig, rabbit, and rat ova. Do they form independently in the area vasculosa or in the allantois, or are they derived from the cardiac rudiments?

It was shown that the development of the primary embryonic vessels and of those in the vitelline area was due to independent vascular rudiments that were quite distinct from the heart.

If the allantoic rudiment of the rat or guinea pig was removed and cultured before the appearance of the heart and great vessels, this rudiment would develop and form vessels.

If the cardiac rudiments were completely destroyed, nearby vascular rudiments were seen to appear. The blood islands of the vitelline region continued to develop into corpuscles containing hemoglobin.

2. Problems of Regulation during the Development of Isolated Blastomeres or Fused Ova

Two types of experiments are possible: the regulation of deficiencies, and the regulation of excesses.

The experiments consist of separating and destroying one or several blastomeres, or of causing two ova to fuse. The resulting ova or pieces of ova are then implanted into the uterus of a female host.

a. The Regulation of Deficiencies. Nicholas and Hall (1942) separated the two primary blastomeres of the rat ovum, first removing the zona pellucida and then separating the blastomeres with fine needles. Each of these blastomeres was implanted into the uterine horn of a pregnant female. More than half of the blastomeres developed normally after implantation. The majority of them reached the cylindrical stage (ova with an ectoplacental cone and an amniotic vesicle), but all the embryos died before the 10th day.

Seidel (1952, 1960) carried out analogous experiments using rabbit ova. One of the four primary blastomeres was destroyed using a fine glass needle. The treated ova were then reimplanted in a rabbit. Whole embryos were obtained (35 cases out of 219 implantations).

Tarkowski (1959) used the same technique to study the development of isolated mouse blastomeres. Out of 175 "half blastomeres" implanted, 54 or 30.8% became embedded in the uterine mucosa. At autopsy, 30 or

17.1% appeared normal. Two periods of intense resorption were noted, one immediately after implantation and the other at the beginning of the second half of gestation. Three females gave birth to young (4 females and 2 males) which had developed from "half-blastomeres."

b. The Regulation of Excesses. The first attempts to fuse ova were carried out by Nicholas and Hall (1942). Pairs of rat ova, fertilized but not segmented, were transplanted into the uterus of an animal of a different strain. The donors were pigmented, the hosts albino. A normal embryo developed, with normal constitution, but it was much larger than a control embryo of the same age.

Tarkowski (1961) repeated this experiment using mice. To ensure success of the experiment the ova in culture were kept in pairs until the blastocyst stage had been reached. The ova were taken at the 8-blastomere stage, the zona pellucida was removed, and they were then associated in pairs in a small drop of fluid surrounded by liquid paraffin. The oil exerted a pressure on the two ova, and they became stuck together.

The medium, based on Whitten's medium (1956, 1957), was composed of bicarbonate-buffered Krebs-Ringer solution containing the following substances in each 130 ml:

2.6 mg of phenol red	A fraction of albumin V
4.0 mg of penicillin and streptomycin	130 mg of glucose
400 mg of beef plasma	

The ova were cultured for 24–40 hours and then implanted either into mouse oviduct or into the uterus after 3 days of pseudogestation.

After a few hours in culture, the ova developed into morulas that showed no trace of their double origin. A small blastocele appeared in some of these ova.

The first autopsies were carried out on the 10th day of gestation; the results are shown in Table II.

From 138 blastocysts implanted, 38 embryos or young were obtained.

The embryos were of normal size.

Of 14 young examined macroscopically, there were 2 female, 9 male, and 3 intersexual individuals.

The 3 intersexual individuals were chimeras, possessing a female genital tract on one side and a male genital tract on the other (Fig. 20).

It must be noted that different strains of mice were used in these experiments. The most interesting combination was provided by the following cross:

LAB Grey + LAB Grey × A₂G

↙   ↘

(Nonpigmented)   (Black eyes and pigmented Agouti fur)

TABLE II

Duration of culture	Time and type of transplantation	Number of hosts, ♀	Total number of blastocysts transplanted	Implant-ations	Embryos or young	Successful transplant-ations
24 Hours	Oviduct 1st day	13	63	22	16	8
	Uterus 3rd day	7	32	18	13	6
36–40 Hours	Uterus 3rd day	7	21	1	1	1
	Uterus 4th day	12	37	10	6[a]	6
	Total	39	153	51 33%	36(38)[a] 21%	21 54%

[a] Twins (development of two blastocysts after transplantation).

The F_1 hybrids had pigmented eyes, while the LAB Grey young did not. Ova for the experiments were taken from mice of different strains, A_2G albinos, LAB Grey, and mice derived from a cross of the two strains.

Tarkowski's experiments demonstrate that it is possible to fuse completely two ova into one blastocyst in culture. The chimeric nature of these embryos is demonstrated by the fact that some are intersexual and that almost all of the embryos derived from the fusion of ova of pigmented and non-pigmented strains developed black pigment.

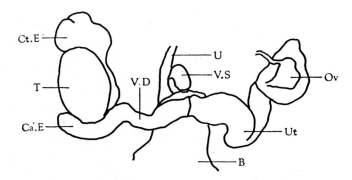

Fig. 20. The genital organs of a chimera. Male on the left, female on the right. B, Bladder; CaE, tail of the epididymis; Ct.E, head of the epididymis; Ov, ovary; T, testis; U, ureter; Ut, uterus; V.D., vas deferens; V.S., seminal vesicle. After Tarkowski (1961).

IV. CONCLUSIONS

The technique of embryo culture has permitted the study of and the solution of many problems, in birds as well as in mammals. Many experiments carried out *in ovo* have been confirmed and extended *in vitro*. Regulation of the blastoderm and of the circulatory system of the extraembryonic area, the study of the organizing center, the localization of rudiments, the positioning of the layers, and the morphogenetic movements have all been studied.

Embryo culture also offers other possibilities for research. The nutritional conditions of the organism may be varied by altering the composition of the medium. Operations that are impossible *in situ* can be carried out in culture. In the case of birds, excision of the germinal crescent coupled with parabiosis has localized the gonocytes in the germinal crescent. It has also been shown that they are carried from the germinal crescent to the gonadial rudiments by the bloodstream. Among the mammals, separation of blastomeres or fusion of ova has shown the capacity for regulation that they possess. These experiments have also shown that it is possible to obtain chimeric individuals from combined ova.

Taken together, these experiments demonstrate the numerous fruitful results obtained by using the techniques of embryo culture. However, these experiments have only begun and it is to be hoped that improvements in culture conditions will permit prolonged survival of the organisms and that other problems can be analyzed using similar methods.

BIBLIOGRAPHY

1. Adams C. E. "Artificial Insemination". 5, *Third International Congress on Animal Reproduction*, Cambridge, 1956.
2. Ancel P. *La chimiotératogénèse chez les Vertébrés* (réalisation des monstruosités par des substances chimiques). Un vol., 1950, Doin, édit., Paris, 1–393.
3. Assheton R. An experimental examination into the growth of the blastoderm of of the chick. *Proc. roy. Soc.*, 1896, **60**, 349–356.
4. Austin C. R. Fertilization of mammalian eggs *in vitro*. *Internatl. Rev. Cytol.*, 1961, **12**, 337–359.
5. Barron P. and Mc Kenzie. The inhibitory action of insulin in the early chick embryo. *J. Embryol. exp. Morph.*, 1962, **10**, No. 1, 88–98.
6. Brachet A. Recherches sur le déterminisme héréditaire de l'œuf des Mammifères. Développement *in vitro* de jeunes vésicules blastodermiques de Lapin. *Arch. de Biol.*, 1913, **28**, 447–503.
7. Brinster R. L. A method for *in vitro* cultivation of mouse ova from two cell to blastocyst. *Exp. Cell. Research.*, 1963, **32**, 205–208.
8. Britt L. G. and Herrmann H. Protein accumulation in early chick embryos grown under different conditions of explantations. *J. Embryol. Exptl. Morph.*, 1959, **7**, 66–72.

9. Chang M. C. Fertilizability of rabbit ova and the effects of temperature *in vitro* on their subsequent fertilization and activation *in vivo. J. exp. Zool.*, 1952, **121**, 351–381.
10. C. da Costa A. and Pires-Soares J. Développement d'embryons de Mammifères *in vitro. C. R. Soc. Biol.*, 1932, **113**, 510.
11. Dauzier L., Thibault Ch. and Wintemberger S. La fécondation *in vitro* de l'œuf de Lapine. *C. R. Acad. Sci.*, 1954, **238**, 844–845.
12. O'Dell D. S. and Mc Kenzie. The action of aminopterin on the explanted early chick embryo. *J. Embryol. exp. Morph.*, 1963, **11**, No. 1, 185–200.
13. Deuchar E. M. Adenosine triphosphatase activity in early somite tissue of the chick embryo. *J. Embryol. and exp. Morph.*, 1960, **8**, No. 3, 251–258.
14. Deuchar E. M. Relation between somite segregation rate and ATP-ase activity in early chick embryo. *J. Embryol. and exp. Morph.*, 1960, **8**, No. 3, 259–267.
15. Deuchar E. M. The effect of an amino acid analog on catheptic activity in somite mesoderm of the chick embryo. *Develop. Biol.*, 1960, **2**, 129–137.
16. Dubois R. Sur l'attraction des cellules germinales primordiales par la jeune région gonadique chez l'embryon de Poulet. *C. R. Acad. Sci.*, 1964, **258**, 3904–3907.
17. Dubois R. Sur l'attraction des éléments germinaux de gonades indifférenciées par le jeune épithélium germinatif chez l'embryon de Poulet, en culture *in vitro. C. R. Acad. Sci.*, 1964, **258**, 5070–5072.
18. Emanuelson H. Biochemically induced effects on morphogenesis of early chick embryos cultivated *in vitro. Klg. fysiogr. Sällstr. Lund Förhandl,*1961, **31**, 169–188.
19. Essenberg J. M. von and Srejda A. J. The effect of the destruction of the germinal crescent on the origin of the germ cells and the development of the gonads in the domestic fowl. *West. J. Surg.*, 1939, **47**, 318–327 (cité d'après D. Simon, 1960).
20. Fell H. B. and Robison R. The growth, development and phosphatase activity of embryonic avian femora and limb buds cultivated *in vitro. Biochem. J.*, 1929, **23**, 767–784.
21. Fraser R. C. Somite genesis in the chick. Partial characterization of stimulatory factors in egg white. *Growth.*, 1957, **21**, 29–44.
22. Fraser R. C. Somite genesis in the chick. (III) The role of induction. *J. exp. Zool.*, 1960, **145**, 151–167.
23. Fraser R. C. Somite genesis in the chick. (IV) Activity of sulfur containing compounds. *J. exp. Zool.*, 1960, **145**, 169–178.
24. Fraser R. C. Somite genesis in the chick. (II) Analysis of nutrients from yolk. *Biol. Bull.*, 1961, **116**, 420–428.
25. Gallera J. Culture *in vitro* des blastodermes de Poulet. Rapports entre les feuillets embryonnaires et le milieu nutritif contenant de la gélose. *Revue Suisse de Zoologie*, 1963, **70**, No. 29, 587–594.
26. Gallera J. and Nicolet G. Quelques commentaires sur les méthodes de culture *in vitro* de jeunes blastodermes de Poulet. *Experientia*, 1961, **17**, 134–135.
27. Grabowsky C. T. The induction of secondary embryos in the early chick blastoderm by grafts of Hensen's node. *Amer. J. Anat.*, 1957, **101**, 101–134.
28. Gräper L. Die primitiventwicklung des Hühnchens nach stereokinematographischen Untersuchungen, kontrolliert durch vitale Farbmarkierung und verglichen mit der Entwicklung anderer Wirbeltiere. *Arch. Entw. Mech.*, 1929, **116**, 382–430.
29. Gregory P. W. The early Embryology of the Rabbit. Publication 407 of the Carnegie Institution of Washington, Contributions to Embryology No. 125, p. 141, 1930 (cité d'après Jolly et Lieure, 1938).

30. Hahn H. P. von and Herrmann H.   Effects of amino acid analogs on growth and catheptic activity of chick embryo explants. *Develop. Biol.*, 1962, **5**, 309–327.

31. Hammond J.   Recovery and culture of tubal mouse ova. *Nature*, 1949, **163**, 28–29.

32. Hara K.   Regional neural differentiation induced by prechordal and presumptive chordal mesoderm in the chick embryo. *Drukkerij Libertas N. V. Utrecht*, 1961, 1–41.

33. Hayashi Y. and Herrmann H.   Growth and glycine incorporation in chick embryo explants. *Develop. Biol.*, 1959, **1**, 437–458.

34. Herrmann H.   Interference of amino acid analogues with normal embryonic development. *J. Embryol. exp. Morph.*, 1953, **1**, 291–295.

35. Herrmann H. and Marchok A.   Gain and loss of protein in explanted chick embryos. *Develop. Biol.*, 1962, **7**, 207.

36. Herrmann H., Rothfels-Konigsberg U. and Curry M. F.   A comparison of the effects of antagonists of leucine and methionine on the chick embryo. *J. exp. Zool.*, 1955, **128**, No. 2, 359–377.

37. Herrmann H. and Schultz P. W.   Incorporation of glycine into the proteins of explanted chick embryos. *Arch. Biochem. Biophys.*, 1958, **73**, 296–305.

38. Jensen P., Lehmann F. E. and Weber R.   Catheptic activity in the regenerating tail of *Xenopus larvae* and its reaction to histostatic substances. *Helv. Physiol. Acta*, 1956, **14**, 188–201.

39. Jolly and Lieure C.   Sur la culture des œufs de Mammifères. *C. R. Soc. Biol.*, 1936, **122**, 723.

40. Jolly J. and Lieure C.   Recherches sur la culture des œufs de Mammifères. *Arch. Anat. micr.*, 1938, **34**, 307–74.

41. Jurand A.   Action of triethano melanine (TEM) on early stages of chick embryos. *J. of Embryol. and exp. Morph.*, 1958, **6**, No. 2, 357–362.

42. Jurand A.   Comparative investigations of the action of two nitrogen mustard derivatives. On the early stages of development of chick embryos. *J. Embryol. and exp. Morph.*, 1960, **8**, 60–67.

43. Jurand A.   Anti-mesodermal activity of a nitrogen mustard derivatives. *J. Embryol. and exp. Morph.*, 1963, **4**, 689–696.

44. McLaren A. and Biggers J. D.   Successful development and birth of mice cultivated *in vitro* as early embryos. *Nature*, 1958, **182**, 877–878.

45. Lewis W. H. and Gregory P. W.   Moving pictures of developing living Rabbit eggs. *Am. Ass. of Anatomist, Ann. Record.*, 1929, **42**, 27.

46. Lutz H.   Sur la production expérimentale de la polyembryonie et des monstruosités doubles chez les Oiseaux. *Arch. Anat. micr. Morph. exp.*, 1949, **38**, 80–144.

47. Lutz H.   L'orientation des axes embryonnaires dans la gémellité expérimentale chez les Oiseaux. *Bull. Biol. France et Belgique*, 1953, **87**, 34–67.

48. Lutz H.   Contribution expérimentale à l'étude de la formation de l'endoblaste chez les Oiseaux. *J. Embryol. exp. Morph.*, 1955, **3**, 59–76.

49. Lutz H.   Association de blastodermes d'Oiseaux. *Anat. Anz. Erg.*, 1962, **109**, 120–125.

50. Lutz H., Departout M., Hubert J. and Pieau Cl.   Contribution à l'étude de la potentialité du blastoderme non incubé chez les Oiseaux. *Develop. Biol.*, 1963, **6**, No. 1, 23–44.

51. Lutz H. and Lutz-Ostertag Y.   Culture *in vitro* du blastoderme non incubé d'Oiseau. Action de l'endoblaste et de l'ectomésoblaste. *C. R. Assoc. des Anat.* 42ᵉ Réunion, 1955, 972–974.

52. Matsumoto T.   On the early localization and history of the so-called primordial germ cells in the chick embryo. *Sc. Rep. Tôhoku, Imp. Univ.*, 1932, **4**, 89–127.

53. Maximow A.   Tissue cultures of young mammalian embryos. *Contr. Embryol.*, 1925, **80**, 16, 47. *Carn. Inst. of Washington Publ.*, No. 361.

54. New D. A. T.   A new technique for the cultivation of the chick embryo *in vitro*. *J. Embryol. exp. Morph.*, 1955, **3**, 326–331.

55. New D. A. T. and Stein K. F.   Cultivation of mouse embryos *in vitro*. *Nature*, 1963, **199**, 297–299.

56. New D. A. T. and Stein K. F.   Cultivation of post-implantation mouse and rat embryos on plasma clots. *J. Embryol. exp. Morph.*, 1964, **12**, No. 1, 101–111.

57. Nicholas J. S. and Hall B. V.   The development of isolated blastomeres of the Rat. *Ana. Rec.*, 1934, **58**, 83.

58. Nicholas J. S. and Hall B. V.   Experiments on developing Rats. (II) The development of isolated blastomeres and fused eggs. *J. exp. Zool.*, 1942, **90**, 441–458.

59. Nicholas J. S. and Rudnick D.   The development of Rat embryos in tissue culture. *Proc. Nat. Acad. Sci.*, 1934, **20**, 656–658.

60. Nicholas J. S. and Rudnick D.   Development of Rat embryos of egg cylinder to head fold stages in plasma cultures. *J. exp. Zool.*, 1938, **78**, 205–232.

61. Nicolet G.   Action du LiCl sur de jeunes blastodermes de Poulet cultivés *in vitro*. *Experientia*, 1961, **17**, 413–414.

62. Nicolet G. and Gallera J.   Dans quelles conditions l'amnios de l'embryon de Poulet peut-il se former en culture *in vitro?* *Experientia*, 1963, **19**, 165–166.

63. Pasteels J.   Étude sur la gastrulation des Vertébrés méroblastiques (III) Oiseaux. (IV) Conclusions générales. *Arch. Biol.*, 1937, **48**, 381–488.

64. Pincus G.   The comparative behavior of mammalian eggs *in vivo* and *in vitro*. (IV) The development of fertilized and artificially activated rabbit eggs. *J. Exp. Zool.*, **82**, 85–130.

65. Pincus G. and Werthessen N. T.   The maintenance of embryo life in ovariectomized rabbits. *Am. J. Physiol.*, 1938, **124**, 484–490.

66. Pincus G. and Werthessen N. T.   The comparative behavior of mammalian eggs *in vivo* and *in vitro*. III: Factors controlling the growth of the rabbit blastocyste. *J. exp. Zool.*, 1938, **78**, 118.

67. Purshottan N. and Pincus G.   *In vitro* cultivation of mammalian eggs. *Anat. Record.*, 1961, **140**, 51–55.

68. Rogers K. T.   Experimental production of perfect cyclopia in the chick by means of LiCl, with a survey of the literature on cyclopia produced experimentally by various means. *Develop. Biol.*, 1963, **8**, 129–150.

69. Romanoff A. L.   Cultivation of the early chick embryo *in vitro*. *Anat. Record*, 1943, **87**, 365–368.

70. Rothfels U.   The effects of some acid analogues on the development of the chick embryo *in vitro*. *J. exp. Zool.*, 1954, **125**, 17–38.

71. Schultz P. W. and Herrmann H.   Effect of a leucine analogue on incorporation of glycine into the proteins of explanted chick embryos. *J. Embryol. Exptl. Morphol.*, 1958, **6**, 262–269.

72. Seidel F.   Die Entwicklungsfähigkeiten isolierter Furchungszellen aus dem Ei des Kaninchens *Oryctolagus cuniculus*. *Wilhelm Roux Arch. f. Entw. Mech. Org.*, 1960, **152**, 43–127.

73. Simon D.   Sur une technique de culture *in vitro* de blastodermes entiers d'embryons de Poulet et sur les interactions expérimentales qu'elle rend possibles. *Arch. Anat. micr. et Morph. exp.*, 1956, **45**, No. 4, 290–301.

74. Simon D.   Contribution à l'étude de la circulation et du transport des gonocytes

primaires dans les blastodermes d'Oiseaux cultivés *in vitro*. *Arch. Anat. micr. Morph. exp.*, 1960, **49**, 93–176.

75. Spratt N. T.   Location of organ-specific regions and their relationship to the development of the primitive streak in the early chick blastoderm. *J. exp. Zool.*, 1942, **89**, No. 1, 69–101.

76. Spratt N. T.   Formation of the primitive streak in the explanted chick blastoderm marked with carbon particles. *J. exp. Zool.*, 1946, **103**, No. 2, 259–304.

77. Spratt N. T.   Development *in vitro* of the early chick blastoderm explanted on yolk and albumin extract saline-agar substrata. *J. exp. Zool.*, 1947, **106**, No. 3, 345–366.

78. Spratt N. T.   A simple method for explanting and cultivating early chick embryos *in vitro*. *Science*, 1947, **106**, 452.

79. Spratt N. T.   Nutritional requirements of the early chick embryo. II: Differential nutrient requirements for morphogenesis and differentiation of the heart and brain. *Anat. Record.* U.S.A., 1948, **101**, 716.

80. Spratt N. T.   Development of the early chick blastoderm on synthetic media. *J. Exp. Zool.*, 1948, **107**, No. 1, 39–64.

81. Spratt N. T.   Nutritional requirements of the early chick embryo. I: The utilization of carbohydrate substrates. *J. of exp. Zool.*, 1949, **110**, No. 2, 272–298.

82. Spratt N. T.   Nutritional requirements of the early chick embryo. II: Differential nutrient requirements for morphogenesis and differentiation of the heart and brain. *J. exp. Zool.*, 1950, **114**, No. 2, 375–402.

83. Spratt N. T.   Nutritional requirements of the early chick embryo. III: The metabolic basis of morphogenesis and differentiation as revealed by the use of inhibitors. *Biol. Bull.*, 1950, **99**, No. 1, 120–135.

84. Spratt N. T.   Localization of the prospective neural plate in the early chick blastoderm. *J. of exp. Zool.*, 1952, **120**, No. 1, 109–130.

85. Spratt N. T.   Metabolism of the early embryo. *Ann. of the N. Y. Acad. of Sci.*, 1952, **55**, No. 2, 40–49.

86. Spratt N. T.   Localization of prospective notochord and somite cells. *J. Exp. Zool.*, 1955, **128**, 121–163.

87. Spratt N. T.   Regulative properties of the chorda and somite centers. *J. Exp. Zool.*, 1957, **135**, 319–353.

88. Spratt N. T.   Some differential enzyme activities of node center cells. *J. Exp. Zool.*, 1958, **138**, 51–80.

89. Spratt N. T.   Nutrient necessities in chick development. Embryonic Nutrition. *The developmental Biology Conference.* Series **1956**. Chicago, 1958, 72–86.

90. Spratt N. T. and Haas H.   Importance of morphogenetic movements in the lower surface of the young chick blastoderm. *J. Exp. Zool.*, 1960, **144**, No. 3, 257–276.

91. Spratt N. T. and Haas H.   Morphogenetic movements in the lower surface of the unincubated and early chick blastoderm. *J. Exp. Zool.*, 1960, **144**, No. 2, 139–158.

92. Spratt N. T. and Haas H.   Integrative mechanisms in development of the early chick blastoderm. I: Regulative potentiality of separated parts. *J. Exp. Zool.*, 1960, **145**, 97–138.

93. Spratt N. T. and Haas H.   Role of morphogenetic movements and regenerative growth in synthetic and topographically disarranged blastoderms. *J. of exp. Zool.*, 1961, **147**, No. 1, 57–94.

94. Spratt N. T. and Haas H.   Role of cell population size and growth potentiality in synthetic systems larger than normal. *J. of exp. Zool.*, 1961, **147**, No. 3, 271–294.

95. Spratt N. T. and Haas H.   Integrative mechanisms in development of the early chick blastoderm. IV: Synthetic systems composed of parts of different develop-

mental age, synchronization of developmental rates. *J. exp. Zool.*, 1962, **149**, 75–102.

96. Stephan F. Contribution expérimentale à l'étude du développement du système circulatoire de l'embryon de Poulet. *Bull. Biol. Fr. Belg.*, 1952, **86**, No. 3, 217–308.

97. Swift Ch. H. Origin and early history of the primordial germ-cells in the chick. *Amer. Journ. Anat.*, 1914, **15**, 483–516.

98. Tarkowski A. K. Experiments on the development of isolated blastomeres of mouse eggs. *Nature*, 1959, **184**, 1286–1287.

99. Tarkowski A. K. Experimental studies on regulation in the development of isolated blastomeres of mouse eggs. *Acta Theriologica*, 1959, **3**, 191–267.

100. Tarkowski A. K. Mouse chimaeras developed from fused eggs. *Nature*, 1961, **190**, 857–860.

101. Thibault Ch. La parthénogénèse expérimentale chez le Lapin. *C. R. Acad. Sci.*, 1947, **224**, 297–299.

102. Thibault Ch. L'activation et la régulation de l'ovocyte parthénogénétique de la Lapine. *C. R. Soc. Biol.*, 1948, **142**, No. 7-8, 495–497.

103. Thomas J. A. Nouveaux procédés de perfusion physiologique et aseptique, permettant la survie prolongée d'organes ou d'organismes pesant plusieurs kilogrammes *J. Physiologie*, 1948, **40**, 123–146.

104. Thomas J. A., Salomon L. and Salomon Lé. La survie des grands fœtus de Mammifères perfusés aseptiquement. *J. Physiologie*, 1948, **40**, 233–250.

105. Vollmar H. Eine methode zur Beobachtung der Entwicklung des Hühnerembryo *in vitro*. *Z. Zellforschung*, 1935, **23**, 566–570.

106. Waddington C. H. Experiments on the development of chick and duck embryos cultivated *in vitro*. *Phil. Trans. Royal Soc. London.* Série B, 1932, **221**, 179–230.

107. Waddington C. H. The development of isolated parts of the chick blastoderm. *J. exp. Zool.*, 1935, **71**, 273–288.

108. Waddington C. H. and Schmidt G. A. Induction by heteroplastic grafts of the primitive streak in birds. *W. Roux' Arch. Entwickl. Mech. Org.*, 1933, **128**, 522–563.

109. Waddington C. H. and Waterman A. J. The development *in vitro* of young rabbit embryos. *J. Anat.*, 1933, **67**, 355–370.

110. Washburn Jr. W. W. A study of the modifications in rat eggs observed *in vitro* and following tubal retention. *Arch. Biol.*, 1951, **62**, 439–458.

111. Wetzel R. Untersuchungen am Hühnchen. Die Entwicklung des Keims während der ersten beiden Bruttage. *Roux' Arch. Entwikl. Mech. Org.*, 1929, **119**, 188–322.

112. White P. R. Cultivation of animal tissues in nutrients of precisely known constitution. *Growth*, 1946, **10**, 231–289.

113. Whitten M. K. Culture of tubal mouse ova. *Nature*, 1956, **177**, 96.

114. Whitten W. K. Culture of tubal ova. *Nature*, 1957, **179**, 1081.

115. Wintemberger S., Dauzier L. and Thibault C. Le développement *in vitro* de l'œuf de la Brebis et de celui de la Chèvre. *C. R. Soc. Biol.*, 1953, **147**, 1971–1974.

116. Wolff Et. La duplication de l'axe embryonnaire et la polyembryonie chez les Vertébrés. *C. R. Soc. Biol.*, 1948, **142**, No. 19-20, 1282–1306.

117. Wolff Et. and Haffen K. Sur les résultats de la culture *in vitro* des gonades embryonnaires des Oiseaux. *C. R. Soc. Biol.*, 1951, **145**, 1388–1391.

118. Wolff Et. and Simon D. L'explantation et la parabiose *in vitro* de blastodermes incubés d'embryons de Poulet. L'organisation de la circulation extra-embryonnaire. *C. R. Acad. Sci.*, 1955, **241**, 1994–1996.

ADDENDUM

I. CULTURE OF AVIAN BLASTODERMS

Much of the work described in the first part of this account has been completed or established in greater detail during the last few years. Investigations on the early developmental stages of the egg will be briefly surveyed, together with the nutritional requirements of the blastoderm, and lastly, the action of various inhibitory factors on blastoderm development.

A. Problems of Morphogenesis

Research into early embryonic development has consisted mainly of studying the inductive properties of Hensen's node and the primitive streak, and on the origin and the role of the entoderm. The results of these experiments show striking analogies with results obtained using amphibians. The potentialities for regulation of blastoderms cultured *in vitro* have been extensively investigated. Valuable research carried out on blastoderms cultured *in vitro* has enabled much to be learned about the origin, localization in the nonincubated blastoderm, and migration of the germ cells.

1. STUDY OF THE ORGANIZING CENTER–NEURAL INDUCTIONS

Gallera (1965a) studied the inductive action of a graft taken from different parts of the early or completed primitive streak (stages 3 and 4 of Hamburger and Hamilton). Four fragments were excised from the region between Hensen's node and the posterior portion of the primitive streak. Each of the grafts was transplanted onto the vitelline entoderm of the operated blastoderm, to the right of the area pellucida. These blastoderms were cultured for periods varying from 40 to 60 hours. The investigations showed that the anterior portion of the primitive streak possessed inductive capacities, but that this capacity diminished in an antero-posterior direction. The age of the blastoderm also had some influence on these induction phenomena. Fragments transplanted only blastoderms at the stage of the completed primitive streak induced only brain, but if the operation was carried out on younger blastoderms, the complete neural rudiment was induced.

Gallera (1965b) attempted to establish the duration of contact necessary for obtaining neural inductions. As an inductor he used the anterior region of the completed primitive streak, including Hensen's node, with the entoderm removed. It was implanted in front of the area pellucida in the vitelline

283

entoderm of a blastoderm with the primitive streak at an intermediate stage of formation. At least 6 hours of contact were required between the inductor and the ectoderm to obtain a nervous structure in the ectoderm. After $8\frac{1}{2}$ hours of contact, cerebral structures had formed. If the inductive action was interrupted, the ectoderm became transformed into a neural plate only when the host embryo underwent neurulation.

Investigations carried out by Leikola and McCallion (1967) led to the same results. These authors used a fragment of liver as a heterologous inductor that was placed in contact with the explanted embryo on Butros' culture medium (1963). This liver fragment was inserted between the entoderm and the ectoderm. An intimate contact is necessary between the inductor (liver) and the ectoderm, and contact of 6 hours was required to obtain formation of a neural plate.

Gallera and Ivanov (1964) investigated the problem of neurogenic competence of the external blastoderm layer, taking the "time" factor into account. They excised the anterior portion of the fully formed primitive streak, i.e., Henson's node and a small portion of material situated below it, and transplanted this graft into blastoderms of various ages, either in the anterolateral region of the area pellucida or in the vitelline entoderm. These experiments showed that once the primitive streak was fully formed, the ectoderm lost its neurogenic competence. Neural inductions were obtained throughout the period of primitive streak formation, while the frequency of medullary inductions fell rapidly after the intermediate stage of primitive streak formation. The degree of development of these neural formations was shown to correspond with the development of the lost embryo's neural rudiment.

Recent work by Gallera (1968), however, has shown that both neural rudiments—i.e., the one induced by the graft and the one in the host blastoderm—appear at the same time, at least when the graft has been carried out at a sufficiently early stage with the ectoderm still competent.

Hensen's node always induces neural rudiments when implanted into the area opaca of chick blastoderm, at various stages of primitive streak formation.

If the graft is taken from the intermediate region of the young primitive streak, a new primitive streak is formed, confirming the work of Vakaet (1964, 1965). However, this secondary neural formation can appear later than that in the host embryo (Gallera, 1969). The latter author concluded that in birds, as in amphibians, it is the ectoderm itself that determines the time of its neuralization, the latter only becoming effective at a specific stage in ectoderm development.

In a recent study, following the work of Hara (1961), Rao (1968) studied the appearance and progress of neural differentiation in the embryonic neurectoderm, these investigations being based on experiments carried out by Eyal-Giladi (1954) using amphibians. Rao removed blastoderms at various stages of development: I to IV (definitive stages in the primitive streak, early and intermediate stages in the formation of the head process). The blastoderms were placed on Hara's medium (see Ch. VI, Hara, 1961) and the entodermal and mesodermal layers were separated from the overlying ectoderm in the anterior region of Hensen's node using fine tungsten needles. The median and lateral portions of the ectoderm were cut into fragments of equal size and were introduced into the coelom of a $2\frac{1}{2}$-day-old host embryo. Differentiation of the nervous system was then observed (prosencephalic, mesencaphalic, and rhombencephalic structures) in each of the grafts. The results were as follows:

Ectodermal transplants taken from the region of the prechordal mesoderm, i.e., the midportion situated in front of the primitive streak, produced a distinctly higher level of neural structures than did the lateral and anterior portions. When the latter were removed at stages I and II they produced no differentiation of neural structures. However, as development progressed the number of neural structures differentiating from the median and lateral zone grafts increased (100% for the posteromedian areas at stage III).

Grafts of the most anterior median portion (presumptive prosencephalic region) gave rise primarily to prosencephalic structures.

Grafts from the posterior median zone (stages III and IV), including part of the presumptive mesencephalon and rhombencephalon, also showed prosencephalic differentiation. More posterior neural structures appeared in these grafts, and this character became more pronounced during the subsequent stages.

Most of the transplants taken from lateral zones produced only prosencephalic differentiations.

The author interpreted these results in terms of the "activation-transformation" hypothesis put forward by Nieuwkoop (1952).

During the first contact, the prechordal mesoderm exerts an activating influence on the neurectoderm, which subsequently extends to the ectoderm as a whole. A neural "activation field" forms and brings about the appearance of prosencephalic differentiations.

These investigations demonstrate the similarities between the processes of neural induction in amphibians and birds.

2. STUDIES ON THE ORIGIN AND INDUCTIVE ROLE OF THE ENTODERM

Investigations in this field have been carried out by Vakaet (1962), Modak (1965), Gallera (1965a,b, 1968), and Gallera and Nicolet (1969). According to the work of Vakaet (1962) and Modak (1965), total ablation of the entoderm in the area pellucida before the stage of the fully formed primitive streak is followed by regeneration of a new entoderm by the primitive streak from invaginated cells.

Nicolet (1965, 1967) confirmed these conclusions. This author labeled the cells of Hensen's node with ^{3}H-thymidine and observed their fate during development. He carried out experiments in which regions from labeled and nonlabeled blastoderms were exchanged. According to his observations, Hensen's node—which contains the presumptive chordal material—participated in formation of the foregut.

The entoderm of the area pellucida arises from invaginated cells in the anterior region of the primitive streak at stage 2 and this phenomenon continues up to stage 4 of Hamburger and Hamilton. However, the vitelline entoderm is formed from the internal margin of the area opaca.

Gallera and Nicolet (1969) showed that the embryonic entoderm in the anterior portion of the primitive streak possesses a powerful inducing activity throughout the period of its invagination, whereas entoderm whose localization is already established and the floor of the foregut are devoid of any inducing activity.

3. Blastodermal Potentialities for Regulation

Investigations on splitting of the blastoderm carried out in duck eggs *in ovo* have shown the extent to which this blastoderm is capable of regulation (see Lutz of this account).

Using Nicolet and Gallera's culture technique (see Ch. VI, Nicolet and Gallera, 1963), Lutz-Ostertag, Beaudenon, and Billaud (1965) explanted the blastoderms from nonincubated hen's egg and demonstrated the existence of a posteroanterior gradient of development, whereas the duck blastoderm is totipotential. The authors attributed this difference in behavior between the chick and the duck blastoderm to a difference in the developmental stages at the time of laying.

Eyal-Giladi and Spratt (1965) carried out transplantation experiments on isolated portions of chick blastoderm at different stages. They used either very early blastoderms from nonincubated winter eggs or older blastoderms from nonincubated summer eggs or from winter eggs incubated for 4–5 hours. They explanted a semicircular central zone onto Spratt and Haas' culture medium (see Ch. VI, Spratt and Haas, 1960) for 3–4 days.

With very early blastoderms (nonincubated winter eggs), central fragments formed an embryo, while at a more advanced stage (nonincubated summer eggs), the fragments lost this capacity. In the course of development this embryogenic capacity was first confined to the entire marginal zone and subsequently to only the posterior part of this same zone. When even older blastoderms were used (stage prior to the formation of the primitive streak, after extension of the endoderm), the central fragments of ectoderm with the underlying entoderm were once more capable of forming an embryo.

The authors concluded that the early chick blastoderm shows the same capacities for development as the duck blastoderm. In both cases the capacity to form an embryo is not initially confined to the marginal zone alone. It is also present in the central region of the early blastoderm but is normally dominated by the posterior marginal zone.

Eyal-Giladi (1969) confirmed these investigations. He folded both incubated and nonincubated early chick blastoderms (up to the stage of the primitive streak) either along their longitudinal axis or else perpendicularly to this axis and studied the subsequent differentiation. The results showed that the longitudinal folding did not modify the capacity for embryonic differentiation, but that blastoderms folded perpendicularly to the axis give rise to various types of embryonic formations. The embryos developed, either conforming with the original posteroanterior orientation of the blastoderm or perpendicularly to the initial posteroanterior orientation. Certain blastoderms showed both types of development, giving rise to crossed embryonic formations.

The author observed that the left side of the blastoderms possessed a greater embryogenic potential than did the right side. Furthermore, in other experiments on very early blastoderms the posterior embryonic center was inactive, whereas with older blastoderms this posterior marginal zone showed an increasing embryogenic capacity. These results confirm the author's previous investigations (Eyal-Giladi and Spratt, 1965).

Spratt and Haas (1967) studied the nutritional requirements of the young chick blastoderm during the process of regulation and attempted to determine whether the composition of the culture medium influenced the blastodermal capacities for regeneration. They compared the results obtained in culture on a variety of nutrient media with those obtained by splitting the blastoderm *in ovo* (see Ch. VI, Lutz' method, 1949).

These experiments were carried out on intact blastoderms and fragments of blastoderms (6, 12, and 20 hours of incubation).

Whole-egg extract provided a very good medium, in all cases producing 100% embryonic formations.

Using an albumin-based extract, there was embryonic development for 90% of whole blastoderms, but only for 40–55% of the explanted blastoderm fragments.

Media containing smaller amounts of nutrient substances inhibited the formation of embryos. White's synthetic medium gave 61% of embryos from whole blastoderms, and on a glucose-based medium only 24% of whole blastoderms produced embryonic axes.

The embryogenic capacity of an early blastoderm fragment explanted *in vitro* depends not only on the stage, size, and intrinsic growth of the blastoderm but also on the nutrient properties of the culture medium.

4. Localization and Migration of Germ Cells

New experiments carried out by Dubois (1965, 1966) have provided further evidence for the earlier hypothesis that the young germinal epithelium exerts a selective attraction on the primordial cells of the germinal crescent and on the primary gonocytes of chick embryo gonads. Dubois showed that this phenomenon of attraction is exercised by means of a diffusible substance which originates in the germinal epithelium and which acts directly on the germinal cells (for details of these experiments see Chapter IV - Differentiation and Intersexuality *in Vitro* by K. Haffen).

Dubois' investigations (1967a,b) afforded some interesting details concerning the origin of the primordial germ cells and their localization in the nonincubated blastula of chick embryo.

The blastodiscs were taken from nonincubated eggs, oriented according to Van Baer's rule (1828), and were placed on Wolff and Haffen's culture medium with the outer layer or ectophyllum laid face down on the medium. After cutting off the anterior quarter of the blastoderm a fragment of eggshell membrane was inserted between the outer and inner layers. Carbon particles placed on the endophyllum were used as a labeling device, and the whole was cultured for 48 hours. Morphogenetic movements pushed the inner layer onto the eggshell membrane in those cases in which the embryonic axis coincided with the axis of orientation. The outer and inner layers were thus separated, and the author observed the differentiation of germinal cells *in vitro* in each of the layers.

In a second series of experiments, the author cultured anterior and posterior blastula fragments, cut off from a diametric strip of tissue, in a fold of vitelline membrane. In this way he was able to observe the behavior of primordial cells in early blastula prior to separation of the layers, and to make a detailed study of gonocyte distribution at the time of the experiment.

The results of these investigations showed that at the time of laying, the primordial germinal cells lie in a transverse band perpendicular to the embryonic axis. They are distinctly predominant in the posterior region. Subsequently, when the egg is incubated, caudocephalic morphogenetic movements push the germinal cells forward into the extraembryonic area of the crescent.

The germinal cells originate in the inner layer (vitelline endoderm) of the nonincubated blastula. They migrate by ameboid movement, leaving the deep vitelline layers, and coming to occupy the entodermal or mesodermal layers of the postgastrula.

5. Development of the Vascular Area *in Vitro*

Using the blastoderm-culture technique, Hell (1964), Deuchar and Dryland (1964), and Manelli, Raunick, Mastrolia, Gardenghi, and Callegarini (1966) studied the development of the vascular area and the differentiation and synthesis of hemoglobin.

B. Nutritional Requirements

Klein, McConnell, and Buckingham (1962) studied the growth of 11- to 13-somite chick embryos which had been cultured for 24 or 48 hours on Hayashi and Hermann's synthetic medium. They showed that, among the amino acids studied, the chick embryo required leucine or lysine primarily, while aspartic acid and proline were not essential.

According to the work of Klein, McConnell, and Riquier (1964), culture of young blastoderms (11–13 somites, 40 hours of incubation) on a medium composed of whole-egg homogenate was particularly successful with high concentrations of oxygen in the air. The best gaseous environment was a mixture of 75% air and 25% oxygen at the beginning of culture (0–24 hours) followed by a mixture of 95% oxygen and 5% carbon dioxide (from 24 to 48 hours). This allowed good embryonic survival, with 86% of the embryos continuing to develop for 72 hours. Under these conditions the levels of protein nitrogen and DNA increased by factors of 18.4 and 12.7, respectively.

C. Action of Various Inhibitory Factors on the Development of Blastoderms

Antibiotics affect early embryonic development. The effects of *actinomycin D* on morphogenesis and nucleic acid metabolism in chick embryo were studied Heilporn-Pohl (1964).

Embryos at the primitive streak stage (10 hours of incubation) or at the stage of the fully formed primitive streak (18 hours of incubation) were explanted using Spratt's method onto a medium containing actinomycin D (0.1–15 μg/ml) and cultured for 5–16 hours. Differentiation of the nervous system was inhibited with the inhibition intensity being the greater the earlier the stage at which treatment was applied. When early neurulas were subjected to the action of actinomycin D the anterior part of the nervous system was normal but the posterior portion showed malformations.

The author also studied nucleic acid metabolism using autoradiographic methods. After observing the incorporation of ^{3}H-uridine into the cells of explanted embryos, it was found that 5 and 8 hours of treatment with actinomycin D inhibited ^{3}H-uridine uptake by 50 and 70–80% respectively. This inhibition took place primarily at the cytoplasmic level. In the treated embryo, as opposed to controls, nuclear radioactivity was higher than that of the cytoplasm. From these experiments the author concluded that actinomycin D inhibits the transfer of nuclear RNA into the cytoplasm.

Another antibiotic, antimycin A, which is a powerful metabolic inhibitor with a specific effect on the succinate-oxidase system has been tested by

Ebert *et al*. Duffey and Ebert (1957) and McKenzie and Ebert (1960) cultured blastoderms using Spratt's method and New's method and obtained the inhibition of heart and somite formation. These effects depended upon the way in which the toxic substance was administered to the embryo, and on whether the explant was laid with the ventral or the dorsal surface down on the culture medium. The heart and the somites were found to be sensitive to the action of antimycin A in doses of $0.01–0.0035 \, \mu g/ml$ of the medium at different stages of development. At stages 4 and 5 the inhibition affected the heart, while the somites were affected at more advanced stages. Reporter and Ebert (1965) in a subsequent investigation isolated a factor from an aqueous extract of chick liver mitochondria, and found that this factor strongly counteracted the effects of antimycin A. The embryos, explanted at stage 5–8 of Hamburger and Hamilton, were subjected to the action of antimycin for 6 hours. When this factor was present in the culture medium, the effects of antimycin A were canceled and the embryonic somites formed normally. The authors inferred from these results that part of the protein might be capable of combining with antimycin A in the embryo. However, this protective effect has not been observed in the case of the cardiac rudiment. The authors showed further that all compounds that interfere with mitochondrial oxidative phosphorylation also affect embryogenesis.

Various inhibitors, e.g., fluorouracil, chloramphenicol, and acetylpyridine, have been found to affect the development of blood vessels in the extraembryonic region to varying degrees, shown by the work of Newburgh, Clark, Wilson, and Scholz (1964). They also observed an inhibition of DNA, RNA, and protein levels in embryos when treated with chloramphenicol $(7.5 \, \mu g/ml$ of the medium), but found an increase after treatment with acetylpyridine $(100 \, \mu g/ml)$. The same number of somites developed in the presence of either inhibitor. Differentiation was thus accomplished even in the absence of growth, taking place at the expense of existing DNA, RNA, and proteins, with degradation of these compounds exceeding synthesis in some cases. In the extraembryonic area, only 5-fluorouracil $(50 \, \mu g/ml$ of medium) inhibited the level of RNA, DNA, and proteins.

Certain enzyme activities have been measured after the action of inhibitors. Different results were obtained for the embryonic and the extraembryonic area. Acetylpyridine affected all enzymes (glucose-6-phosphatase, 6-phosphogluconic dehydrogenase, and isocitric dehydrogenase) in the extraembryonic area, but those of the embryo itself were not affected. Buckingham and Herrmann (1967) found that embryos explanted at the 11- to 13-somite stage and cultured in the presence of 3-acetylpyridine $(100 \, \mu g/ml)$ for 24 hours showed a growth inhibition. Measurements of protein nitrogen and studies of ^{14}C-glycine incorporation into treated embryos were used as criteria of growth.

The level of protein nitrogen diminished in the central nervous system and in the lateral mesoderm when the embryos were treated with acetylpyridine.

Reporter and Ebert (1965) and Bowman (1967) tested the effect of 2,4-dinitrophenol, an inhibitor of oxidative phosphorylation, on the *in vitro* development of chick embryos. Concentrations of 10^{-4} to $2 \times 10^{-3}M$ were used. Dinitrophenol in concentration of 10^{-4} to $2 \times 10^{-3}M$ caused degeneration and sometimes complete absence of the nervous system, with reduction or inhibition in the number of somites, while the heart, notochord, and blood islands were unaffected.

Billett, Collini, and Hamilton (1965), and Colombo, Notarniola, Micciarelli, and Pinamonti (1964) studied the effects of chloramphenicol, which was found to inhibit closure of the posterior part of the neural tube and the formation of blood islets in the vascular area. The anomalies were accompanied by a reduction in the surface area of the blastoderm and the vascular zone. The teratological reaction is due to an inhibition of protein synthesis.

Various sulfhydryl-group inhibitors have been tested on blastoderms explanted *in vitro*, at the stage of the primitive streak and the head process. Among these are chloroacetophenone (Lakshmi, 1962; Lakshmi and Mulkerkar, 1963), chloropicrin (Joshi, 1968), and colchicine (Diwan, 1966). The latter affects cell division, probably by acting on the sulfhydryl groups of the spindle proteins.

The authors studied the action of these substances on embryonic morphogenesis and on the inductive capacity of Hensen's node. After treatment, the latter was grafted into a host blastoderm, using Waddington's method.

All the experiments showed that morphogenesis was disturbed. The cerebral region and the nervous system were specifically affected and were malformed. Depending on the dose used, the inductive capacity of Hensen's node diminished and even disappeared. With increasing dosage, a decrease in the number and quality of induced neural structures was observed.

Some protection against the effects of colchicine was obtained after treatment with cysteine hydrochloride.

II. *IN VITRO* CULTURE OF MAMMALIAN EGGS

A. Culture and Nutritional Requirements

Many workers have investigated the nutritional requirements of eggs from the 2-cell to the blastocyst stage (see general articles by New, 1966; Brinster, 1968; Nalbandov and Cook, 1968). According to Brinster (1968), the medium generally used for the culture of mammalian eggs consists of a solution of Krebs-Ringer bicarbonate with a sodium bicarbonate buffer, a gaseous atmosphere of 5% CO_2, a pH of about 7.4, protein at a concentration of 1–10 mg/ml, glucose (1 mg/ml), and pyruvate in concentrations of $5 \times 10^{-4}M$.

Other media have been tried, but the development of eggs explanted *in vitro* proceeded no further than the blastocyst stage.

The conditions for blastocyst development have recently been analyzed by Daniel (1969) and by Bitton-Casimiri and Psychoyos (1968, 1969). Daniel demonstrated the presence of a specific glucoprotein (blastokinin) in the uterine secretion of rabbits during the preimplantation phase that might control growth and differentiation of the blastocyst. This factor stimulated the synthesis of nucleic acids and proteins; the action was inhibited by actinomycin D. In addition, rabbit blastokinin stimulated the *in vitro* growth of resting blastocysts from mammals with delayed implantation.

According to Bitton-Casimiri and Psychoyos, the uterus contains a factor that plays a part in the phenomena of dissolution of the zona pellucida in the rat blastocyst, this liberation taking place later *in vitro* than *in vivo*. The authors compared the specific activities of RNA in resting and in normal blastocysts, and found that 2 hours after removal from the uterus ^{3}H-uridine uptake by blastocysts from animals with delayed implantation was 75% lower than that of normal blastocysts. However, 22 hours after removal the radioactivity of delayed blastocysts was 20 times higher than that observed 2 hours after removal from the uterus. The authors concluded that the RNA synthetic activity of blastocysts subjected to delayed implantation was repressed, but that this repression was released when the blastocysts were removed from the uterine environment.

Rat embryos removed at stages after implantation have been cultured successfully by New (1967) in a "circulating" medium. The culture medium was composed of homologous serum equilibrated with a gaseous mixture of 95% oxygen and 5% carbon dioxide. Fifty percent of embryos explanted at 7- to 15-somite or 22- to 28-somite stages reached 30- to 35-somite and 40- to 46-somite stages, respectively. During these periods of culture the embryos synthesized considerable quantities of protein: 0.3–0.5 and 1.0–1.5 mg. Embryos removed at the 45-somite stage did not develop. Using this culture method, Givelber and Di Paolo (1968) obtained survival and growth of 8-day-old hamster embryos for 48 hours.

Using radioactive precursors incorporated into the culture medium, Mintz (1964, 1965), Ellem and Gwatkin (1968), Woodland and Graham (1969), and Brinster (1969) studied the synthesis of nucleic acids and proteins during embryonic development from the 2-celled to the blastocyst stage. Mintz (1964) and Silagi (1963) tested the action of actinomycin D on the development of normal embryos and t^{12}/t^{12} mutants and on their RNA synthesis. Mutant embryos died at the morula stage and showed a deficiency in cytoplasmic and nucleolar RNA levels. With increasing doses of actinomycin $10^{-6}–10^{-5}M$, the development of normal and mutant eggs was inhibited. The nucleoli were most strongly affected and there was a distinct decrease in

RNA synthesis, while protein synthesis was resistant to treatment at these doses.

The successful culture of early mammalian embryos has made it possible not only to investigate the metabolism and nutritional requirements of young embryos, but also to carry out valuable experiments on these early stages by combining two methods: culture followed by implantation into a host organism.

B. Experimental Research on Mammalian Eggs

1. FUSION OF EGGS

Investigations on the fusion of mammalian eggs and the production of chimeras have been carried out by Mintz (1962a,b,c, 1963, 1964a,b,c, 1965a,b,c, 1967) and Tarkowski (1962, 1964a,b, 1968; also see Ch. VI, Tarkowski, 1961).

Mouse eggs were freed of the zona pellucida, either by mechanical means (Tarkowski, 1962) or by digestion with pronase (Mintz, 1962). Two or more eggs, at stages 8–32, were associated and then cultured *in vitro* until they had reached the blastocyst stage.

The culture medium used by Mintz (1964a) was as follows: 50% calf fetus serum; 50% Eagle's solution containing 0.002% of phenol red; lactic acid at a concentration of 1.0 mg/ml of medium. The pH was adjusted to 7.

The author used a culture chamber that permitted the maintenance of a constant gaseous atmosphere (5% carbon dioxide in air). The technique developed by Tarkowski has been described earlier.

After culture, the embryos were grafted into the oviduct or uterus of a pseudogestational mouse, where they continued to develop until birth. Some of them became adult. Mintz (1965a) obtained 34% survival at birth. Other associations of various types have been carried out: (1) fusion of normal eggs, one of them labeled with ^{3}H-thymidine so that the fate of cells could be observed (Mintz, 1965b); (2) association of eggs of differing genetic constitution.

Egg cytoplasm can show different types and degrees of granulation. For example, Mintz (1965b) used eggs from strain C57BL/6 with large granules and eggs strain Icr with fine granules. A third association, fusion of normal eggs and eggs from lethal mutants, was carried out by Mintz (1963, 1964).

The homozygous t_{12}/t_{12} mutants died in the uterus before reaching the blastocyst stage. At the morula stage, a characteristic deficiency of RNA was observed, both in the cytoplasm and the nucleolus. However, the mosaics arising from the fusion of normal and mutant blastomeres developed into blastocysts.

All these experiments show the great lability of the mouse egg during segmentation.

a. *Study of Pigmentation.* Coat pigmentation provides a method of distinguishing strains. The combination of eggs of strain C57BL/6 non-Agouti and C3Hf Agouti produced mice showing three types of pigmentation: black, Agouti, and dappled. In a recent experiment Mintz (1967) studied the distribution of pigmentation in mosaic mice. The observations were carried out on a total of seven combinations of genotypes, homozygous for the melanocyte. Some of the animals developed from these associations had uniformly colored coats, while others showed a characteristic pattern of pigmentation: large transverse stripes of regularly alternating color, which covered the head (three stripes), the body (six stripes), and the tail (eight stripes).

After studying the distribution of melanocytes in the coat, the author concluded that all the melanocytes in the adult coat arise from a cellular clone of 34 primordial melanoblasts arranged as two longitudinal chains in the dorsal region, each chain being made up of 17 melanoblasts. This distinct separation down the middle of the back seems to indicate that the two sides are established autonomously. In these chains, the genes determining pigment differentiation are active in the young embryo and then become stabilized. Each clone of melanoblasts is derived from the proliferation of a single cell.

The problem of pigmentation in mouse chimeras has also been studied by Tarkowski (see the first part of this account). The investigations have recently been supplemented by studies on coat pigmentation and pigmentation of the external layer of the retina, and by karyological examination of the bone marrow (Tarkowski, 1964; Mystkowska and Tarkowski, 1968).

Of a total of nine adult mice arising from a combination CBA-T_6T_6/CBA-p, seven showed characteristics of chimerism. CBA/HT_6T_6 have two small chromosomes in their cells by which they can be distinguished from cells of a normal karyotype. Pigmentation is of the Agouti type. The type CBA-p with pink eyes has a light coat and its karyotype is normal. According to the author's observations, both types of pigment cell were present in the coat and the retina but the participation of the two cell types varied from one individual to another. Karyological examination of bone marrow cells led to the same conclusions.

b. *Study of Sexuality.* Mintz (1965b) and Tarkowski (1964a,b, 1968) studied the sexual development of these chimeric animals and obtained hermaphroditic mice. Mintz described a 2-month-old subject with a mosaic character in which the external appearance was male, while the mouse showed primarily female characteristics on the right side (ovotestis, oviduct, and uterus) and a male apparatus on the left.

Tarkowski (1964), and Mystkowska and Tarkowski (1968) extended the previous investigations. Nine of 14 neonates obtained by fusion between eggs of strains CBA-p and CBA-T_6T_6 attained maturity. The distribution of the sexes in the nine adult individuals and the three neonates that were sexually identified was as follows: 9 males♂♂, 1 male♂, and 2 females♀♀.

The hermaphrodite showed an ovotestis on the right side, composed of both ovarian and testicular tissue, while the reproductive apparatus on the left was of the male type. In one neonate mouse the authors found typical oocytes in the growth phase within the male genital cords.

The authors noted the high proportion of male subjects in their experiments. Cytological examinations revealed that some of these males were sexual chimeras, possessing a mosaic of sex chromosomes.

2. Action of Various Factors on Embryonic Development

Seidel showed that destruction of one or two blastomeres scarcely disturbed the normal development of the rabbit embryo. Daniel and Takahashi destroyed some of the blastomeres in rabbit eggs at the 2-, 4-, 8-, and 16-blastomere stages using a laser. Culture *in vitro* was then carried out to determine the segmentation capacity of the blastomeres surviving the treatment. It was found that embryos developed normally in all cases, despite the presence of injured blastomeres.

Benoit studied the regulatory capacity of $7\frac{1}{2}$-day-old mouse gastrulas after X-ray irradiation of the axial region, either in front of or behind Hensen's node. The embryos were cultured for 24–42 hours on a liquid medium based on foal serum. Those with best development reached the 12- to 15-somite stage. These experiments show that the older gastrula has a certain capacity for regulation after irradiation. However, the author observed certain deficiences in the cephalic neurectoderm and the lateral plate mesoderm although the notochord always developed. Last, despite the effects of irradiation, neurogenic induction did occur and a nervous system was formed.

Using New and Stein's technique Turbow (1965) cultured 5- to 14-somite rat embryos and treated them with 0.05–0.4% solutions of trypan blue. He observed the appearance of various malformations: edema, dilatation of the heart and pericardium, retardation of growth, and deterioration of cardiovascular function. Compounds related to trypan blue had no teratogenic or toxic action.

BIBLIOGRAPHY

1. Benoit J.   Irradiations localisées *in vitro* de gastrulas de Souris. *C. R. Acad. Sci.*, 1969, **268**, 371–374.
2. Billett F. S., Collini R. and Hamilton L.   The effects of D- and L-threo-chloramphenicol on the early development of the chick embryo. *J. Embryol. exp. Morph.*, 1965, **13**, 341–356.

3. Bitton-Casimiri V. and Psychoyos A. Développement du blastocyste du Rat *in vitro*. *C. R. Acad. Sci.*, 1968, **267**, 762–764.

4. Bitton-Casimiri V. and Psychoyos A. Captation *in vitro* d'un précurseur d'acide ribonucléique (ARN) uridine-5 ^{3}H par le blastocyste du Rat; différences entre blastocystes normaux et blastocystes en diapause. *C. R. Acad. Sci.*, 1969, **268**, 188–190.

5. Bowman P. The effect of 2,4-dinitrophenol on the development of early chick embryos. *J. Embryol. exp. Morph.*, 1967, **17**, 425–431.

6. Brinster R. L. Culture of mammalian embryos. *J. Anim. Sci.*, 1968, Suppl. 27. Also see Nalbandov and Cook (1968).

7. Brinster R. L. Metabolism of pre-implantation mammalian embryos. *Research in Reproduction*, 1969, **1**, 2–3.

8. Buckingham B. J. and Herrmann H. The effect of 3-acetylpyridine on the explanted chick embryo. *J. Embryol. exp. Morph.*, 1967, **17**, 239–246.

9. Butros J. Differentiation in explanted fragments of early chick blastoderms. I. Culture techniques. *J. exp. Zool.*, 1963, **152**, 57–66.

10. Colombo G., Notarniola L., Micciarelli A. and Pinamonti S. Gli effetti del chloramfenicolo su embrioni di pollo expiatati *in vitro*. *Acta Embryol. Morph. exp.*, 1964, **7**, 89.

11. Daniel J. C. Jr. Maternal control of nucleic acid and protein synthesis in the mammalian embryo prior to implantation. VI° Congrès International d'Embryologie, Paris, 1968. *Ann. Embryol. Morph.* Suppl. 1–1969, 276.

12. Daniel J. C. and Takahashi K. Selective laser destruction of rabbits' blastomeres and continued cleavage of survivors *in vitro*. *Exp. Cell Research*, 1965, **39**, 475–482.

13. Deuchar E. and Dryland A. Effects of methyl norvaline on synthesis of haemoglobin in the area vasculosa of the chick embryo. *Nature*, 1964, **201**, 832–833.

14. Diwan B. A. A study of the effects of colchicine on the process of morphogenesis and induction in chick embryos. *J. Embryol. exp. Morph.*, 1966, **16**, 245–257.

15. Dubois R. Sur l'attraction exercée par le jeune épithelium germinatif sur les gonocytes primaires de l'embryon de Poulet, en culture *in vitro:* démonstration à l'aide de la thymidine tritiée. *C. R. Acad. Sci.*, 1965, **260**, 5885–5887.

16. Dubois R. L'attraction exercée par le jeune épithélium germinatif sur les cellules germinales de l'embryon de Poulet est un phénomène d'ordre chimiotactique: démonstration en culture *in vitro*. *C. R. Acad. Sci.*, 1966, **262**, 2623–2626.

17. Dubois R. Sur l'origine et l'amoeboïdisme des cellules germinales de l'embryon de Poulet en culture *in vitro* et leur localisation dans le germe non incubé. *C. R. Acad. Sci.*, 1967a, **265**, 497–500.

18. Dubois R. Localisation et migration des cellules germinales du blastoderme non incubé de Poulet d'après les résultats de cultures *in vitro*. *Arch. Anat. micr. Morph. exp.*, 1967b, **56**, 245–264.

19. Duffey L. M. and Ebert J. D. Metabolic characteristics of heart-forming areas of the early chick embryo. *J. Embryol. exp. Morph.*, 1957, **5**, 324–339.

20. Ellem K. A. O. and Gwatkin R. B. L. Patterns of nucleic acid synthesis in the early mouse embryo. *Develop. Biol.*, 1968, **18**, 311–330.

21. Eyal-Giladi H. Dynamic aspects of neural induction in amphibia. *Arch. Biol.*, *Liége*, 1954, **65**, 179–259.

22. Eyal-Giladi H. Differentiation potencies of the young chick blastoderms as revealed by different manipulations. I. Folding experiments and position effects of the culture medium. *J. Embryol. exp. Morph.*, **21**, 177–192.

23. Eyal-Giladi H. and Spratt N. T. Jr.   The embryo-forming potencies of the young chick blastoderm. *J. Embryol. exp. Morph.*, 1965, **13**, 267–273.
24. Gallera J.   Excision et transplantation des différentes régions de la ligne primitive chez le Poulet. *Bull. Assoc. Anat. Paris*, 1965*a*, **125**, 632–639.
25. Gallera J.   Quelle est la durée nécessaire pour déclencher des inductions neurales chez le Poulet? *Experientia*, 1965*b*, **21**, 218–219.
26. Gallera J.   Induction neurale chez les oiseaux. Rapport temporel entre la neurulation du blastoderme hôte et l'apparition d'une ébauche neurale induite par un fragment de la ligne primitive. *Rev. Suisse Zool.*, 1968, **75**, 227–234.
27. Gallera J.   Évolution intrinsèque de l'ectoblaste et induction neurale chez les Oiseaux. VIᵉ Congrès International d'Embryologie, Paris, 1968. *Ann. Embryol. Morph.* Suppl. 1–1969, 273.
28. Gallera J. and Ivanov I.   La compétence neurogène du feuillet externe du blastoderme de Poulet en fonction du facteur "temps." *J. Embryol. exp. Morph.*, 1964, **12**, 693–711.
29. Gallera J. and Nicolet G.   Le pouvoir inducteur de l'endoblaste présomptif contenu dans la ligne primitive jeune de Poulet. *J. Embryol. exp. Morph.*, 1969, **21**, 105–118.
30. Givelber H. M. and Di Paolo J. A.   Growth of explanted eight day hamster embryos in circulating medium. *Nature*, 1968, **220**, 1131–1133.
31. Heilporn-Pohl V.   Effets de l'actinomycine D sur la morphogenèse et le métabolisme des acides nucléiques chez l'embryon de Poulet. *J. Embryol. exp. Morph.*, 1964, **12**, 439–446.
32. Hell A.   The initial synthesis of haemoglobin in deembryonated chick blastoderms. I. Metabolism of the blastodisc cultured *in vitro*. II. The effect of metabolic inhibitors on the blastodisc cultured *in vitro*. *J. Embryol. exp. Morph.*, 1964, **12**, 609–619, 621–632.
33. Joshi S. S.   Effect of chloropicrin on the early development of chick embryo. *Arch. Entw. Mech. Org.*, 1968, **160**, 237–242.
34. Klein N. W., McConnell E. and Buckingham B. J.   Growth of explanted chick embryos on a chemically defined medium and effects of specific amino acid deficiencies. *Develop. Biol.*, 1962, **5**, 296–308.
35. Klein N. W., McConnell E. and Riquier D. J.   Enhanced growth and survival of explanted chick embryos cultured under high levels of oxygen. *Develop. Biol.*, 1964, **10**, 17–44.
36. Lakshmi M. S.   I. The effect of chloracetophenone on chick embryos cultured *in vitro*. II. The effect of chloracetophenone on the inducing capacity of Hensen's node. *J. Embryol. exp. Morph.*, 1962, **10**, 373–382, 383–388.
37. Lakshmi M. S. and Mulkerkar L.   Paper chromatographic study of the role of sulphur containing amino acids in the process of induction in the chick embryo. *Experientia*, 1963, **19**, 155–156.
38. Leikola A. and McCallion D. J.   Time required for heterogenous induction in chick embryo ectoderm. *Experientia*, 1967, **23**, 869.
39. Lutz-Ostertag Y., Beaudenon Th. and Billaud M. C.   Culture *in vitro* de blastodermes non incubés d'oiseaux et développement de parties isolées. *C. R. Soc. Biol.*, 1965, **159**, 1489–1491.
40. McKenzie J. and Ebert J. D.   The inhibitory action of antimycin A in the early chick embryo. *J. Embryol. exp. Morph.*, 1960, **8**, 314–320.
41. Manelli H., Raunick L., Mastrolia L., Gardenghi G. and Callegarini C.   Cell and hemoglobin differentiation in explants of the area vasculosa in the chick embryo. *Acta Embryol. Morph. exp.*, 1966, **9**, 169–186.

42. Mintz B. Formation of genotypically mosaic mouse embryos. *Amer. Zool.*, 1962*a*, **2**, 310.

43. Mintz B. Incorporation of nucleic acid and protein precursors by developing mouse eggs. *Amer. Zool.*, 1962*b*, **2**, 189.

44. Mintz B. Experimental study of the developing mammalian egg: removal of the zona pellucida. *Science*, 1962*c*, **138**, 594–595.

45. Mintz B. Growth *in vitro* of t^{12}/t^{12} lethal mutant mouse eggs. *Amer. Zool.*, 1963, **3**, 317.

46. Mintz B. Formation of genetically mosaic mouse embryos and early development of lethal t^{12}/t^{12} normal mosaics. *J. exp. Zool.*, 1964*a*, **157**, 273–292.

47. Mintz B. Gene expression in the morula stage of mouse embryos, as observed during development of t^{12}/t^{12} lethal mutants *in vitro*. *J. exp. Zool.*, 1964*b*, **157**, 267–272.

48. Mintz B. Synthetic process and early development in the mammalian egg. *J. exp. Zool.*, 1964*c*, **157**, 85–100.

49. Mintz B. Genetic mosaicism in adult mice of quadriparental lineage. *Science*, 1965*a*, **148**, 1232–1233.

50. Mintz B. Experimental genetic mosaicism in the mouse. *Ciba Found. Symp. Preimplantation Stages of Pregnancy*, 1965*b*, pp. 194–207.

51. Mintz B. Nucleic acid and protein synthesis in the developing mouse embryo. *Ciba Found. Symp. Preimplantation Stages of Pregnancy*, 1965*c*, pp. 145–155.

52. Mintz B. Gene control of mammalian pigmentary differentiation. I. Clonal origin of melanocytes. *Proc. Nat. Acad. Sci.*, 1967, **58**, 344–351.

53. Modak S. P. Sur l'origine de l'hypoblaste chez les oiseaux. *Experientia*, 1965, **21**, 273–274.

54. Mystkowska E. T. and Tarkowski A. K. Observations on CBA-*p*/CBA-T_6T_6 mouse chimeras. *J. Embryol. exp. Morph.*, 1968, **20**, 33–52.

55. Nalbandov A. V. and Cook B. Reproduction (*in vitro* culture of eggs and embryos). *Ann. Rev. Physiol.*, 1968, **30**, 245–278.

56. New D. A. T. "The Culture of Vertebrate Embryos," 245 pp. Academic Press (Logos), New York, 1966.

57. New D. A. T. Development of explanted rat embryos in circulating medium. *J. Embryol. exp. Morph.*, 1967, **17**, 513–525.

58. Newburgh R. W., Clark A., Wilson A. and Scholz M. Effect of various inhibitors on several enzymes and other biochemical substances in chick embryo explants. *J. Embryol. exp. Morph.*, 1964, **12**, 219–227.

59. Nicolet G. Étude autoradiographique de la destination des cellules invaginées au niveau du nœud de Hensen de la ligne primitive achevée de l'embryon de Poulet. *Acta Embryol. Morph. exp.*, 1965, **8**, 213–220.

60. Nicolet G. La chronologie d'invagination chez le Poulet. Étude à l'aide de thymidine tritiée. *Experientia*, 1967, **23**, 576–577.

61. Nieuwkoop P. D. Activation and organization of the central nervous system in amphibians. I. Induction and activation. II. Differentiation and organization. III. Synthesis of a new working hypothesis. *J. exp. Zool.*, 1952, **120**, 1–108.

62. Rao B. R. The appearance and extension of neural differentiation tendencies in the neurectoderm of the early chick embryo. *Arch. Entw. Mech. Org.*, 1968, **160**, 187–236.

63. Reporter M. C. and Ebert J. D. A mitochondrial factor that prevents the effects of antimycin A on myogenesis. *Develop. Biol.*, 1965, **12**, 154–184.

64. Silagi S. Some aspects of the relationship of RNA metabolism to development in normal and mutant mouse embryos cultivated *in vitro*. *Exp. Cell Research*, 1963, **32**, 149–152.

65. Spratt N. T. and Haas H.   Nutritional requirements for the realization of regulative (repair) capacities of young chick blastoderms. *J. exp. Zool.*, 1967, **164**, 31–46.

66. Tarkowski A. K.   Studies on mouse chimeras developed from eggs fused *in vitro*. The 13th Annual Meeting of the Tissue Culture Association, Washington, D.C., 1962.

67. Tarkowski A. K.   Patterns of pigmentation in experimentally produced mouse chimaeras. *J. Embryol. exp. Morph.*, 1964a, **12**, 575–585.

68. Tarkowski A. K.   True hermaphroditism in chimeric mice. *J. Embryol. exp. Morph.*, 1964b, **12**, 735–757.

69. Turbow M. M.   Trypan blue induced teratogenesis of rat embryos cultivated *in vitro*. *J. Embryol. exp. Morph.*, 1965, **15**, 387–395.

70. Vakaet L.   Some new data concerning the formation of the definitive endoblast in the chick embryo. *J. Embryol. exp. Morph.*, 1962, **10**, 38–57.

71. Vakaet L.   Diversité fonctionnelle de la ligne primitive du blastoderme de Poulet. *C. R. Soc. Biol.*, 1964, **158**, 1964–1966.

72. Vakaet L.   Résultats de la greffe de nœud de Hensen d'âge différent sur le blastoderme de Poulet. *C. R. Soc. Biol.*, **159**, 232–233.

73. Woodland H. R. and Graham C. F.   RNA synthesis during early development of mouse. *Nature*, 1969, **221**, 327–332.

CHAPTER VII

ORGAN CULTURE
IN THE INVERTEBRATES

C. Ziller-Sengel

INSTITUT D'EMBRYOLOGIE ET DE TÉRATOLOGIE EXPÉRIMENTALE
DU COLLÈGE DE FRANCE ET DU C.N.R.S.
PARIS, FRANCE

I. INTRODUCTION

Culture of invertebrate tissues *in vitro* is not as well developed as for the vertebrates. Cell culture of invertebrate tissues has progressed in recent years but organ culture is still in its infancy. Most of the work discussed in this chapter has been carried out in recent years.

The previous lack of progress was essentially due to technical obstacles. The great variety of invertebrate species makes it difficult to find a culture medium that is suitable for each case. The composition of the "milieu interieur" varies from one group to another, and even from one species to another. This is not true for the vertebrates. The sterility of the cultures must also be considered. The internal environment of the invertebrates is very constant. Most species carry bacteria and generally each organ must be sterilized in some way or another before it is explanted onto the culture medium.

Nevertheless, although research is still in its early stages, it is already possible to see that organ culture of invertebrate tissues is a method likely to show as much success as has been obtained with the culture of vertebrate tissues at the present time. Different problems of invertebrate physiology have been tackled indirectly by organ culture, and this chapter will deal with most of the main fields of biology; that is, morphogenesis and differentiation in regeneration and embryonic development, endocrinology, reproduction, genetics, and physiology.

The opportunities offered by this technique for the study of the ability of organs to survive and function outside of the intact organism will be considered. These purely technical experiments are interesting in that they open up the way for experimental research.

The application of organ culture techniques to the study of sexuality will

301

be considered. Much progress has been made recently in this field using organ culture, particularly as it has kept pace with endocrinological research. Organ culture techniques have also been used for the study of hormonal effects, both in vertebrates and in many groups of invertebrates.

Organ culture can be used to good effect in the study of embryogenesis, in the study of the endocrinology of development, and in genetics, particularly in insects.

Many invertebrates possess the capacity for regeneration. Organ culture techniques have made it possible to study certain aspects of morphological regeneration. These four aspects of work on invertebrates will be considered.

II. EXPERIMENTAL TECHNIQUES FOR THE SURVIVAL AND FUNCTION OF VARIOUS ORGANS *IN VITRO*

It is essential to determine the conditions required by each organ for survival and function *in vitro*. It is still not clear what these conditions are among any of the invertebrate groups.

Thomas (68–70) was one of the first workers to change from cell culture to organ culture techniques, and he was able to maintain the survival of explanted organs from many invertebrate species. Survival (3–6 months), marked growth, and some activity *in vitro* were obtained when the "free urns" of *Sipunculus* were cultured. These organs had long been considered to be parasites, but Thomas was able to show, using *in vitro* culture, that they were true epithelial formations freely derived from the coelom. He also showed that certain organs from coelenterates, annelids, crustaceans, and especially echinoderms were able to survive in the simple medium, sea water. Tube feet and pedicellaria from starfish survived and showed *in vitro* activity (tube feet, 5–20 days, and pedicellaria, 3 months). The pedicellaria showed remarkable vitality and muscular activity. It seemed probable that they acquired nutrients in solution through the integuments. They carried out calcium metabolism. In contrast, organs from other groups of echinoderms tended to dedifferentiate *in vitro* under the same conditions. It is possible that this dedifferentiation was due to an exhaustion of the reserves and to the absence of a nervous system.

Bevelander and Martin (9) were able to culture pieces of the mantle of the marine mollusk *Pintata radiata* using mollusk plasma. The mantle functioned normally *in vitro*. There was secretion of conchiolin and the characteristic prismatic layer of the shell was formed.

Fischer-Piette (23, 24) cultured organs from crustaceans. Normal activity of lobster lymphatic gland in culture was obtained. The mitotic count was constant and lymphocytes were produced for 11 days. Demal (16) explanted various insect organs, such as pieces of aorta from *Calliphora* and salivary glands from *Drosophila* larvae. The media employed were based on Wolff and Haffen's medium and contained a physiological saline solution with added nutrient fluids such as chick embryo extract, insect hemolymph, and a synthetic solution. The hanging drop technique was used, and on the medium containing embryo extract the pieces of aorta survived and contractions persisted. Hemolymph was found to totally unsuitable. The salivary glands survived perfectly *in vitro* and did not show the degeneration that they normally undergo in the larva *in vivo*. Demal stressed the favorable effects of embryo extract in these experiments. Larsen (44) observed beating in the embryonic heart of *Blatta in vitro*. On a nutrient medium the pieces of heart survived for more than 260 days and the contractions continued as long as the fragments lived.

Organ culture techniques have recently been applied to the marine invertebrates. These techniques are similar to those developed by Wolff and Haffen (75) for the culture of avian embryonic organs. Sengel (63) explanted several organs from the bivalve mollusk *Barnea candida* and from the ascidian *Ciona intestinalis*. The two media used were derived from those of Wolff and Haffen. The composition of the simplest medium was:

> 7 Parts of 10% agar in Gey's solution
> 6 Parts of sterile sea water with added penicillin

Another medium was enriched with a nutrient fluid:

> 7 Parts 1% agar in Gey's solution
> 4 Parts of sea water
> 2 Parts chick embryo extract

The branchial lamella and the intestinal diverticula of *Barnea* were explanted, as well as the ovary and the heart of *Ciona*. All these organs retained their characteristic structure and remained healthy during the 7 days of culture. Ciliary activity of the branchial lamella and intestinal diverticula of *Barnea* continued throughout the period of culture, as did the contractions of the heart in *Ciona*.

Analogous observations were carried out by Em. Wolff (73, 74) on organs explanted from young specimens of *Limulus (Xiphosura polyphemus)*. The technique was the same as that used by Sengel. The following nutrient fluids were added to the medium:

> *Limulus* lymph
> *Limulus* lymph serum
> chick embryo extract
> chicken plasma
> Parker's solution 199

The dorsal vessel, intestine, nervous system, liver, and gonads were cultured for 4–14 days. The normal structure was retained *in vitro*. Wolff noted that contractions of the dorsal vessel persisted only on a nutrient medium. Some development of neurons *in vitro* was also observed.

Streiff and Peyre (67) also used Wolff and Haffen's technique to culture, *in vitro*, organs from the gastropod mollusk *Calyptraea sinensis*. The medium used was composed of agar, sea water, and egg albumin. All the organs explanted were perfectly preserved, and there was no necrosis. The organs used were the ocular tentacle, the penis, the ovary, the testis, the seminal vesicle, the intestine, and the hepatopancreas. The normal activity of most of the organs continued *in vitro*. Throughout the 17 days of culture the ocular tentacle showed a reflex contraction on stimulation. The penis also remained mobile. Nucleolar activity and RNA synthesis were noted in the ova, while cell division and spermatogenesis occurred in the testis. The intestinal mucous cells functioned normally.

It can be concluded from these experiments that the culture techniques used encouraged normal functional activity *in vitro* as well as survival of the explanted differentiated organs.

The physiologist is able to utilize the technique of explantation with subsequent survival, and in fact experiments on the physiology of explanted organs have already been carried out, but mainly using vertebrate species.

In 1934, Pantin (56) studied *in vitro* the contractions of muscles taken from the crab *Carcinus moenas*, using a perfusion technique. Ripplinger and Joly (58) used the heart muscle of *Helix pomatia* and found that the isolated heart could survive on an appropriate medium. If a homogenate of nerve fibers was added to the medium, cardiac contractions were maintained for 48–72 hours. Snail hemolymph also showed activity as a heart stimulator. After fractionation of the hemolymph, Ripplinger and Joly were able to show that it was the dialyzable fraction and not the protein fraction that acted on the explanted heart. Does the hemolymph dialyzate contain specific heart-stimulating compounds like the nerve homogenate, or does it act merely because of its better ionic composition? *In vitro* culture may provide the answer.

Further experiments on the survival of organs in culture have already been carried out in the course of other research. During a study of the parasites of the mollusk *Planorbis*, Benex (3, 4) obtained the *in vitro* survival of tentacles of this species. The medium used consisted of a physiological solution, antibiotics, and nutrients (glucose, amino acids, yeast extract, *Planorbis* muscle extract, and *Planorbis* blood). The tentacles scarred over in a few hours and survived for about 4 weeks. For the first week they retained their mobility and showed much spontaneous muscular activity.

Then they dedifferentiated. However, survival could be prolonged and dedifferentiation retarded under the influence of the nervous system.

In order to study the physiology of the embryonic development in parthogenesis in the worm *Eisenia foetida*, André (1) defined media whose physical characteristics and nutrient properties were as close as possible to those of the natural medium. The first medium contained a homogenate of cocoons in a physiological saline solution with added glucose. This liquid progressively solidified and coated the ova and explanted embryos, thus reproducing the natural conditions. A second medium contained the nutrient contents of older embryos and was a sirupy, rather viscous fluid. These media supported segmentation and development of the embryos up to the time of hatching.

III. THE USE OF CULTURE TECHNIQUES FOR RESEARCH INTO SEXUALITY

Experiments regarding the survival of organs *in vitro* suggest further work that can be carried out on the study of the function of explanted organs, their capacity for differentiation, and the factors influencing this differentiation. The gonads are among the most interesting organs in invertebrates, as in the vertebrates. Differentiation occurs in the gonads throughout the life of the animal and this differentiation is not irreversible, as can be seen from experiments on sexual inversion in vertebrates. In many invertebrates sexual inversion is spontaneous and normal. There are hermaphrodite species where the individuals are male at certain times and female at others. In other species the sex is determined once for all. Sexual differentiation and the modifications occurring in the region of the genital glands are under the control of hormonal factors. The gonads are thus chosen for experimentation but research into sexual endocrinology, which is advanced in the vertebrates, is just beginning in the invertebrates. *In vitro* organ culture has already been carried out in different groups.

A. Sexual Differentiation *in Vitro*

Several authors have attempted to obtain the occurrence of sexual differentiation, that is, spermatogenesis and oogenesis during culture, in the absence of specific endocrine secretions. Germinal cells were taken at various definite stages in their development and an attempt was made to determine if the cells were able to follow and complete their differentiation when isolated from the parent organism.

Work on insects (16, 46, 47) and on mollusk (13) confirmed that differentiation did continue. Several other workers had already obtained sexual differentiation *in vitro* using isolated germinal cells from insects, but this was considered to be cell culture rather than organ culture of the gonads.

Demal (16) cultured the germinal zone of both ovary and testis from larvae of *Calliphora*, using his standard medium based on embryo extract. The tissues survived and differentiation began. The stage at which the gonads were taken was important and better developed gonads survived longer in culture.

Lender and Duveau-Hagège (46, 47) explanted larval gonads from both sexes of *Galleria mellonella* (Lepidoptera). The solid medium used was derived from that of Wolff and Haffen and had the following composition:

A physiological saline solution adopted for insects, with agar and
    trehalose (2 parts)
50% Chick embryo extract in saline solution (2 parts)
Horse serum (1 part)
Penicillin and streptomycin

The ovaries and testes were taken from the last larval stage. One gonad from each animal was fixed immediately to serve as control, and the other gonad was explanted and cultured for 2–7 days.

Testis. The testis of *Galleria* is composed of four utricles and these retained their characteristic appearance *in vitro*. The stage of differentiation reached by the male germinal cells at the time of explantation was variable. The characteristic zones containing the different stages were as follows:

1. The germinal zone containing spermatogonia (Plate 1, Fig. 1). Mitoses were seen in the spermatogonia both *in vivo* and *in vitro*.

2. A zone where the spermatogonia are transformed into spermatocytes. These enter meiosis and become grouped together in cysts. In culture, the cysts were well preserved and many meioses were seen in them (Plate 1, Figs. 2 and 3).

3. The distal end of the utricle contained the various stages of spermatogenesis (spermatids, mature spermatozoa). All these stages were clearly seen in culture (Plate 1, Fig. 4). The appearance of new stages of development indicated differentiation of the male germinal cells, but this only took place if the testes contained cysts at the time of explantation (that is, spermatocytes undergoing the first maturation division). The cystic stage was critical and could not be induced *in vitro* if it had not already begun *in vivo*. All other stages of spermatogenesis could be obtained from spermatocytes in culture, that is, spermatids and spermatozoa.

Ovary. In most cases, only the early stages of oogenesis were present in the ovary at the time of explantation (Plate II, Fig. 1).

Each ovary contained a zone of oogonia and a zone of oocytes in the prophase of meiosis. There is little growth of the oocytes during this, the

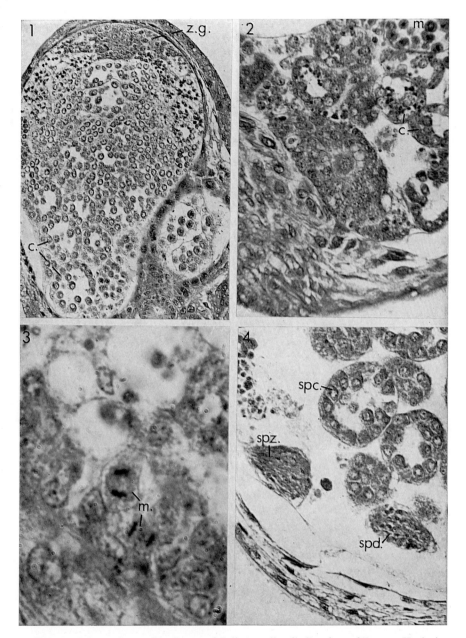

Plate I. Culture of testes from larvae of *Galleria mellonella* (Lender and Duveau-Hagège).

Fig. 1.   Control testis at the time of explantation. c, Cysts; z.g., germinal zone ($\times$ 160).
Fig. 2.   Cultured testis showing cysts in meiosis. c, Cysts; m, meiosis ($\times$ 320).
Fig. 3.   Meiosis in a cyst from a cultured testis. m, Meiosis ($\times$ 1200).
Fig. 4.   Spermatogenesis in a cultured testis. spc, Spermatocytes; spd, spermatids; spz, spermatozoa ($\times$ 400).

307

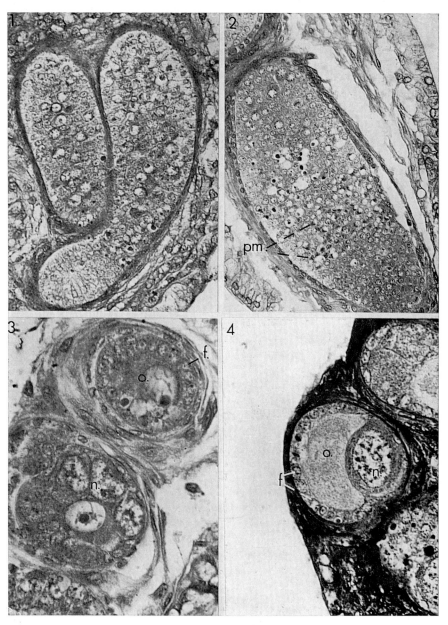

Plate II. Culture of ovaries from larvae of *Galleria mellonella* (Lender and Duveau-Hagège).

FIG. 1.   Control ovary at the time of explantation. (× 240).

FIG. 2.   Cultured ovary showing the "bouquet" stage. p.m., Prophase of meiosis. (× 200).

FIG. 3.   Cultured ovary showing the organization of follicles. (× 430).

FIG. 4.   Differentiated follicle from a cultured ovary. f, Follicular cells; n, nurse cells; o, oocyte. PAS technique (× 520).

"bouquet" stage, so-called because of the appearance of the nuclear chromatin at the time of meiotic prophase (Plate II, Fig. 2). Follicular and nurse cells are already clearly distinguishable from the germinal cells, and are mixed among the oogonia and oocytes. After 6–7 days of culture marked growth of the oocytes had occurred, and the initial diameter of 15 μ was increased to 45 μ. The nurse cells had differentiated and their cytoplasm could be distinguished from that of the oocytes by increased basophilia. At the end of the ovariole, differentiation of the follicular cells and normal organization of the follicles were obtained in culture. Follicular cells were seen around an oocyte together with 3–5 nurse cells (Plate II, Figs. 3 and 4). In many cases, cytoplasmic bridges were seen, linking the nurse cells with the oocyte. It was possible to demonstrate histologically that nutrient materials passed from the trophocyte to the oocyte. The phase of considerable growth of the oocyte had begun in culture. This stage precedes yolk formation but it was difficult to confirm whether true yolk formation had occurred since yolk is difficult to demonstrate histochemically.

Duveau-Hagège (20) was able to reproduce similar results when studying the larval and adult ovaries of the cockroach *Periplaneta americana*.

Survival and differentiation of gonads *in vitro* has been shown to be possible. Male and female gametogenesis have occurred in the absence of insect hormones. In the species investigated, the secretions of the corpora allata, in particular, do not seem to be essential to gametogenesis. Lender and Duveau-Hagège have suggested that insect hemolymph did not improve their culture conditions and chick embryo extract was shown to be indispensable, as in Demal's experiments. Further *in vitro* culture will no doubt show whether or not embryo extract contains compounds that encourage the development of the gametes.

Using the gastropod mollusk *Patella vulgata*, Choquet (13) obtained survival and differentiation of the gonads in organ culture. The medium used was based on that of Sengel for marine invertebrates. As well as chick embryo extract, the medium contained egg albumin and horse serum. When fragments of testis or ovary were explanted onto this medium, they scarred over after 8–10 days and survived for more than 3 months. The fragments were transferred to fresh medium every 4 days. There was no pycnosis. The pieces became surrounded by a newly formed epithelial layer that protected them and made possible the change of medium. Both male and female germinal cells developed normally. At the time of explantation, the fragments of tissue from both sexes had the same appearance. The germinal elements could not be identified as either spermatogonia or oogonia. After 20 days of culture, the male fragments were seen to contain both spermatogonia and spermatocytes. These differentiated into flagellate spermatozoa after 36 days. In the female explants, cells with a diameter of 10 μ could be seen at the time of explantation. After 36 days these had developed into oocytes with a diameter of 25 μ. They became more basophilic and entered the stage preceding yolk formation. At the end of culture, oocytes were obtained, with a diameter of 40 μ and containing intracytoplasmic yolk granules. Hence, true yolk production had taken place *in vitro*.

B. Study of Sexual Endocrinology *in Vitro*

Examples of sexual differentiation in the absence of hormones have been described in some invertebrate species. We shall now turn to some experiments designed to study the various influences on sexual differentiation *in vitro*.

Durchon and Schaller (19) used organ culture techniques to investigate the endocrinology of polychaete annelids. The polychaetes do not have well-differentiated gonads. The sex cells are formed by proliferation of cells in the walls of the coelom. These then fall into the coelomic cavity, where they undergo gametogenesis. Whole parapodia containing sex cells were cultured rather than gonads. In many species of polychaetes, the parapodia undergo marked morphological change at the time of sexual maturity. The normal bristles or chaetae become replaced by oarlike bristles. The worm passes from the immature atoke to the sexually mature epitoke stage. Experiments carried out *in vivo* (18) suggest that metamorphosis in this worm is under endocrine control. There is a cerebral hormone, secreted in the region of the prostomium, that can inhibit gametogenesis and also epitoky. Absence of this hormone induced maturation of the sex cells and metamorphosis of the atoke form into the epitoke form. *In vitro* culture was used to confirm these results. Durchon and Scaller explanted parapodia from various species of *Nereis, Platynereis*, and *Perinereis*, using a medium modified from that of Wolff and Haffen.

Composition of the medium:

> 1% Agar dissolved in 1% of glucose in sea water (7 parts)
> 1% Glucose in sea water (3 parts)
> 50% Egg albumin in 1% glucose in sea water (3 parts)
> Horse serum (1 part)
> 50% Chick embryo extract in 1% glucose in sea water (1 part)
> Penicillin, streptomycin

The explants were transplanted every 4 days. The parapodia scarred after 3–5 days and survived for 8–21 days depending on the species. The parapodia showed spontaneous contractions and an active blood circulation throughout the culture period. Histological examination showed that the tissues survived perfectly, remaining healthy and preserving their normal appearance. Most important was the observed differentiation of the parapodia in culture. On the described hormone-free medium parapodia taken from the atoke stage differentiated the typical oarlike swimming bristles, characteristic of the epitoke stage. Microscopic examination showed also the development of the spermatocytes present in the parapodium at the time of explantation. Maturation divisions were seen from the 4th day of culture, and spermatozoa escaped from the nephridial pore on the 5th day. Thus, in the absence of the hormone from the prostomium, an atoke parapodium underwent the characteristic transformation into the epitoke form. Heteronereid bristles developed and gametogenesis occurred. To find what would happen in the presence of the cerebral hormone, Durchon and Schaller explanted two parapodia from the same male specimen of *Nereis*. One parapodium was explanted onto the hormone-deficient medium and the other was explanted together with the prostomium. The parapodium and the prostomium quickly fused together, and it was seen that gametogenesis was prevented in the presence of the prostomium. After culture for 1 month, the spermatocytes contained in the coelom of the parapod still appeared as they did at the time of explantation; the spermatocytes had not differentiated into spermatozoa. Organ culture *in vitro* has thus demonstrated the inhibiting effect of the hormone from the prostomium.

Organ culture techniques have also been used to study sexual endocrinology in crustaceans (5–8). The humoral mechanism of the crustaceans have been partially elucidated. An endocrine gland has been found in male crustaceans (11, 12). This androgenic gland produces a hormone that determines spermatogenesis in the gonads. When the hormone is absent, the gonads develop into the female type. The female type is thus the anhormonal neutral type, and the presence of differentiated testes depends on the presence and functioning of the androgenic gland.

Berreur-Bonnenfant explanted functional adult male testes from *Orchestia gammarella*, either alone or in association with the androgenic gland. The isolated testis survived for 30–45 days on Wolff and Haffen's medium, adapted for crustaceans and containing chick embryo extract. When chick embryo extract was absent from the medium, the testes emptied and became pycnotic after 4 days of culture. When the medium contained embryo extract, morphological and histological structure was unaltered and normal spermatogenesis occurred. The differentiated spermatozoa could not be released and accumulated in the testis. When a testis was cultured together with the androgenic gland, the percentage of successful cultures was increased and there was prolonged survival of the testis. The germinal zone was maintained in good condition, whereas that in the testis cultured alone was emptied by the 30th day after explantation (Plate III, Figs. 1 and 2). These results demonstrated the effect of the androgenic hormone on the testis, especially in the region of the germinal zone. Males of *Talitrus* and

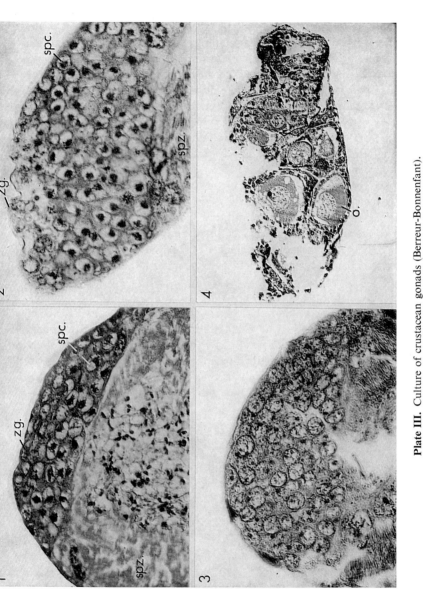

Plate III. Culture of crustacean gonads (Berreur-Bonnenfant).

Fig. 1. Testis from *Orchestia gammarella*, cultured in association with the androgenic gland. Presentation of the germinal zone. Fig. 2. Testis from *Orchestia gammarella*, cultured without the androgenic gland. Degeneration of the germinal zone. spc, Spermatocytes; spz, spermatozoa; zg., germinal zone. Fig. 3. Testis of *Anilocra physodes* at the time of explantation. Fig. 4. Testis of *Anilocra physodes* cultured without the androgenic gland. Ovarian differentiation. o, Oocytes.

Anilocra show spontaneous sexual inversion with oogenesis occurring in the testis at certain times of the year. This is undoubtedly due to a decrease in the concentration of the androgenic hormone in the organism. Berreur-Bonnenfant obtained differentiation of oocytes in the germinal zone of testes cultured alone in the absence of the androgenic gland (Plate III, Figs. 3 and 4). Ovarian autodifferentiation occurred on a hormone-deficient medium *in vitro*. This also takes place normally *in vivo*. Thus the role of the androgenic hormone in crustaceans has been demonstrated *in vitro*. It inhibits oogenesis and the maintenance of spermatogenesis.

Some indication has been given of the possible interactions between hormones or trophic substances and sexual glands in other groups of invertebrates where the endocrine systems are still poorly understood. Work has been carried out on ascidians (64, 65) and on mollusks (33).

The ascidians possess a complex formed by the subneural gland, the nerve ganglion, and the ciliated funnel. The role of this complex is still poorly understood—attempts have been made to compare it with the vertebrate pituitary. Sengel and Kieny investigated the response of the ascidian gonads to a direct hormonal effect similar to the gonadotrophic effect of the pituitary. They thought that this effect might be mediated by the neural gland complex. Male and female gonads of the ascidian *Molgula manhattensis* were explanted alone or in association with the complex. Two media were used, one non-nutrient (agar and sea water) and one nutrient (with added horse serum, chicken plasma, *Limulus* serum, chick embryo extract, or Parker's solution 199). The somatic elements of the gonads survived unchanged on all of these media, both nutrient and nonnutrient, and in combination with the complex and without it. The germinal elements became completely necrotic on the nonnutrient medium and partly necrotic on the nutrient media. Gonocytes, both male and female, survived when the explants were cultured in association with the complex (Plate IV, Figs. 1 and 2). Moreover, the various stages of maturation of the oocytes were obtained (Plate IV, Figs. 3 and 4). The male cells survived without differentiating. It seems that the complex exerts a positive effect on the survival and to a certain extent on the differentiation of the sex cells. Whilst the favorable effect of the complex was more pronounced than the effect of the various nutrient media, it could not be concluded that the complex had a specific effect, corresponding to the normal function of this complex in the intact animal. The effect may have been only a nonspecific nutrient one.

In some cases, it had been thought that trophic factors may have been responsible for the determination of the sex cells. Gomot and Guyard (1964) studied this in the Gasteropod mollusk *Helix aspera*, using organ culture techniques. The hermaphrodite glands from 2-month snails were explanted onto various organic and inorganic media. On nonnutrient media (containing

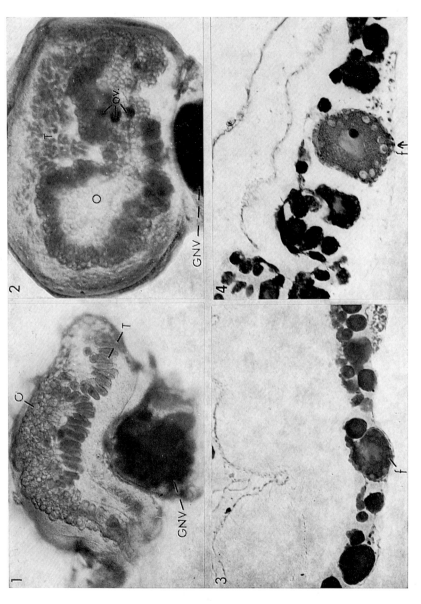

Plate IV. Culture of gonads from *Molgula manhattensis* (Sengel and Kieny).

agar and physiological saline) the sex cells survived for 10–15 days. The spermatogonia present at the time of explantation matured into spermatocytes and then died. The oocytes grew, became surrounded by follicular cells, and then degenrated. When an organic medium based on chick embryo extract or snail hemolymph was used, the survival proved to be much better. The male cells survived for 25 days and the female gametes for 50 days. Hemolymph permitted differentiation of spermatozoa and organization of oocytes and follicular cells into follicles. It was probable that the hemolymph contained trophic factors necessary for sexual differentation.

IV. ORGAN CULTURE APPLIED TO ENDOCRINOLOGICAL RESEARCH IN EMBRYOGENESIS AND GENETICS

Organ culture has been applied to the study of sexual determination in several invertebrate species, and the technique has also been used to study the role of hormones during the larval development in insects, particularly with regard to the genetics of the group.

The imaginal disks of insect larvae are the embryonic rudiments of the adult organs, and these can survive, develop, and differentiate *in vitro* (26, 15, 17). Frew obtained the beginning of differentiation of the segmented limbs from the imaginal disks in the legs of *Calliphora* larvae. Demal and Leloup obtained development of legs and eyes from the imaginal disks of *Calliphora* and *Drosophila*. In all these experiments, the differentiation of the disks occurred only in the presence of an extract of, or the lymph from, the pupal stage of the insect. Thus, certain specific substances seem to be necessary for the development of the imaginal rudiments.

Kuroda and Yamaguchi (43) found that the differentiation of the imaginal disks in culture could be used to study, *in vitro*, the effects of the cephalic complex on the oculo-antennal disk of *Drosophila*. These experiments were concerned with insect embryological development, genetics, and endocrinology. Metamorphosis and more particularly the differentiation of the imaginal disks are under the control of the cephalic complex, that is, a complex composed of the brain and Weissmann's ring. In mutants, where the morphology of some organ is affected, it is necessary to determine whether the mutant

---

FIG. 1.   Association between a young, undifferentiated gonad and the neural gland complex after 7 days of culture (macroscopic appearance). GNV, Complex; O, ovary; T, testis ($\times$ 17).

FIG. 2.   Association between a gonad and the complex. The number of ova released into the ovarian cavity has increased during the 7 days of culture (macroscopic appearance). GNV, Complex; O, ovary; ov, ova; T, testis ($\times$ 12.5).

FIG. 3.   Ovary at the time of explantation, with a follicle beginning to differentiate (histological appearance). f, Follicle ($\times$ 200).

FIG. 4.   Adjacent ovary after 7 days of culture, with a follicle considerably increased in size and differentiated. f, Follicle ($\times$ 200).

gene acts directly on the imaginal disk of this organ, or whether the gene acts first on the cephalic complex, which then exerts a secondary effect on the development of the disk. Kuroda and Yamaguchi investigated this problem in the bar gene of *Drosophila*. This gene reduces the size of the eyes and alters their shape. They cultured *in vitro* the cephalic complex and the oculo-antennal disk from third-stage larvae of the normal, wild, Oregon strain and from the mutant bar strain. The explants were cultured in physiological saline solution, with added casein hydrolyzate, amino acids, vitamins, and glucose, using the hanging drop technique. When cultured alone, the oculo-antennal disk of the Oregon strain showed a little growth and organization, and the cellular masses destined to form the ommatidia differentiated after 17 hours of culture. However, when these disks were cultured with the cephalic complex from the same strain, growth and differentiation were very good. The ocular disk was transformed into an almost normal eye with ommatidia. When the ocular disk of the Oregon strain was cultured with the cephalic complex of the bar strain, it developed into the bar form. There was a little increase in the size of the disk and a few ommatidia differentiated. However, the antennal disk grew and differentiated normally, indicating that the bar cephalic complex must act specifically on the eye rudiment causing it to assume the bar form.

The effects of the Oregon and bar cephalic complexes on the bar imaginal disks were then compared. In the presence of the bar cephalic complex, the bar ocular disk scarcely grew in the anteroposterior axis; this lack of growth is characteristic of the bar strain. However, the antennal disk showed marked growth. The Oregon cephalic complex had a striking effect on the bar ocular disk. There was a considerable increase in size, and the ommatidia differentiated and formed a normal eye. Thus, the bar disk can develop into an Oregon eye when exposed to the influence of the Oregon cephalic complex.

It can therefore be supposed that the effect of the gene is initially exerted on the brain and Weissmann's ring. These then influence the growth and differentiation of the disk by means of hormonal secretions.

Further experiments were carried out by Horikawa (37, 38) and by Fujio (27, 28). Horikawa studied *in vitro* the synthesis of pigment in the ocular disks of third-stage *Drosophila* larvae. Substances were added to the medium that were known to be intermediates in the synthesis of the pigment, that is, tryptophan, kynurenine, and hydroxykynurenine. The synthesis of pigment in the disks being cultured took place in the presence of each of these three metabolites. The further the metabolite was from the end product of synthetics, the longer it took for the pigment to appear (72 hours for tryptophan, 30–55 hours for kynurenine, and 5–15 hours for hydroxykynurenine). Moreover, the time at which the pigment appeared varied according to whether the disks were derived from the Oregon strain or from some eye color mutant. These experiments show that all the enzymes necessary for pigment synthesis are already present in the disk of a third-stage larva.

Fujio showed that various chemical compounds, such as urea, stimulate the development of the oculo-antennal disks in some strains of larvae, whilst they are inactive in other strains. He also demonstrated that *in vitro* development of disks could occur on media which had previously had cephalic complexes grown upon them. The success of the cultures was due to substances present in the medium that had diffused out from the cephalic complexes. These substances could exert their effect in the absence of the cephalic complex.

In *Drosophila*, treatment with X-rays retarded pupation or inhibited the imaginal molt. It is possible that these developmental disturbances were due to damage in the cephalic complex and particularly in Weissmann's ring. However, the X-rays may have damaged the imaginal disks themselves. In 1960, Horikawa and Sugahara (39) used *in vitro* culture to resolve this problem. Irradiated imaginal disks and nonirradiated cephalic complexes were associated together on the medium. Nonirradiated imaginal disks were then associated with irradiated cephalic complexes. An eye disk grew and differentiated normally after heavy irradiation (20 kr) if it was cultured together with a healthy cephalic complex. In contrast, an irradiated cephalic complex (5–15 kr) prevented the differentiation of a healthy ocular disk. Growth was not affected but when a higher dose of irradiation was used (20 kr), neither growth nor differentiation of the optic disk occurred. Thus, the principal effect of X-rays is to disturb the function of the cephalic complex and its action on the development of the disks. Moreover, if the ocular disk was irradiated with very high doses (greater than 25 kr) it degenerated even if it was associated with a healthy cephalic complex. The sensitivity of the disks for different organs (wing, leg, testis, and so on) is seen to vary. These experiments show that there is differential sensitivity of the *Drosophila* larval rudiments to the effect of X-rays, the cephalic complex being the most sensitive organ.

Gottschewski (34, 35) carried out a detailed study of the morphogenesis of *Drosophila* ocular disks *in vitro*. The various stages of development were described in great detail for disks from the normal strain and from a series of mutant strains. A synthetic culture medium was used, composed of amino acids, vitamins, enzymes, sugars, mineral salts, purines and pyrimidines, peptides, and proteins). The prinicpal conclusions reached were the same as those quoted above. *In vitro* development of the optic disks from third-stage larvae is only possible in the presence of the corpora allata, corpora cardiaca, and the pericardiac gland, that is, Weissmann's ring. The cerebral bulb and optic lobe were also indispensable, particularly for the development of the "navette" or hemispherical stage. If the bulb was lacking, the disk remained in the navette form, but despite this ommatidia still differentiated.

Gottschewski and Querner (36) suggested that only ocular disks taken toward the end of the third larval stage could develop *in vitro*. Younger disks, taken during the second stage or at the beginning of the third stage, scarcely developed, even when associated with the cephalic complex in culture. It was suggested that during these early stages there may be a barrier preventing the passage of materials from Weissmann's ring and the other glands into the ocular disk. However, this does not seem to be the case, as further experiments have shown the passage of fluorescent materials from the cephalic complex to the disk in culture.

Work has also been carried out on the molting of the grasshopper *Melanopus differentialis* (51). Whole embryos, the anterior or posterior halves of embryos, and isolated metathoracic limbs were explanted before the first molt and were cultured using the hanging drop technique. Two normal embryonic molts occurred in both whole embryos and half-embryos in culture. The isolated limbs accomplished one molt. Since molting occurred as often in the posterior halves and limbs as in the anterior halves or whole embryos, it was concluded that the neuroendocrine system of the head was not necessary for the accomplishment of the molts. In this species, the embryonic development is controlled by the epidermal tissue and not by the hormonal centers.

V. ORGAN CULTURE APPLIED TO EXPERIMENTS ON REGENERATION

During the process of regeneration, a tissue, an organ, or an organ complex has certain points in common with an embryonic rudiment or a young embryo. Like the embryonic rudiment, regenerating tissue contains elements with multiple morphogenetic potentialities. These totipotent elements differentiate into given cell types under the influence of the surroundings and following predetermined interactions. It is tempting to remove these tissues from the normal influences that occur *in vivo* during the course of development, and, by culturing them *in vitro*, to isolate them so that their total intrinsic potentialities can be defined. *In vitro* culture has been successful in the study of the potentialities of vertebrate embryonic organs. The method has also been applied to the study of larval rudiments in insects. Regeneration experiments involving explanting of tissues or pieces of organisms that possess multiple morphogenetic potentialities have been carried out on groups of relatively primitive invertebrates, that is, sponges, coelenterates, flat worms, and earthworms. One case of regeneration in an insect tissue will also be mentioned.

Classical work on regeneration was carried out by Wilson (71), Huxley (41, 42), Galtsoff (29, 30), and Fauré-Frémiet (21, 22), and more recently by Curtis (14), Ganguly (31), Borojevic (10), Humphreys (40), and Moscona (50). These workers all experimented with sponges where dissociation and re-association of the cells is followed by regeneration and reconstitution of a whole organism (see the chapter by Sigot).

Experimental dissociation of tissues has been carried out in the coelenterates. The intrinsic properties of the ectodermal and endodermal layers of the animal can be determined by separating the layers from one another and then culturing them. The results obtained vary according to the species investigated. *Eudendrium* and *Pennaria* reconstituted hydrants from dissociated cells, while *Leptogorgia* did not (72). Papenfuss and Bokenham (57) cultured separately the endoderm and ectoderm of *Hydra*. Neither of these layers reconstituted a whole animal. In contrast, Normandin (55) obtained a normal *Hydra* from endoderm alone, whilst Steinberg (66) and Zwilling (76) induced ectodermal fragments from *Aurelia* and *Cordylophora* to reconstitute whole animals. Controversy has arisen regarding the participation of the interstitial cells in these reconstitutions, and the question of the potentialities of the two layers remains open.

A series of *in vitro* experiments has been devoted to regeneration in planarians. Most species in this Platyhelminthes group possess a particularly high capacity for regeneration. Almost any piece of a planarian can reconstitute a whole animal. The planarians appear to be like the sponges and coelenterates in this respect, and it was an obvious step to repeat in the planarians the dissociation and reassociation experiments that had been carried out on the tissues of sponges *in vitro*.

Freisling and Reisinger (25) pressed adult planarians through a silk sieve into Holtfreter's solution. Small spheres of living tissue or restitution bodies (spheres) were obtained from the suspension of cells. Studies were made on the potentialities for differentiation and the movements of these spheres. The spheres were shown to have been derived from small pieces of intact, ciliated epidermis, to which were attached masses of mesenchymal tissue. The suspension also contained pieces of separate epidermis and mesenchyme, but these separate tissues were unable to form restitution bodies. Contact between epidermis and mesenchyme seemed to be necessary for the morphogenesis of these spheres. The restitution bodies developed according to their own properties, and at a constant rate. Initially the cells in the center of the sphere underwent histolysis, and then formed a syncytium. The external layer was ciliated. Fluid-filled spaces appeared in the syncytium, and the spheres increased in volume. Spontaneous invagination of the external layer sometimes occurred and this was thought to be a process of pseudogastrulation. A mouth appeared, opening into a large intestinelike cavity with a ciliated lining. This development was not analogous with the normal embryonic development of planarians nor with their regenerative development. Active movements of the spheres occurred, with the speed of movement increasing when the temperature was increased. However, neuroactive substances such as narcotics and excitants did not affect the speed of this rotatory movement. The ciliary movements of Planaria were thus shown to be autonomous and not dependent on the nervous system.

An analogous experiment was carried out by Ansevin and Buchsbaum (2). Planaria of the species *Dugesia tigrina* were minced mechanically or dissociated using Versene. The isolated cells were cultured on solid or liquid media based on Holtfreter's solution and a Planaria tissue extract. On a solid gelatine medium, considerable cellular migration was seen, which resulted in the formation of sheets of cells. Sometimes there was differentiation of intestinal tissue. On a liquid medium restitution bodies differentiated, as in Freisling and Reisinger's experiments.

From these experiments it was concluded that dissociated Planaria cells cannot reconstitute tissue with a normal structure, nor can they reform a whole organism, at least under the culture conditions used up to now. This is in contrast to the tissues of sponges and coelenterates.

Experiments were carried out using undissociated pieces of planarian tissues (52–54). Organ growth with membrane formation occurred only on a solid medium. On a liquid medium, only cell culture took place.

Seilern Aspang (59, 60) showed that planarian tissues explanted in culture (that is, tissue from the pharynx and from young embryos) could not retain an organized structure unless they could extend in three dimensions. On a coverslip, where the culture could only grow in two dimensions, the tissues tended to spread out and dissociate. In the case of adult tissues the culture often became cellular. An embryo cultured on a cover glass did not dissociate into cells, but into many embryonic rudiments. Two-dimensional culture induced a kind of polyembryony.

In 1960, Sengel (61, 62) obtained an organ culture of young regeneration blastemas from the planarian species *Dugesia lugubris* and *Dugesia tigrina*. The blastemas were 3 days old and still undifferentiated at the time of explantation. They were composed of a mass of regenerating cells (neoblasts). These all had the same appearance and were covered by a thin epidermal layer. The buds could not survive when isolated in water. The aim of these experiments was to establish the intrinsic potentialities of blastemas when they were separated from the intact organism and thus removed from its influences. The medium used was a modification of Wolff and Haffen's medium:

1% Agar solution in Holtfreter's saline solution (5 or 6 parts)

1% Glucose in Holtfreter's solution (4 parts)
9-Day chick embryo extract diluted to 50% in Holtfreter's
    solution (3 parts)

This solid medium allowed true organotypical culture of the blastemas, which survived for periods ranging from 10 days to 3 weeks and differentiated according to their presumptive fate. Two kinds of blastema were explanted; anterior regenerating buds and posterior regenerating buds. The former were destined to produce heads, the latter tails. In culture, the buds differentiated into heads or tails respectively, the period of delay being about the same as *in vivo*. In all the blastemas explanted there was epidermal differentiation with the appearance of subepidermal pigmentation. Functional muscle cells appeared within the parenchyma. Normal eyes and a well-formed brain appeared in the cephalic blastema (Plate V, Figs. 1, 2, and 3). It was easy to associate several blastemas on one culture medium where they rapidly fused at their cut surfaces. The association of several cephalic blastemas resulted in a head with supernumerary brains and eyes. Several caudal blastemas fused to form a kind of lobed tail. The association of a cephalic blastema with a caudal blastema was more interesting. Besides the differentiation previously mentioned (that is, the formation of epidermis, pigment, muscles, and eyes and brain in the anterior part), a pharynx and a three-branched digestive tract were also formed. This three-branched gut is characteristic of the triclad turbellarians. Thus, a small planarian with all its principal organs can be developed from undifferentiated cells (Plate V, Fig. 4). The main conclusion to be drawn from these experiments is that the regenerating blastemas are already determined at the time of explantation. Although separated from the basis of this determination, they cannot express any potentialities other than those that they would have shown *in vivo*.

These results obtained on blastemas cultured *in vitro* were partly reproduced by Manelli and Negri (48) using *Planaria torva*.

The tissues or the blastemas from other animals able to regenerate, such as annelids and some arthropods, have not been used to such an extent for organ culture, but earthworms (32) and insects (49) have been tried.

Gay explanted pieces of *Lumbricus herculeus* on an acid agar medium based on Tyrode's solution, with added amino acids, glucose, and earthworm extract. Scarring occurred normally and a sort of blastema was formed, composed of dedifferentiated muscle cells. It was not a normal regeneration blastema and did not differentiate. The endoderm disappeared and the clitellum involuted.

Marks and Reinecke cultured *in vitro* the regenerating limb structures from the nymph of the cockroach *Leucophaea maderae*. Survival and development were observed on a nutrient medium based on bactopeptone. Cell culture

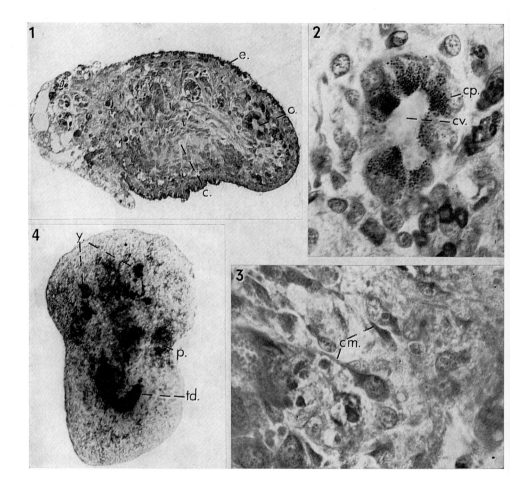

Plate V. *In vitro* differentiation of regeneration blastemas from *Dugesia lugubris* (Sengel).

FIG. 1. Cephalic blastema cultured for 8 days, showing differentiation. c, Brain; e, epidermis; o, eye (× 120).

FIG. 2. Differentiated eye in a cephalic blastema after 8 days of culture. c.p., Pigment cells; c.v., visual cells (× 562).

FIG. 3. Differentiated muscle cells in a blastema after 8 days of culture. c.m., Muscle cells. (× 562).

FIG. 4. Association of a cephalic blastema with a caudal blastema after culture for 15 days (macroscopic appearance). p, Pigment; t.d., digestive tube; y, eyes (× 50).

and organized formations were obtained and deep, spherical vesicles appeared, formed from a layer of epithelial cells interwoven with fibrous cells. These vesicles formed as buds along the edge of the explant from which they sometimes became detached. Their structural appearance and activity showed some resemblance to young, regenerating buds. Two types of activity were noted in the vesicles:

1. There was absorption of relatively large amounts of the external medium into the vesicles, which increased in size.

2. A gelatinous, sometimes granular material was secreted onto the surface of the epithelium of the vesicles. This secretory process was similar to the beginning of cuticle formation.

These two activities were also seen in the early stages of normal regeneration. This was perhaps a form of regeneration in culture *in vitro*.

VI. CONCLUSIONS

The study of these examples of organ culture in invertebrates gives an impression of expansion both in the number and diversity of the species chosen, in the techniques, in the types of media, and above all in the types of experiments, the problems posed, and the directions taken by the researchers. It is difficult to draw any general conclusions from this work and this is not only due to the fact that organ culture in invertebrates is still in the early stage. Organ culture has not only solved certain set problems, but has also opened up many other fields of investigation.

Some of the main points that can be derived from this work relate to the various methods used in these experiments. The technique first described in 1952 by Wolff and Haffen for the culture of avian embryonic organs and accepted for vertebrates, has now been successful in the field of organ culture in vertebrates. This is due mainly to the simplicity of this technique, which can be adapted for very different animal tissues, such as those of a planarian, an insect, and a bird.

The main points arising from the *in vitro* experiments are as follows. Most of the organs studied functioned normally *in vitro* and on a variety of media, from the simplest, such as sea water, to the most complex, either natural or synthetic.

The study of sexuality has produced several concrete facts. The gonads of some species differentiate in the absence of hormones, whereas in other species, sexual differentiation depends on the presence of specific trophic factors or hormonal material. Complex endocrine mechanisms have been elucidated, such as those found in polychaetes and crustaceans.

The experiments on the *in vitro* development of the imaginal disks of insects show the great importance of the cephalic complex and in particular of Weissmann's ring, during molting. These experiments show that the gene effect is manifested initially in the region of the cephalic complex.

Regenerating cells or tissues in the process of regeneration are able to survive and differentiate *in vitro*. Thus, cells of the sponges or coelenterates, or young planarian blastemas, can give rise to whole animals or at least differentiated structures in culture. It is thus possible to study some of the mechanisms of regeneration outside the intact organism, and some of the factors that influence this special kind of development and morphogenesis.

BIBLIOGRAPHY

1. André F.   La culture des œufs et des embryons du Lombricien *Eisenia foetida. Sav. Bull. Soc. Zool.*, 1962, **87**, 153.
2. Ansevin K. and Buchsbaum R.   Observations on planarian cells cultivated in solid and liquid media. *J. exp. Zool.*, 1961, **146**, 153.
3. Benex J.   La survie d'explants de planorbes (*Australorbis glabratus*) en milieu synthétique, antiseptique et nutritif. *C. R. Acad. Sci.*, 1961, **253**, 734.
4. Benex J.   Sur la dédifférenciation des tentacules de planorbes en survie: rôle de la présence d'éléments nerveux sur le retard de cette dédifférenciation. *C. R. Acad. Sci.*, 1964, **258**, 2193.
5. Berreur-Bonnenfant J.   Essai de culture *in vitro* de gonades de Crustacé. *Bull. Soc. Zool.*, 1962, **87**, 377.
6. Berreur-Bonnenfant J.   Survie et activité des gonades et de la glande androgène des mâles d'*Orchestia gammarella* en culture organotypique. *C. R. Acad. Sci.*, 1963, **256**, 2244.
7. Berreur-Bonnenfant J.   Autodifférenciation ovarienne dans les gonades mâles de Crustacés en culture *in vitro. Bull. Soc. Zool.*, 1963, **88**, 235.
8. Berreur-Bonnenfant J.   La culture *in vitro* de gonades de Crustacés et son intérêt pour l'étude endocrinologique. *Gen. comp. Endocr.*, 1963, **3**, 11.
9. Bevelander G. and Martin J.   Culture of mantle tissue of marine Molluscs. *Anat. Rec.*, 1949, **105**, 604.
10. Borojevic R.   Essai de reconstitution du choanoderme à partir d'une suspension choanocytaire d'Éponge Acalcaire. *C. R. Acad. Sci.*, 1963, **257**, 961.
11. Charniaux-Cotton H.   Découverte chez un Crustacé Amphipode (*Orchestia gammarella*) d'une glande endocrine responsable de la différenciation des caractères primaires et secondaires mâles. *C. R. Acad. Sci.*, 1954, **239**, 780.
12. Charniaux-Cotton H.   La glande androgène de quelques Crustacés Décapodes et particulièrement de *Lysmata sedicaudata* à hermaphrodisme protandrique fronctionnel. *C. R. Acad. Sci.*, 1958, **246**, 2814.
13. Choquet M.   Culture organotypique de gonades de *Patella vulgata* L. (Mollusque Gastéropode Prosobranche). *C. R. Acad. Sci.*, 1964, **258**, 1089.
14. Curtis A. S.   Pattern and mechanism in the reaggregation of Sponges. *Nature*, 1962, **196**, 245.
15. Demal J.   Différenciation d'ébauches imaginales de Diptères en culture *in vitro. Bull. Acad. Roy. Belg.*, 1955, **5**, 1061.
16. Demal J.   Problèmes concernant la morphogenèse *in vitro* chez les Insectes. *Bull. Soc. Zool.*, 1962, **86**, 522.

17. Demal J. and Leloup A. M.   Essai de culture *in vitro* d'organes d'Insectes. *Ann. Epiphyties*, 1963, **14**, No. hors série III, 91.

18. Durchon M.   Recherches expérimentales sur deux aspects de la reproduction chez les Annélides Polychètes: l'épitoquie et la stolonisation. *Ann. Sc. Nat. Zool.*, 1952, **14**, 119.

19. Durchon M. and Schaller F.   Application de la méthode de culture organotypique aux recherches endocrinologiques chez les Annélides Polychètes. *C. R. Acad. Sci.*, 1963, **256**, 5615.

20. Duveau-Hagège J.   La culture organotypique d'ovaire de *Periplaneta americana* Linné. *C. R. Acad. Sci.*, 1963, **256**, 5429.

21. Fauré-Frémiet E.   Le mécanisme de la formation des complexes à partir de cellules d'Éponges dissociées. *C. R. Soc. Biol.*, 1925, **93**, 618.

22. Fauré-Frémiet E.   Morphogenèse expérimentale (reconstitution) chez *Ficulina ficus* L. *Arch. Anat. micr.*, 1932, **28**, 1.

23. Fischer-Piette E.   Le tissu lymphocytogène des Crustacés étudié en survie *in vitro*. *C. R. Soc. Biol.*, 1929, **102**, 764.

24. Fischer-Piette E.   Culture de tissus de Crustacés. La glande lymphatique du Homard. *Arch. Zool. exp. gén.*, 1933, **74**, 33.

25. Freisling M. and Reisinger E.   Zur Genese und Physiologie von Restitutionskörpern aus Planariengewebsbrei. *Roux' Arch. Entw. Mech.*, 1958, **150**, 581.

26. Frew J. C. H.   A technique for the cultivation of insect tissues. *J. exp. Biol.*, 1928, **6**, 1.

27. Fujio Y.   Studies on the development of eye-antennal discs of *Drosophila melanogaster* in tissue culture. I: Effects of facet-increasing substances upon the growth and differentiation of eye-antennal discs. *Jap. J. Genet.*, 1960, **35**, 361.

28. Fujio Y.   Studies on the development of eye-antennal discs of *Drosophila melanogaster* in tissue culture. II: Effects of substances secreted from the cephalic complexes upon eye-antennal discs of eye-mutant strains. *Jap. J. Genet.*, 1962, **37**, 110.

29. Galtsoff P. S.   Regeneration after dissociation (an experimental study on Sponges). I: Behaviour of dissociated cells of *Microciona prolifera* under normal and altered conditions. *J. exp. Zool.*, 1925, **42**, 183.

30. Galtsoff P. S.   Regeneration after dissociation (an experimental study on Sponges). II: Histogenesis of *Microciona prolifera* Verr. *J. exp. Zool.*, 1925, **42**, 223.

31. Ganguly B.   The differentiating capacity of dissociated Sponge cells. *Roux' Arch. Entw. Mech.*, 1960, **152**, 22.

32. Gay R.   Cultures d'organes de Lumbricides sur milieu gélosé synthétique. *Ann. Epiphyties*, 1963, **14**, No. hors série III, 61.

33. Gomot L. and Guyard A.   Évolution en culture *in vitro* de la glande hermaphrodite de jeunes Escargots de l'espèce *Helix aspera*. Müll. *C. R. Acad. Sci.*, 1964, **258**, 2902.

34. Gottschewski G.   Ueber das Wachstum von Drosophila Augen. Imalginalscheiben *in vitro*. *Naturwissensch.*, 1958, **45**, 400.

35. Gottschewski G.   Morphogenetische Untersuchungen an *in vitro* wachsenden Augenanlagen von *Drosophila melanogaster*. *Roux' Arch. entw. Mech.*, 1960, **152**, 204.

36. Gottschewski G. and Querner W.   Beobachtungen an explantierten frühen Entwicklungstadien der Augenanlage von *Drosophila melanogaster*. *Roux' Arch. entw. Mech.*, 1961, **153**, 168.

37. Horikawa M.   Developmental-genetic studies of tissue + cultured eye-discs of *Drosophila melanogaster* I: Growth, differentiation and tryptophan metabolism. *Cytologia*, 1958, **23**, 468.

38. Horikawa M.   Developmental-genetic studies of tissue cultured eye-antennal discs of *Drosophila melanogaster*. II: Effects of the metamorphic hormone (cephalic

complex) upon the growth and differentiation of eye-antennal discs and strain differences in relation to the metamorphic hormone. *Jap. J. Genet.*, 1960, **35**, 76.

39. Horikawa M. and Sugahara T.   Studies on the effects of radiation in living cells in tissue culture. I: Radio-sensibility of various imaginal discs and organs in larvae of *Drosophila melanogaster*. *Rad. res.*, 1960, **12**, 266.

40. Humphreys T.   Chemical dissolution and *in vitro* reconstruction of Sponge cell adhesions. I: Isolation and functional demonstration of the components involved. *Devel. Biol.*, 1963, **8**, 27.

41. Huxley J. S.   Differences in viability in different types of regenerates from dissociated Sponges, with a note on the entry of somatic cells by spermatozoa. *Biol. Bull.*, 1921, **40**, 127.

42. Huxley J. S.   Further studies on restitution-bodies and free tissue culture in *Sycon*. *Quart. J. Micr. Sci.*, 1921, **65**, 293.

43. Kuroda Y. and Yamaguchi K.   The effects of the cephalic complex upon the eye discs of *Drosophila melanogaster*. *Jap. J. Genet.*, 1956, **31**, 97.

44. Larsen W.   The maintenance of embryonic cockroach heart fragments *in vitro*. *Life Sci.*, 1963, **8**, 606.

45. Lender T. and Duveau J.   Le développement de la gonade larvaire de *Galleria mellonella* Linné après transplantation ou ligature de la larve. *C. R. Acad. Sci.*, 1960, **250**, 3511.

46. Lender T. and Duveau-Hagège J.   Survie et différenciation des gonades larvaires de *Galleria mellonella* en culture organotypique. *C. R. Acad. Sci.*, 1962, **254**, 2825.

47. Lender T. and Duveau-Hagège J.   La survie et la différenciation en culture *in vitro* des gonades de larves de dernier âge de *Galleria mellonella* (Lépidoptère, Pyralididae). *Devel. Biol.*, 1963, **6**, 1.

48. Manelli H. and Negri A.   Colture *in vitro*, di blastemi rigenerativi di *Planaria torva*. *Boll. Zool.*, 1962, **29**, 787.

49. Marks E. P. and Reinecke J. P.   Regenerating tissues from the Cockroach leg: a system for studying *in vitro*. *Science*, 1964, **143**, 961.

50. Moscona A.   Studies on cell-aggregation: demonstration of materials with binding-activity. *Proc. Nat. Acad. Sci. U.S.A.*, 1963, **49**, 742.

51. Mueller N. S.   An experimental analysis of molting in embryos of *Melanopus differentialis*. *Devel. Biol.*, 1963, **8**, 222.

52. Murray M.   Cultivation of Planarian tissues *in vitro*. *J. exp. Zool.*, 1927, **47**, 467.

53. Murray M.   The calcium-potassium ratio in culture media for *Planaria dorotocephala*. *Phys. Zool.*, 1928, **1**, 137.

54. Murray M.   *In vitro* studies of Planarian parenchyma. *Arch. exp. Zellf.*, 1931, **11**, 656.

55. Normandin D. K.   Regeneration of *Hydra* from the enzymatically isolated endoderm. *Dissert. Abstr. U.S.A.*, 1963, **23**, 3045.

56. Pantin C. F.   On the excitation of Crustacean muscle. *J. exp. Biol.*, 1934, **11**, 11–27.

57. Papenfuss E. J. and Bokenham N. A.   The fate of the ectoderm and endoderm of *Hydra* when cultured independently. *Biol. Bull.*, 1939, **76**, 1.

58. Ripplinger J. and Joly M.   Rôle des constituants de l'hémolymphe sur l'activité du cœur d'*Helix pomatia*. *C. R. Soc. Biol.*, 1961, **155**, 825.

59. Seilern-Aspang F.   Polyembryonie in der Entwicklung von *Planaria torva* (M. Schultz) auf Deckglaskultur. *Zool. Anz.*, 1957, **159**, 193.

60. Seilern-Aspang F.   Zum Problem von Organisationsvorgängen bei drei-dimensionalem Wachstum in Gewebekulturen. *Zool. Anz.*, 1958, **160**, 1.

61. Sengel C.   Culture *in vitro* de blastèmes de régénération de Planaires. *J. Emb. exp. Morph.*, 1960, **8**, 468.

62. Sengel C.   Culture *in vitro* de blastèmes de régénération de la Planaire *Dugesia lugubris*. *Ann. Epiphyties*, 1963, **14**, No. hors série III, 173.

63. Sengel P.   Survie en culture *in vitro* de divers organes d'Invertébrés marins adultes. *C. R. Acad. Sci.*, 1961, **252**, 3666.

64. Sengel P. and Kieny M.   Action de divers liquides nutritifs et du complexe "glande neurale-ganglion nerveux-organe vibratile" sur les gonades de *Molgula manhattensis* (Tunicier Ascidiacé) cultivées *in vitro*. *C. R. Acad. Sci.*, 1962, **254**, 1682.

65. Sengel P. and Kieny M.   Culture de gonades de *Molgula manhattensis*, isolées ou associées au complexe formé par la glande neurale, le ganglion nerveux et l'organe vibratile. *Ann. Epiphyties*, 1963, **14**, No. hors série III, 95.

66. Steinberg S. N.   The regeneration of whole polyp from ectodermal fragments of scyphostoma larvae of *Aurelia aurita*. *Biol. Bull.*, 1963, **124**, 337.

67. Streiff W. and Peyre A.   Survie en culture *in vitro* d'organes de *Calyptraea sinensis*. L. (Mollusque Prosobranche). *C. R. Acad. Sci.*, 1963, **256**, 292.

68. Thomas J. A.   La culture des vésicules énigmatiques et des urnes du Siponcle. *C. R. Soc. Biol.*, 1932, **110**, 451.

69. Thomas J. A.   La survie d'organites de Stellérides *in vitro*. *C. R. Acad. Sci.*, 1941, **213**, 85.

70. Thomas J. A.   La dédifférenciation des organites d'Echinodermes, en survie *in vitro*. *C. R. Acad. Sci.*, 1941, **213**, 252.

71. Wilson H. V.   On some phenomena of coalescence and regeneration in Sponges. *J. exp. Zool.*, 1908, **5**, 245.

72. Wilson H. V.   On the behaviour of the dissociated cells in Hydroids, *Alcyonaria* and *Asterias*. *J. exo. Zool.*, 1911, **11**, 280.

73. Wolff Em.   Culture organotypique de tissus de jeunes Limules (*Xiphosura polyphemus*). *Bull. Soc. Zool.*, 1962, **87**, 120.

74. Wolff Em.   Sur l'explantation *in vitro* de fragments d'organes de Limules (*Xiphosura polyphemus*). *Ann. Epiphytes*, 1963, **14**, No. hors série III, 113.

75. Wolff Et. and Haffen K.   Sur une méthode de culture d'organes embryonnaires *in vitro*. *J. exp. Rep. Biol. Med.*, 1952, **10**, 463.

76. Zwilling E.   Formation of endoderm from ectoderm in *Cordylophora*. *Biol. Bull.*, 1963, **124**, 368.

ADDENDUM

Organ culture of invertebrate tissues and organs has continued to develop since the initial period of intensive study during the years 1960–1963 [see the main article and Sengel (76)]. Of the various lines of research arising at this time, two have proved particularly valuable. There have been many detailed investigations on sexual differentiation and endocrinology in diverse groups of animals (worms, molluscs, echinoderms, crustaceans, myriapods, and insects), and on the other hand a large number of publications have been devoted to research on morphogenesis in *in vitro* culture, embryonic and larval development of insects, and regeneration in various groups. Apart from these two important problems, organ culture has been used to study other specific aspects: physiological and cytological investigations, parasitism, genetics, and the search for media of a composition favorable to one or other function of the explanted organ or tissue. We shall deal initially with these somewhat diverse studies that cover a wide field of results and experimental animals. The account will be brief as much of the work consists of preliminary experiments and development of techniques. The rest of the account will consist of two main sections, one dealing with the study of sexual differentiation and endocrinology and the other with research on embryonic, larval, and regenerative morphogenesis.

I. DEVELOPMENT OF TECHNIQUES ADAPTED TO SPECIFIC PROBLEMS

Molluscs have been the most extensively used animals. Work using the tentacles of *Planorbis* was begun in 1961, and Benex continued these studies between 1964 and 1969 (2–6), with the aim of analyzing parasitic specificity, by studying the experimental infection of *Planorbis* tentacles with miracidia of *Schistosoma mansoni* in *in vitro* culture. Mollusc organs maintained alive *in vitro* have a tendency to become dedifferentiated and the author therefore attempted to discover what factors would favor survival and retard dedifferentiation. Various sulfonamides, such as *p*-aminobenzoic acid, retard dedifferentiation of *Mytilus* organs for several days.

A number of other workers also tried to perfect media and techniques of *in vitro* culture in order to study parasitic infections. Among these were Perkins and Menzel (67) working with oyster tissues, Burch and Cuadros (12) with snail cells and tissues, and Vianey-Liaud and Lancastre (81) with explants from *Australorbis*. Further work on molluscs was carried out by

Kenny (43) who produced a chemically defined medium for culturing oyster heart tissue, and Hollande (42) who studied the secretory synthetic mechanism in the multifid glands of *Helix pomatia* when maintained *in vitro*.

The lumbricoid worms have been studied, using organ culture techniques, by Duprat, Izoard, and Meunier (26) using Wolff and Haffen's culture method (see main article, Ref. 75) and the prochordates were similarly studied by Ghiani, Orsi, and Relini (33).

Last, several workers have studied certain aspects of insect physiology using *in vitro* culture: Larsen obtained growth of insects in organ culture (48) and David and Rougier (21) observed the pulsation of the explanted dorsal vessel of a coleopteran. Rezzonico-Raimondi, Ghini, and Dolfini (69) noted that the cephalic ganglia of wild heterozygous *Drosophila* survived better in culture than did those of the homozygous flies. Schaller and Meunier (71) used organ culture to study neurosecretion in the brain and subesophageal ganglion of the odonate insect *Aeschna cyanea*. In order to observe giant chromosomes more easily, Cannon (15) developed a chemically defined medium for culturing insect salivary glands from *Sciara coprophila*. The development of chromosomes took place normally for 24 hours *in vitro*, with the formation and condensation of puffs, and with DNA synthesis.

II. SEXUAL DIFFERENTIATION AND ENDOCRINOLOGY

In 1963, Durchon and Schaller used organ culture techniques to study the sexual endocrinology and polychaete annelids, a problem Durchon had been investigating since 1952. These *in vitro* studies conducted by Durchon *et al.* produced some valuable results. It should be recalled that the sexual maturation of polychaete worms is subject to the control of a cerebral hormone that inhibits gametogenesis and epitoky. When a nereid parapodium was cultured alone *in vitro* using a hormone-free medium, gametogenesis began and heteronereid metamorphosis was observed. On the contrary, when the parapodium was associated in culture with a prostomium, the cerebral hormone exerted its inhibitory influence on gametogenesis and epitoky (27). Dhainaut (25), Durchon and Dhainaut (30), Durchon and Boilly (28), and Durchon, Boilly, and Dhainaut (29) studied the action of the cerebral hormone at the cellular level. Organ culture was found to be particularly valuable for this type of investigation as the gametes could be observed in a hormone-free environment (culture of parapodia alone), or alternatively in the presence of the cerebral hormone (parapodium cultured with prostomium). Dhainaut (25) used autoradiographic methods to study, in culture, the effects of the inhibitory hormone on the male gametes: the spermatocytes from parapodia cultured alone incorporated ^{3}H-thymidine actively from the beginning of culture, i.e., when the parapodium was separated from the prostomium. This incorporation reflects the major DNA synthesis corresponding to gametogenesis. On the other hand, in a parapodium associated with a prostomium, incorporation by the spermatocytes of the labeled precursor was very slow and continued throughout culture. In this case DNA synthesis corresponded to the spermatogonial mitoses, while spermatogenesis was inhibited by the prostomial hormone. These experiments show that this hormone acts as a regulator of DNA synthesis within the gametocytes.

Durchon and Dhainaut (30) and Durchon and Boilly (28) studied the behavior of oocytes. They cultured parapodia from female *Nereis*, either in the presence or absence of the prostomium, and studied the microscopic and ultramicroscopic structure of the oocytes which had or had not been inhibited by the cerebral hormone. In the isolated parapodia the oocytes grew, increasing in diameter by 40–100 μ in 10–20 days of culture. Signs of active RNA synthesis were present. There was an accumulation of concentric lamallae at the nuclear periphery which were in fact fibrils of ribonucleoprotein. This was not observed in oocytes cultured with a prostomium. Thus, in this instance, the cerebral hormone acts as a regulator of RNA synthesis. Malecha (58) also obtained gametogenesis and heteronereid metamorphosis when isolated segments from the epitoke species *Nereis succinea* were cultured. Associated *in vitro* with a prostomium of *Nereis diversicolor*, a nonepitoke species (the heterograft not being possible *in vivo*), inhibition of gametogenesis and epitoky were obtained in the same way as when associated with a prostomium of the same species.

Berjon, Andre, and Meunier (8) and Berjon (7) also studied sexual endocrinology in the lumbricoid worm *Eisenia foetida* (Oligochaeta). They first showed that the cerebral endocrine organ retained its structure and function in organ culture when an agar medium based on that of Wolff and Haffen was used. The neurosecretory cells showed all the signs of normal synthetic activity. Berjon subsequently studied in culture the endocrine action of cerebral ganglia from mature animals on fragments of clitellum from immature, premature, and mature animals. Culture of clitellar fragments, either alone or associated with cerebral ganglia, confirmed the existence of a factor responsible for clitellar turgescence and provided information on its mode of action on the tegumental secretory cells.

Malecha (57, 59) showed that in the Hirudinea, the endocrine influences are the reverse of those observed in the polychaete annelids. Testes of *Hirudo medicinalis* were cultured alone or in association with the peripharyngeal nerve mass, using a medium based on that used by Sengel for Planaria. At the beginning of culture, the testis contained spermatogonia and spermatocytes. When cultured alone, spermatogenesis did not occur in the testis. Germ cell differentiation was observed in culture if the testes were associated with the peripharyngeal nerve mass. It can thus be concluded that the presence of the peripharyngeal nerve mass is essential for the occurrence of spermatogenesis in *Hirudo*.

Before 1964 there had been little research on the sexual endocrinology of molluscs. Gomot and Guyard (34) began a series of investigations, culturing organs from the hermaphrodite snail *Helix aspersa*. A semisolid physiological medium, similar to that of Wolff and Haffen's, was used, with or without the addition of various nutrients. Gomot and Guyard (34) and Guyard and Gomot (41) showed the importance of trophic factors in the gametogenesis of *Helix*. On a non-nutrient physiological medium the gonad survived without differentiating while the addition of nutrient substances permitted gametogenesis. Spermatogonia developed to the spermatocyte I stage in the presence of chick embryo extracts, and as far as the spermatozooid stage in the presence of snail hemolymph. Hemolymph also favored the growth of oocytes. The experiments of Guyard and Gomot (41), Guyard (38–40), and Griffond (37) showed that gametogenesis of gastropods is influenced not only by trophic but also by hormonal factors which originate from the cephalic nerve complex. The latter, when associated with the gonad, favored sexual differentiation. In the presence of a cerebral ganglion from an adult snail in the female stage, the juvenile ovotestis of *Helix aspersa* showed female differentiation. On a hormone-free synthetic medium, female autodifferentiation of the gonadal rudiment was observed. This is also seen in the gastropod *Viviparus viviparus* in which the sexes are separate. If the testis of this gastropod is explanted onto a hormone-free medium, it produces oocytes (37). The phenomenon here is comparable to that observed in Crustacea, in which female differentiation is an autodifferentiation that can take place without hormonal influence.

Molluscan sexual endocrinology was also studied by Streiff and Peyre (see main article, Ref. 67) and Streiff (78, 79), who developed media suitable for culturing various organs from the marine gastropod *Calyptrea sinensis*. Results obtained by Streiff in 1966 (80) on the mechanism of sexual differentiation in this protandrous hermaphrodite are similar to those obtained by Gomot, Guyard, and Griffond. Gonads or gonadal rudiments of young individuals in the male stage were cultured for 20 days using Wolff and Haffen's method. In a hormone-free medium, the explants became transformed directly into ovaries. The germinal cells in the process of spermatogenesis underwent cytolysis, and intense oogenesis was observed. However, in a medium containing male hemolymph, spermatogenesis in the explanted gonads progressed normally. In *Calyptrea* the neuter form is thus the female form. Masculinizing hormonal factors are necessary for male sexual differentiation.

Choquet (16–18) studied another gastropod mollusc, *Patella vulgata*. Organ culture was used to investigate the reproductive development. The gonad survived for up to 3 months *in vitro* and showed normal gametogenesis. Having achieved favorable experimental conditions, Choquet demonstrated that, in *Patella*, in the gonad is subject to two hormonal influences, one originating in the cerebral ganglion and the other in the tentacles. If gonads in the male stage were cultured alone, spermatogenesis was observed from the beginning of culture. In association with the cerebral ganglion, spermatogenesis was more abundant. The cerebral ganglion thus appears to stimulate mitoses of male germ cells. Association with the tentacles, on the other hand, inhibited gonadal activity. This same inhibitory effect occurred with the cerebral ganglion–tentacle complex. Thus, depending on whether one or the other influence is predominant during the cycle, the gonad will either be in a phase of spermatogenesis or of reproductive quiescence. This functional duality explains the alternation of resting periods with periods of sexual activity during the year.

Richard (70) showed the effect of the photoperiod on female reproductive maturation in the Cephalopod mollusc *Sepia officinalis*. The optic gland seems to play an important role in the mechanism. Durchon and Richard (31) studied the endocrine role of the optic gland in organ culture. In the organism the optic gland is normally inhibited by the brain. When placed in culture, it is no longer subject to this cerebral inhibition and enters a phase of secretory activity. If the ovary is associated in culture with an optic gland that has been activated in this way, mitoses are more numerous and oocyte growth is superior to that in an ovary cultured alone.

To investigate the factors that determine the differential development of the germinal cells in the hermaphrodite echinoderm *Asterina gibbosa*, Delavault and Bruslé (23) and Bruslé (11) developed a culture technique for the gonads of this asteroid. After 18–40 days of culture, using Wolff and Haffen's method, the explanted glands were still intact. Neither spermatogenesis nor oogenesis was disturbed, and the mitoses and meioses were normal. During culture a moderate spermatogenesis preceded the appearance of young oocytes; a sexual change from male to female activity was observed. *In vivo* the gonad normally shows predominantly female characteristics and spermatogenesis occurs only from time to time under the influence of certain factors. Culture of gonads isolated from the organism tends to reduce spermatogenesis and promote oogenesis.

Berreur-Bonnenfant made further studies, using *in vitro* culture, on the factors that determine sexual differentiation in Crustacea. This author showed that the androgenic gland was necessary for maintaining testicular activity for a certain time, and that the brain also had an effect that was exercised via the molting hormone. The simultaneous presence of the molting and androgenic hormones acting together is essential for proper functioning of the germinal zone of the testis (9, 10).

Young larval gonads from the myriapod *Lithobius forficatus* remain undifferentiated during the three first intermolts. When cultured in a hormone-free medium they did not differentiate, but if grafted into individuals which were or were not differentiated sexually, they developed into ovaries (85).

Several workers have studied insect sexual differentiation using organ culture, the main work having been done by Leloup and Lender *et al.* Leloup (50) cultured male and female gonads from protonymphs, nymphs, and very young imagos of the dipteran *Calliphora erythrocephala* on a liquid medium. The medium closely resembled hemolymph in composition, and good survival and active differentiation of germinal cells was obtained.

Duveau-Hagège (32) and Lender and Duveau-Hagège (52) continued their earlier investigations (see main article, Refs. 46 and 47), using *Galleria mellonella* (Lepidoptera) and the cockroach *Periplaneta americana*. In culture both species showed normal testicular spermatogenesis and the beginnings of vitellogenesis in the ovaries. Extracts of adult insect organs (head or abdomen) had a favorable influence. Lender and Laverdure (55) and Laverdure (49) also studied the influence of extracts on the culture of ovaries from the coleopteran *Tenebrio molitor*. Extracts of the fat body, association with the cephalic complex, and addition of glucose in the place of trehalose all favored the survival and growth of oocytes and vitellogenesis.

III. *IN VITRO* STUDIES ON EMBRYONIC, LARVAL, AND REGENERATIVE MORPHOGENESIS

Most studies have concentrated on developing *in vitro* culture methods for whole or fragmented insect embryos. Insect embryogenesis is difficult to study using the usual *in vivo* surgical methods because of the very small size of the embryos, and it is easier to make observations and perform experiments in culture. The media used vary, and the hanging-drop technique is the method most frequently used (75). Lender and Fisher successfully applied Wolff and Haffen's technique, using an agar medium, to insect embryos. Vignau maintained the eggs of *Carausius* in paraffin oil, under an atmosphere of pure oxygen, and obtained survival of the eggs for more than 2 months.

The results of these investigations are largely in agreement. Almost all of the authors stressed the importance of the yolk and the embryonic appendages. However, development can take place to some extent without the yolk or egg membranes under the favorable conditions provided by the culture media (Ref. 47, *Bombyx mori;* Ref. 22, *Calliphora erythrocephala;* Ref. 36, *Scapsipedus marginatus;* Refs. 53 and 54, *Periplaneta americana;* Ref. 82, *Carausius morosus*). It is usually necessary to remove the egg membranes either for purposes of observation or for contact with the medium. In *Miastor* the egg membranes are permeable, and Counce (19) cultured the embryos successfully without removing the surrounding membranes. Almost all the experiments show that a certain stage of development must be attained—usually gastrulation—before subsequent differentiation can take place (22, 35, 44, 54). Segmentation, morphogenetic movements, and differentiation have been observed by all the authors. Ectoderm has been found to differentiate better than endoderm or mesoderm (22, 53, 54). Healing and, to some extent regeneration or regulation have been found to occur in insect embryos cultured *in vitro* (36, 45, 46). Lesseps (56) dissociated the embryos of *Drosophila* and found that the cells became reaggregated in categories.

Insect larval organs, particularly the imaginal disks, have been studied for a long time, using *in vitro* culture, primarily to investigate the hormonal influences on larval development. *In vitro* culture of imaginal rudiments, either alone or associated with endocrine organs, on hormone-free or hormone-containing media, has clearly constituted a useful system for such research. During the 1950's and 1960's valuable results were obtained using these methods (see main article). Since then, several workers have obtained development and sometimes metamorphosis of imaginal disks *in vitro*. Association with the cephalic complex (20, 72–74) or the presence of ecdysone in the medium (13, 66, 77), or both, always seems to be necessary for differentiation to take place. Courgeon (20) found that mitotic activity in the oculo-antennal disks of *Calliphora* depends on the cephalic complex. Ocular and antennal disks have been the most frequently studied, although Oberlander and Fulco (66) did obtain the growth and partial metamorphosis of the olar disks of *Calliphora*. In Sengel and Mandaron's experiments (77), leg, eye, and antennal disks of *Drosophila* differentiated completely and evaginated in the liquid culture medium that contained ecdysone. Demaure (24) cultured various larval organs of *Lucilia sericata* in a medium based on that of Wolff and Haffen. The salivary glands maintained their secretory activity for 2 weeks, the cephalic complexes survived for 10 days, and the imaginal annulus of the proventriculus showed development in culture. Miciarelli, Sbrenna, and Colombo (65) studied the formation of cuticle from larval epidermis of *Schistocerca gregaria* cultured *in vitro*. Only when the explants were taken after the multiplication of epidermal cells was a new complete cuticle comprising both exo- and endocuticle synthesized *in vitro*.

Burnett *et al.* and Marcel, among other, attempted to analyze the morphogenetic factors involved in regeneration. Burnett, Ruffing, Zongker, and Necco (14) studied the growth and differentiation of explants of the Hydroid *Tubularia* in culture. These authors considered that *in vitro* culture provides a means of working with a chemically defined medium, more suitable for chemical embryological studies than the environment provided by the organism *in vivo*. Cultures of cell sheets were obtained from fragments of coenosarc on the medium derived by these authors. Cell divisions were observed, and migrations of interstitial cells which formed aggregates of 4–8 cells. These cell masses subsequently differentiated, the interstitial cells becoming trasformed into cnidoblasts.

Marcel (60, 61) turned to the inductive and inhibitory morphogenetic factors intervening in the regeneration of the oligochaete annelid *Eisenia foetida*. Wolff and Haffen's method was used, with Sengel's medium for planarian blastemas. The author studied the effect of associations between fragments and organs of *Eisenia*, and also the action of crushed organ preparations incorporated into the medium. Marcel (60) first showed that regeneration of the pharynx in *Eisenia* is induced by the cerebral ganglia. Cerebral nervous tissue was found to exert an inhibitory effect on cephalic regeneration (61). This inhibitory factor, demonstrated in crushed preparations of nervous tissue, was found to be distributed along the nerve chain following a cephalo-caudal gradient. The nervous tissue also contained a trophic substance, which antagonized the inhibitory substance to varying degrees. The morphogenetic effects in cephalic regeneration depend on the equilibrium established between these two actions. This mechanism is comparable to that demonstrated by Wolff (83), Lender (51), and Wolff, Lender, and Ziller-Sengel (84) in the regeneration of planarians.

Marks and Reinecke (63, 64) continued their experiments on the cockroach, begun in 1964. They were able to culture regenerating legs, using an appropriate nutrient medium (62, 63), and to study the effect of endocrine glands on the *in vitro* regeneration of the leg. The regenerating tissues were cultured in association with explants of brain, prothoracic gland, and corpus allatum. The interactions observed *in vitro* were comparable to those that occur during regeneration of the leg *in vivo*. Healing and growth of the regenerated tissues were found to be hormone-dependent.

IV. CONCLUSIONS

Work on the culture of invertebrate organs covers such a wide field that it is impossible to give a full or concise account, and only the main points of certain broad lines of research are presented here. *In vitro* culture is a technique which has made it possible to approach the extremely diverse problems posed by animal physiology. This is true not only of vertebrate physiology but also of that of invertebrates. *In vitro* culture has proved valuable to the many workers investigating the lower animals, as shown by the number of publications and the interesting results that have been obtained. The widespread interest in this sphere is indicated by the many scientific meetings devoted to the culture of invertebrate tissues and organs in recent years. The Montpellier Congress in 1962 was followed by a colloquium at the Zoological Society of France in 1963, an International Congress at Milan in 1967, and a French-speaking colloquium at Clermont-Ferrand in 1968.

While the immense and varied world of the insects is still the most important source of experimental material for invertebrate organ culture, there have recently been important developments in research dealing with other invertebrates, particularly worms and molluscs, which have provided valuable information on reproductive endocrinology.

BIBLIOGRAPHY

1. Benex J.   Sur la dédifférenciation des tentacules de Planorbes en survie: rôle de la présence d'éléments nerveux sur le retard de cette dédifférenciation. *C. R. Acad. Sci.*, 1964, **258**, 2193–2196.
2. Benex J.   Recherches sur l'infection expérimentale de tentacules de Planorbes en survie, par des miracidiums de *Schistosoma mansoni*. (Application à l'analyse de la spécificité parasitaire.) Thèse, Université de Paris, 1965.
3. Benex J.   Action comparée de certains sulfamides à noyau pyrimidique, sur des explants de Mollusques maintenus en culture organotypique. *C. R. Acad. Sci.*, 1965, **261**, 5233–5236.
4. Benex J.   Substances susceptibles d'augmenter la survie d'explants maintenus en culture organotypique. *C. R. Acad. Sci.*, 1967, **265**, 571–574.
5. Benex J.   Action de divers types de sulfamides dans la survie d'explants de *Mytilus edulis*. *C. R. Acad. Sci.*, 1969, **268**, 158–161.
6. Benex J.   Survie et respiration des explants maintenus en culture *in vitro*. *C. R. Acad. Sci.*, 1969, **268**, 842–844.
7. Berjon, J. J.   Application de la culture organotypique sur milieux artificiels à la discrimination des fonctions endocrines des ganglions cérébroïdes du Lombricien *Eisenia foetida*. *C. R. Acad. Sci.*, 1965, **260**, 6212–6214.
8. Berjon J. J., Andre F. and Meunier J. M.   Culture organotypique sur milieux artificiels de la région endocrine du cerveau du Lombricien *Eisenia foetida*. *C. R. Soc. Biol.*, 1965, **159**, 139–141.
9. Berreur-Bonnenfant J.   La culture *in vitro* d'organes de Crustacés. *Bull. Soc. Zool.*, 1964, **89**, 59–64.
10. Berreur-Bonnenfant J.   Actions des cerveaux de mâle et de femelle sur le testicule du Crustacé Amphipode *Orchestia gammarella* en culture *in vitro*. *Bull. Soc. Zool.*, 1967, **91**, 327.
11. Bruslé J.   Différenciation des gonades hermaphrodites d'*Asterina gibbosa* en culture *in vitro*. *C. R. Acad. Sci.*, 1966, **263**, 1514–1516.
12. Burch J. B. and Cuadros C.   A culture medium for snail cells and tissues. *Nature*, 1965, **206**, 637–638.
13. Burdette W. J., Hanley E. W. and Grosch J.   The effect of ecdysones on the maintenance and development of ocular imaginal discs *in vitro*. *Texas Rep. Biol. Med.*, 1968, **26**, 173–180.
14. Burnett A. L., Ruffing F. E., Zongker J. and Necco A.   Growth and differentiation of *Tubularia* cells in a chemically defined physiological medium. *J. Emb. exp. Morph.*, 1968, **20**, 73–80.
15. Cannon G. B.   Culture of Insect salivary glands in a chemically defined medium. *Science*, 1964, **146**, 1063.
16. Choquet M.   Culture organotypique de gonades de *Patella vulgata* (Mollusque Gastéropode Prosobranche). *C. R. Acad. Sci.*, 1964, **258**, 1089–1091.
17. Choquet M.   Recherches en culture organotypique sur la spermatogenèse chez *Patella*

vulgata. Rôle des ganglions cérébroïdes et des testicules. *C. R. Acad. Sci.*, 1965, **261**, 4521–4524.

18. Choquet M. Gamétogenèse *in vitro* au cours du cycle annuel chez *Patella vulgata* en phase mâle. *C. R. Acad. Sci.*, 1967, **265**, 333–335.

19. Counce S. J. Culture of insect embryos *in vitro*. *Ann. N.Y. Acad. Sci.*, 1966, **139**, 65–78.

20. Courgeon A. M. L'activité mitotique, en culture organotypique, dans les disques oculo-antennaires de larves de *Calliphora erythrocephala* (Insecte Diptère). *C. R. Acad. Sci.*, 1969, **268**, 950–592.

21. David J. and Rougier M. Influence du pH du milieu sur la fréquence des battements et la durée de survie du vaisseau dorsal explanté de *Cybister lateralimarginalis* (Coléoptère Dytiscide). *C. R. Acad. Sci.*, 1965, **261**, 1394–1396.

22. Davis C., Krause J. and Krause G. Morphogenetic movements and segmentation of posterior egg fragments *in vitro* (*Calliphora erythrocephala*, Diptera). *Roux' Arch. Entw. Mech.*, 1968, **161**, 209–240.

23. Delavault R. and Bruslé J. Survie, en culture *in vitro*, de gonades d'une étoile de mer hermaphrodite, *Asterina gibbosa*. *Bull. Soc. Zool.*, 1966, **90**, 361–364.

24. Demaure J. C. Culture *in vitro* d'organes larvaires de Diptères. *C. R. Soc. Biol.*, 1968, **162**, 224–227.

25. Dhainaut A. Étude, en culture organotypique, de l'influence de l'hormone cérébrale des Néréidiens sur les synthèses de DNA au cours de la spermatogenèse. *C. R. Acad. Sci.*, 1964, **259**, 461–464.

26. Duprat P., Izoard F. and Meunier J. M. Cultures organotypiques de parois du corps de Lombriciens. *C. R. Acad. Sci.*, 1965, **260**, 7018–7021.

27. Durchon M. Résultats de cultures organotypiques chez les Annélides et les Mollusques Gastéropodes. *Bull. Soc. Zool.*, 1964, **89**, 45–48.

28. Durchon M. and Boilly B. Étude ultrastructurale de l'influence de l'hormone cérébrale des Néréidiens sur le développement des ovocytes de *Nereis diversicolor* (Annélide Polychète) en culture organotypique. *C. R. Acad. Sci.*, 1964, **259**, 1245–1247.

29. Durchon M., Boilly B. and Dhainaut A. Recherches en culture organotypique sur l'action de l'hormone cérébrale des Néréidiens (Annélides Polychètes). *C. R. Soc. Biol.*, 1965, **159**, 106–109.

30. Durchon M. and Dhainaut A. Influence de l'hormone cérébrale des Néréidiens sur la croissance des ovocytes. Étude en culture organotypique. *C. R. Acad. Sci.*, 1964, **259**, 917–919.

31. Durchon M. and Richard A. Étude, en culture organotypique, du rôle endocrine de la glande optique dans la maturation ovarienne chez *Sepia officinalis* (Mollusque Céphalopode). *C. R. Acad. Sci.*, 1967, **264**, 1497–1500.

32. Duveau-Hagège J. La culture *in vitro* des gonades de *Galleria mellonella* et de *Periplaneta americana*. Développement et vitellogenèse. *Bull. Soc. Zool.*, 1964, **89**, 66–69.

33. Ghiani P., Orsi L. and Relini G. Strutture di protocordati in coltura organotypica. *Atti Accad. Ligure Sci. Lettere*, 1964, **20**, 93–105.

34. Gomot L. and Guyard A. Évolution en culture *in vitro* de la glande hermaphrodite de jeunes Escargots de l'espèce *Helix aspersa*. *C. R. Acad. Sci.*, 1964, **258**, 2902–2905.

35. Grellet P. Culture *in vitro* d'embryons de *Scapsipedus marginatus* (Orthoptère Grillide). *C. R. Acad. Sci.*, 1965, **260**, 5100–5103.

36. Grellet P. Rôle des annexes embryonnaires dans l'œuf de *Scapsipedus marginatus* (Orthoptère Grillide) cultivé *in vitro*. *C. R. Acad. Sci.*, 1965, **260**, 5881–5884.

37. Griffond B. Survie et évolution, en culture *in vitro*, des testicules de *Viviparus viviparus*, Gastéropode Prosobranche à sexes séparés. *C. R. Acad. Sci.*, 1969, **268**, 963–965.

38. Guyard A.   Féminisation de la glande hermaphrodite juvénile d'*Helix aspersa* associée *in vitro* au ganglion cérébroïde d'Escargot adulte ou de Paludine femelle. *C. R. Acad. Sci.*, 1967, **265**, 147–149.

39. Guyard A.   Élaboration d'un milieu synthétique enrichi destiné à la culture d'organes de Mollusques. *C. R. Acad. Sci.*, 1969, **268**, 162–164.

40. Guyard A.   Autodifférenciation femelle de l'ébauche gonadique de l'Escargot *Helix aspersa* cultivée sur milieu anhormonal. *C. R. Acad. Sci.*, 1969, **268**, 966–969.

41. Guyard A. and Gomot L.   Survie et différenciation de la gonade juvénile d'*Helix aspersa* en culture organotypique. *Bull. Soc. Zool.*, 1964, **89**, 48–56.

42. Hollande E.   Évolution des grains de sécrétion dans les cellules des glandes multifides d'*Helix pomatia*, maintenus en survie expérimentale. *C. R. Acad. Sci.*, 1968, **267**, 1054–1057.

43. Kenny M. T.   The *in vitro* maintenance of oyster cardiac tissue in undefined and chemically defined media. *Diss. Abstr.*, 1965, **25**, 3762.

44. Koch P.   *In vitro*-Kultur und entwicklungsphysiologische Ergebnisse an Embryonen der Stabheuschrecke *Carausius morosus*. *Roux' Arch. Entw. Mech.*, 1964, **155**, 549–593.

45. Krause G.   Zum Verhalten explantierter Larvalgeweben und Embryonanlagen des Seidenspinners *Bombyx mori* in hängenden Tropfen. *Zool. Anz.*, 1963, **26**, 190–199.

46. Krause G.   Uber das Vermögen median durchschnittener Keimanlagen von *Bombyx mori* sich *in ovo* und sich *in vitro* zwillingsartig zu entwicklen. *Z. Naturforsch.*, 1965, **20**, 334–339.

47. Krause G. and Krause J.   Schichtenbau und Segmentierung junger Keimanlagen von *Bombyx mori* (Lepidoptera) *in vitro* ohne Dottersystem. *Roux' Arch. Entw. Mech.*, 1964, **155**, 451–510.

48. Larsen W. P.   Growth in an insect organ culture. *J. Insect Physiol.*, 1967, **13**, 613–619.

49. Laverdure A. M.   Culture *in vitro* des ovaires de *Tenebrio molitor* (Coléoptère). Importance de la composition du milieu sur la survie, la croissance et la vitellogenèse. *C. R. Acad. Sci.*, 1967, **265**, 505–507.

50. Leloup A. M.   Cultures organotypiques de gonades d'Insecte *(Calliphora erythrocephala)*. *Bull. Soc. Zool.*, 1964, **89**, 70–77.

51. Lender T.   Factors in morphogenesis of regenerating freshwater Planaria. *Adv. Morphogenesis*, 1962, **2**, 305–331.

52. Lender T. and Duveau-Hagege J.   Influence du milieu de culture sur le développement *in vitro* des ovaires de larves et nymphes de *Galleria mellonella* (Lépidoptère). *C. R. Soc. Biol.*, 1965, **159**, 104–106.

53. Lender T. and Fisher K. R.   La culture *in vitro* d'embryons de *Periplaneta americana* privés de leur vitellus. *C. R. Acad. Sci.*, 1965, **261**, 244–245.

54. Lender T. and Fisher K. R.   La survie et la différenciation *in vitro* des embryons de la Blatte *Periplaneta americana* (Dictyoptère). *Bull. Soc. Zool.*, 1965, **90**, 591–597.

55. Lender T. and Laverdure A. M.   Culture *in vitro* des ovaires de *Tenebrio molitor* (Coléoptère). Croissance et vitellogenèse. *C. R. Acad. Sci.*, 1967, **265**, 451–454.

56. Lesseps R. J.   Culture of dissociated *Drosophila* embryos: aggregated cells differentiate and sort out. *Science*, 1965, **148**, 502.

57. Malecha J.   Culture organotypique d'Hirudinées. *C. R. Soc. Biol.*, 1966, **159**, 1674–1675.

58. Malecha J.   Transformation hétéronéréidienne et gamétogenèse chez *Nereis succinea* (Annélide Polychète) en culture organotypique. *C. R. Acad. Sci.*, 1967, **265**, 613–615.

59. Malecha J.   Étude en culture organotypique de l'influence endocrine de la masse nerveuse péripharyngienne sur la maturation testiculaire chez *Hirudo medicinalis*. *C. R. Acad. Sci.*, 1967, **265**, 1806–1808.

60. Marcel R.   Rôle inducteur du cerveau au cours de la régénération du pharynx chez *Eisenia foetida* (Annélide Oligochète). *C. R. Acad. Sci.*, 1966, **262**, 2470–2472.

61. Marcel R.   Effets inhibiteur et trophique dans la régénération céphalique de *Eisenia foetida* (Annélide Oligochète). *Ann. Emb. Morph.*, 1968, **1**, 417–426.

62. Marks E. P. and Reinecke J. P.   Regenerating tissues from the Cockroach leg: a system for studying *in vitro*. *Science*, 1964, **143**, 961–963.

63. Marks E. P. and Reinecke J. P.   Regenerating tissues from the Cockroach leg: nutrient media for maintenance *in vitro*. *J. Kansas Entomol. Soc.*, 1965, **38**, 179–182.

64. Marks E. P. and Reinecke J. P.   Regenerating tissues from the Cockroach *Leucophaea maderae:* effects of endocrine glands *in vitro*. *Gen. comp. Endocr.*, 1965, **5**, 241–247.

65. Miciarelli A., Sbrenna G. and Colombo G.   Experiments on *in vitro* cultures of larval epiderm of desert locust *(Schistocerca gregaria)*. *Experientia*, 1967, **23**, 64–66.

66. Oberlander H. and Fulco L.   Growth and partial metamorphosis of imaginal discs of the greater wax moth, *Galleria mellonella, in vitro*. *Nature*, 1967, **216**, 1140–1141.

67. Perkins F. O. and Henzel R. W.   Maintenance of oyster cells *in vitro*. *Nature*, 1964, **204**, 1106–1107.

68. Remy-Philippe.   Comportement en culture du tractus génital du Crabe *Carcinus moenas*. *Bull. Acad. Soc. Lorraine Sci.*, 1967, **6**, 348–352.

69. Rezzonico-Raimondi G., Ghini C. and Dolfini S.   Comparative observations on the behaviour *in vitro* of cephalic ganglia of wild homozygous and heterozygous Drosophilae. *Experientia*, 1964, **20**, 440–441.

70. Richard A.   Rôle de la photopériode dans le déterminisme de la maturation génitale femelle du Céphalopode *Sepia officinalis*. *C. R. Acad. Sci.*, 1967, **264**, 1315–1318.

71. Schaller F. and Meunier J.   Résultats de cultures organotypiques du cerveau et du ganglion sous-oesophagien d'*Aeschna cyanea* (Insecte Odonate). Survie des organes et évolution des éléments neuro-sécréteurs. *C. R. Acad. Sci.*, 1967, **264**, 1441–1444.

72. Schneider I.   Differentiation of larval Drosophila eye-antennal discs *in vitro*. *J. exp. Zool.*, 1964, **156**, 91–104.

73. Schneider I.   Inadvisability of using the raft technique for Drosophila organ culture. *Drosophila Inform. Serv.*, 1965, **40**, 74–75.

74. Schneider I.   Histology of larval eye-antennal discs and cephalic ganglia of Drosophila cultured *in vitro*. *J. Emb. exp. Morph.*, 1966, **15**, 271–279.

75. Seidel F. and Koch P.   Untersuchungen zur Kultur von Insektenembryonen *in vitro*. *Embryologia*, 1964, **8**, 200–222.

76. Sengel P.   Utilisation de la culture organotypique pour l'étude de la morphogenèse et de l'endocrinologie chez les Invertébrés. *Bull. Soc. Zool.*, 1964, **89**, 10–41.

77. Sengel P. and Mandaron P.   Aspects morphologiques du développement *in vitro* des disques imaginaux de la Drosophile. *C. R. Acad. Sci.*, 1969, **268**, 405–407.

78. Streiff W.   Survie d'organes de Mollusques marins en culture *in vitro*. Présentation des milieux A6, A7, A7c et B2. Améliorations apportées à la technique de culture. *Gen. comp. Endocr.*, 1963, **3**, No. 98.

79. Streiff W.   Survie d'organes de Mollusques marins en culture *in vitro*. Résultats obtenus sur les milieux A6, A7, A7c et A8c. *Bull. Soc. Zool.*, 1964, **89**, 56–59.

80. Streiff W.   Autodifférenciation ovarienne chez un Mollusque Prosobranche hermaphrodite protandre *Calyptrea sinensis*. *C. R. Acad. Sci.*, 1966, **263**, 539–542.

81. Vianey-Liaud M. and Lancastre F.   Utilisation d'un milieu diphasique pour la culture organotypique d'explants d'*Australorbis glabratus* (Pulmoné Basommatophore). *C. R. Acad. Sci.*, 1968, **266**, 1317–1319.

82. Vignau J.   Mise au point d'une méthode de culture des œufs du Phasme *Carausius morosus* privés d'exochorion. *C. R. Acad. Sci.*, 1967, **265**, 1504–1507.

83. Wolff E.   Recent researches on the regeneration of Planaria. *In* "Regeneration," 20th Growth Symp., pp. 53–84. Ronald Press, New York, 1962.

84. Wolff E., Lender T. and Ziller-Sengel C.   Le rôle de facteurs auto-inhibiteurs dans la régénération des Planaires. *Rev. Suisse Zool.*, 1964, **71**, 75–98.

85. Zerbib C.   Expériences de greffes et essais de culture *in vitro* de tronçons de corps contenant la gonade indifférenciée de jeunes larves du Myriapode Chilopode *Lithobius forficatus*. *Bull. Soc. Zool.*, 1966, **91**, 344.

CHAPTER VIII

IN VITRO REASSOCIATION
OF DISSOCIATED CELLS

Michel Sigot

INSTITUT D'EMBRYOLOGIE ET DE TÉRATOLOGIE EXPÉRIMENTALE
DU COLLÈGE DE FRANCE ET DU C.N.R.S.
PARIS, FRANCE

I. INTRODUCTION

The essential character of organ culture is the maintenance of the organized structure possessed by the explant at transplantation. Work using organ culture has been carried out during investigations into cellular reaggregation. The explant is disorganized into a mass of completely separate cells. Culture of this mass permits a study of the reorganization of the dissociated cells.

The starting point for these experiments was the desire to investigate the behavior of cells whose topographic relationships had been completely disrupted. Would they conserve and manifest their potentialities? Most work since that carried out by Wilson has been concerned with this problem. These experiments have shown that the cells have certain properties, unsuspected until recently—for example, regarding reaggregation and the ability of similar cells to recognize one another.

The principal morphological studies of the phenomenon of reaggregation will be reviewed, and an attempt will be made to show how the phenomenon is interpreted at the present time.

II. MORPHOLOGICAL ASPECTS OF REAGGREGATION

Wilson (39) was the first to obtain the reconstitution *in vitro* of previously dissociated organisms. His experiments were the result of observing the phenomena of degeneration and spontaneous regeneration in certain sponges (*Microciona prolifera*, for example).

Under the conditions that induce degeneration most of the body of the sponge will die, but in certain regions cells that are still alive begin to aggregate together into masses of undifferentiated tissue. These spherical masses resemble gemmules and possess powers of regeneration, forming new sponges when they are isolated.

Wilson induced artificial degeneration and, once it had begun, macerated the sponge, allowing the living cells and cell masses to escape. These cells and cell masses then fused together and produced a new sponge. Complete dissociation of a healthy sponge was then attempted as follows. A piece of sponge was finely minced and pressed through a silk sieve. The meshes of the sieve were so fine that only single cells would pass through. The dissociated cells fell into a container containing sea water and were collected on glass coverslips. After a few days, small aggregates formed on the coverslips and these proved to be true miniature sponges.

Wilson extended his research to study reaggregation in different species of coelenterates and echinoderms and found that the reconstitution of an organism or of an organ varied from one group to another and from one species to another.

Galtsoff (11, 12) also studied the phenomenon of reaggregation in sponges and demonstrated the presence of five cell types in cell suspensions derived from them. These five cell types are (1) archeocytes, (2) pinacocytes, (3) desmocytes, (4) collencytes, and (5) choanocytes. The formation of aggregates was due to the mobility and mutual adhesion of the archeocytes but pinacocytes were also necessary for the formation of a complete sponge.

The process of reaggregation has been found to occur in two phases:

1. A phase in which the cells aggregate together in a random fashion after the occurrence of collisions. These cells form small masses that grow by the continued arrival and adhesion of motile cells;

2. A phase during which the mass becomes fixed to the substratum. The cells become regrouped according to their affinities and functions, to reconstitute the organism from which they were derived. This regrouping of the cells is due to chance, with the cells in the mass sliding over one another in random fashion. When two cells of the same type meet they adhere together, remain attached, and lose their mobility. If two dissimilar cells meet, no adhesion occurs and the cells separate.

Galtsoff demonstrated the importance of calcium and magnesium ions in cellular adhesion. This property was the basis of Holtfreter and Moscona's techniques for dissociation.

Fauré-Frémiet (8–10) worked with the sponge *Ficulina ficus* and examined more closely the reconstitution of sponges *in vitro*. He showed that aggregates could not develop until they had become fixed to a solid substratum. Fixation was due to the thigmotactic properties of the archeocytes. These cells formed a mesothelial layer that became closely applied to the substratum, thus inducing adhesion of the whole mass. The archeocytes then multiplied actively and formed bundles of fusiform cells. These bundles formed a framework on which the other cell types became organized. The collencytes were the source of the loose mesenchyme and the dermal covering. The choanocytes formed small spherical masses, which soon became organized into an open ciliated basketwork. Canals appeared as irregular lacunae in the mesenchyme, and became lined by the collencytes. It seems that the current of water created by the choanocytes played a major part in the formation of the canals. The current also had an important function in maintaining the integrity of the culture by imposing upon it a mechanomorphic modeling.

Fauré-Frémiet summarized the following general ideas, based on his own work and that of others.

1. It is a general phenomenon that the dissociated cells of a tissue become "active" and show ameboid movements enabling them to regroup themselves. As the regrouping proceeds, the ameboid movement is lost and there is a return to the stable "quiescent" stage that preceded dissociation.

2. The basis of all research into the dissociation of tissues depends on the ability of cells to retain their original potentialities and return to their original state after mechanical handling and subsequent dedifferentiation. It must be presumed that the different kinds of cells reaggregate in such a way that they occupy the same positions as they occupied in the normal tissue. There would be, as Huxley said, utilization of the leftovers; the destiny of the cells is not a function of their position, but their eventual position is a function of their nature.

Experiments on sponges suggest another hypothesis. In the reaggregates, the different cell types are produced from a single group of cells, the archeocytes. They are not produced from different elements separated by dissociation. These cells are totipotent and are comparable with the neoblasts or regeneration cells. In other words, it could be presumed that the reconstitution of a sponge from a cellular suspension represents true regeneration. In support of this hypothesis can be cited the fact that the regrouping of cells during the reconstitution of a sponge is mainly the effect of the archeocytes. In their absence, reorganization does not occur.*

3. It is necessary to explain the cohesion that keeps a culture of sponge cells together, limits the tendency for expansion, and preserves the unity of the mass. This cohesion within the structure is definitely associated with the organization of the tissues making up the culture. It is doubtful if it is connected with the formation of the intercellular material, spongine, since

---

* It is also possible that there are two phenomena occurring at the same time, and that there is some true regeneration during the process. This question has not yet been tackled; the work carried out has ignored the process of regeneration and has concentrated on the particular phenomenon of cellular adhesion and selective adhesion.

this is formed late in the culture. These properties must be looked for within the protoplasm of the assembled cells.

All experiments on cellular dissociation had been carried out using invertebrates. Holtfreter was the first to carry out this type of experiment using amphibians. Holtfreter (14–18) demonstrated that it is possible to isolate embryonic cells without damaging their ability to differentiate. These cells reaggregate, become regrouped, and recommence their differentiation.

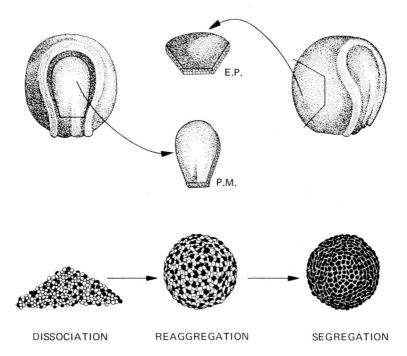

DISSOCIATION   REAGGREGATION   SEGREGATION

FIG. 1.   Combination of cells from presumptive epidermis (E.P.) and medullary plate (P.M.). The excised explants are dissociated and then cultured. The epidermal cells are shown black; the medullary plate cells white. The dissociated cells reaggregate to form a spherical mass. After reaggregation, the cells segregate and only epidermal cells are seen on the surface. The medullary plate cells have migrated to the center. After Townes and Holtfreter.

The technique used to dissociate the amphibian cells was a chemical method, not a mechanical one like that used for the sponges.

The cells were made to dissociate in a physiological saline solution lacking calcium ions, and at an alkaline pH.

In 1955, Holtfreter and Townes (33) published the results of a study into the selective regrouping of the cells in a neurula (33) using the same chemical technique for the dissociation.

In order to differentiate between the various cell types, cellular associations were carried out between two differently pigmented species (*Amblystoma punctatum* and *Triturus torosus*). The following is a brief précis of their experiments in combining different cell types.

1. *Ectodermal Derivatives.* A piece of the presumptive medullary plate and a piece of the presumptive epidermis were dissociated and mixed. The cells aggregated together in random fashion, the mass became spherical,

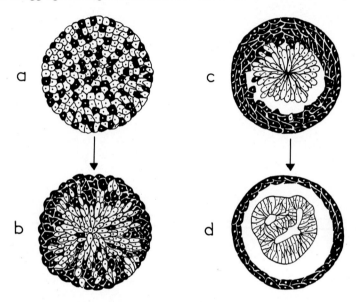

FIG. 2.   Segregation of cells from medullary plate and presumptive epidermis. Diagrammatic sections illustrating four successive stages in segregation. (a) Initial stage; the two cell types are mixed. (b) The beginning of sorting out. (c) The two cell types have separated. (d) The epidermal cells have reconstituted an epidermis and the neural cells have formed a neural tube. After Townes and Holtfreter.

and then the two cell types separated completely. The neural cells showed a tendency to move to an internal position, while the epidermal cells moved to the outside and tended to form a covering layer. The neural cells reconstituted a neural tube (Figs. 1–3).

When the cells from the medullary fold were added to the preceding mixture an intermediate layer formed around the neural tube. This intermediate layer was composed of mesenchyme, melanophores, and ganglion cells and a chorion appeared on the surface of the epidermis (Fig. 4).

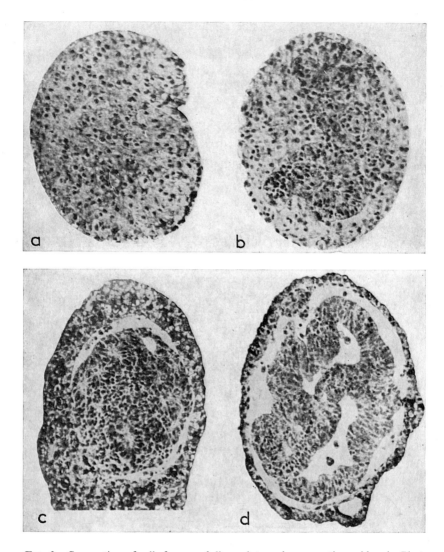

FIG. 3. Segregation of cells from medullary plate and presumptive epidermis. Photomicrographs of histological sections corresponding to Fig. 2a–d. After Townes and Holtfreter.

2. *Ectodermal and Endodermal Derivatives* (Fig. 5). Dissociated endoderm together with medullary plate: the endoderm completely surrounded the neural cells.

Endoderm together with medullary plate and medullary fold: under the influence of the epidermis and the mesenchyme which had differentiated

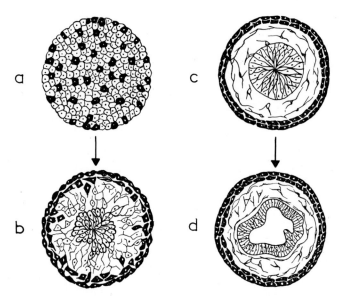

FIG. 4.   Segregation of cells from medullary plate, presumptive epidermis, and medullary fold. Diagrammatic sections illustrating four successive stages in segregation. The cells of the medullary fold form an intermediate layer between the epidermis and the neural tube. After Townes and Holtfreter.

from the medullary fold, the mass of neural cells became hollow, moved into a lateral position, and became surrounded by the epidermis.

3. *Mesodermal and Endodermal Derivatives* (Fig. 6). The endodermal cells showed a centrifugal tendency in relation to the mesodermal cells.

4. *Mesodermal, Endodermal, and Epidermal Derivatives* (Fig. 6).   This was the preceding together with the epidermis. In this case the presence of the ectoderm prevented the mesoderm from becoming embedded in the endoderm. (The ectoderm normally prevents the endoderm from forming a covering layer.) As usual, the epidermis formed the covering layer.

5. *Combinations of Ectoderm with Mesodermal Derivatives.*   Epidermis plus ventrolateral mesoderm: the epidermis surrounded the mesodermal derivatives which form a chorion, mesenchyme, and blood cells (Fig. 7).

Medullary plate together with the roof of the archenteron and the epidermis. The cells of the medullary plate developed into a neural formation which took up a central position.

These experiments have shown that cells regroup according to their affinities, and that newly formed tissues are able to separate following the same topographic relationships that they occupied in the embryo.

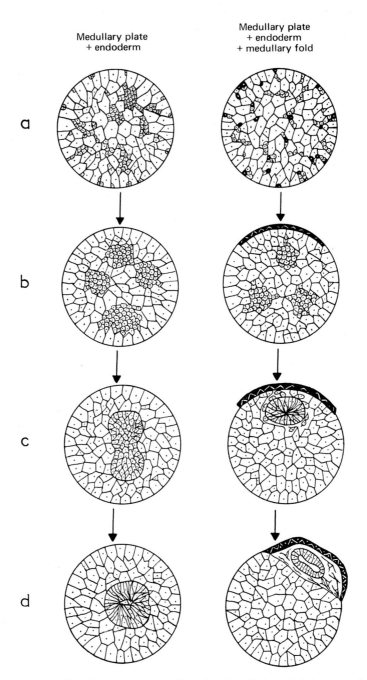

Medullary plate
+ endoderm

Medullary plate
+ endoderm
+ medullary fold

a

b

c

d

FIG. 5. Segregation of cells from ectodermal and endodermal derivatives. On the left, segregation of a mixture of cells from the medullary plate and the endoderm. The endoderm surrounds the neural cells. On the right, the cells of the medullary fold were added to the previous mixture; they form an epidermis and mesenchyme that prevents the neural cells from being buried among the endodermal cells. The formation of a neural tube has been induced. After Townes and Holtfreter.

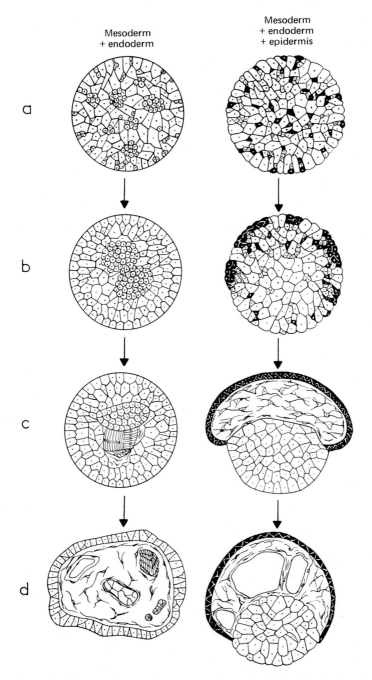

FIG. 6. On the left, segregation of a mixture of mesodermal and endodermal cells. The mesodermal cells migrate into a central position. On the right, epidermal cells added to the preceding mixture prevent the mesodermal cells from being enclosed by the endoderm. After Townes and Holtfreter.

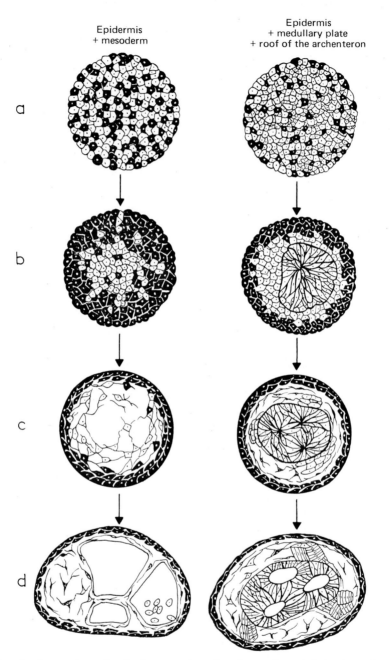

FIG. 7. Segregation of cells from ectodermal and mesodermal derivatives. On the left there is a segregation of a mixture of epidermal and mesodermal cells. The epidermis surrounds the mesodermal cells. On the right, there is a segregation of a mixture of cells from the medulla, epidermis, and the roof of the archenteron. The cells of the medullary plate migrate to a central position and form a neural tube. The cells of the roof of the archenteron form an intermediate layer. After Townes and Holtfreter.

Extending further the field of research into dissociation, Moscona (22) showed that it was possible to dissociate the tissues of chick embryos. The proteolytic enzyme trypsin was used to dissolve the intercellular material.

Moscona's technique involved first placing the tissues in Tyrode's solution, lacking calcium and magnesium. The tissues were then incubated in an identical solution containing 3% of trypsin. Cellular dissociation was achieved by shaking and by suction with a pipet. The suspended cells were washed 2 or 3 times with Tyrode's solution lacking calcium and magnesium, then with normal Tyrode's solution, and were finally placed on a nutrient culture medium.

This method was based on the following properties:

1. The cohesion of cells is decreased in liquids deficient in calcium and magnesium,

2. Under certain conditions, alkaline media induce hydration and swelling of certain cellular materials.

3. Tissues treated in this way are more sensitive to breakdown of the intercellular material by trypsin and they can then be separated by simple rinsing.

Using this technique, Moscona was able to show that dissociated cells from limb bud or the mesonephros were able to sort themselves out, differentiate according to their histological type, and reconstitute the initial tissue.

In other experiments Moscona (1956) used heterotypical combinations between two organs (limb bud and mesonephros):

a. Dissociation of the lateral mesoderm of a 28-somite chick embryo (stage 16). At this stage, the lateral mesoderm contains the limb bud and presumptive mesonephros as undifferentiated cell masses. After several days of culture *in vitro*, the aggregate contained cartilage cells and mesonephric tubules. The differentiation produced in culture corresponded to the normal differentiation of these cells during organogenesis. Dissociation did not destroy the potentialities of the cells.

b. Mixture of cells from the limb bud and mesonephros of a 3–5 day chick embryo. The rudiments are well formed at this stage. The cells regrouped themselves in the center of the aggregates and formed cartilaginous and mesonephric formations (Fig. 9).

Cells of the same type possess a kind of "memory," which is not destroyed by dissociation. The cells regroup themselves preferentially according to their initial type.

In 1957 Moscona tried to define these effects further by using older tissues, derived from two different species (mouse and chicken). The cell types were easily distinguished since the nuclei of the mouse cells were larger than those of the chicken, and their staining reactions were different (21).

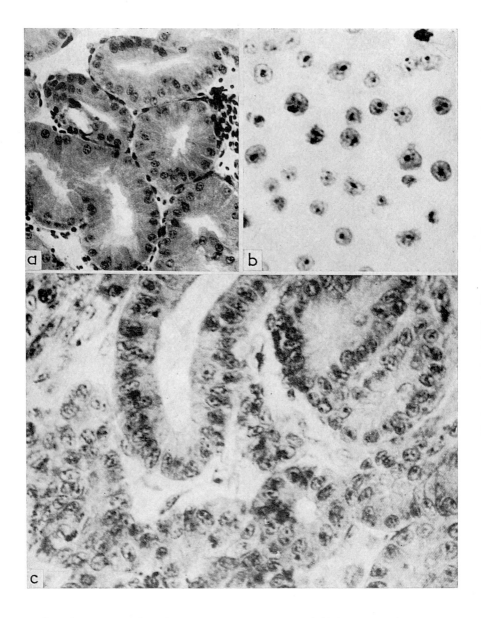

FIG. 8.   Reaggregation of cells from the mesonephros of chick embryo.   (a) Mesonephros before dissociation.   (b) Cells dissociated from the mesonephros.   (c) The cells
have reformed characteristic mesonephric structures.   After Moscona.

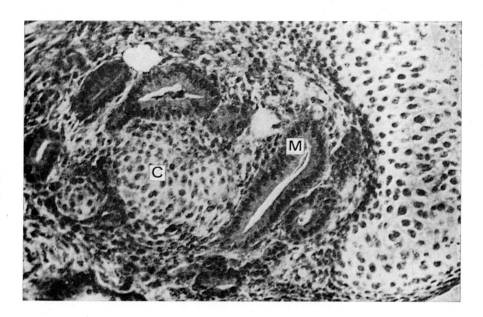

F<small>IG</small>. 9. Segregation of cells from limb bud and mesonephros of chick embryo. The two cell types have separated and have formed cartilaginous (C) and mesonephric (M) structures. After Moscona.

The results of these experiments are as follows:

1. *Isotypical combinations.* A mixture of cartilage cells from the limb buds of 4-day chick embryos and 12-day mouse fetuses (Fig. 10a,b,c). After 6 days of culture there was no segregation within the aggregates. The cartilage cells from the two species had differentiated in the midst of the same ground substance.

Similar results were obtained with a mixture of cells from the liver of 5-day chick embryos and 13-day mouse fetuses. The culture resulted in a mixed aggregate (Fig. 10d).

2. *Heterotypical combinations.* Cells from chicken liver together with cells from mouse cartilage (Fig. 11a): The two types of cells separated into two concentric layers, a nucleus of mouse cartilage and a cortex of chicken liver.

Cells from 4-day chick embryo mesonephros and cartilage cells from 12-day fetal mice (Fig. 11b): Reconstitution of the initial structure (mesonephric tubules and cartilaginous nodules) was seen, the tissues being randomly in the aggregate.

Thus, there was no incompatibility between the tissues of the two different species. The persistence of this tolerance has not been investigated.

The experiments using isotypical combinations, which resulted in chimeric aggregates composed of chicken and mouse tissues, were similar to those carried out by Wolff (40) in 1954. Wolff's experiments involved associating in culture pieces of embryonic testis or pieces of lungs and embryonic bronchi

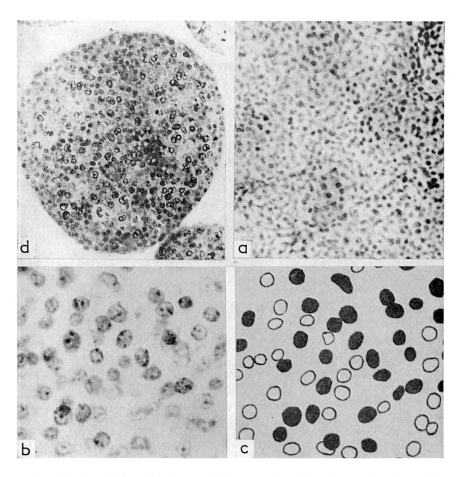

FIG. 10. Isotypical combinations. (a) Reaggregation of a mixture of cartilage cells from chicken and mouse limb buds. No segregation. (b) The same section at a higher magnification. Compare with Fig. 10c. (c) Diagrammatic representation of Fig. 10b showing the distribution of mouse nuclei (black) and chicken nuclei (white). (d) Reaggregation of a mixture of cells from chicken and mouse liver. The chicken cells (pale staining nuclei) and mouse cells (dark staining nuclei) are scattered at random in the aggregate. After Moscona.

from chickens and mice (Fig. 12). The tissues penetrated into one another and there was a change in the primitive structures which resulted in the formation of chimeric organs.

These two types of experiments, the isotypical combinations carried out by Moscona, and those of Wolff, pose the problem of the affinities between homologous cells from two species, affinities that can be manifested in the absence of dissociation. Homologous cells have a structural relationship that overcomes the genetic relationship. When they come into contact, they recognize one another as belonging to the same tissue family and combine their common properties to reconstitute a single organ.

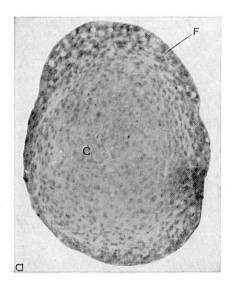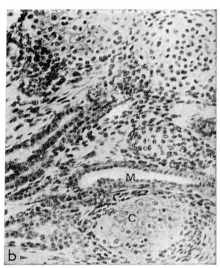

FIG. 11.   Heterotypical combinations.   (a) Reaggregation of a mixture of cells from chicken liver and mouse cartilage. The two cell types have separated, with the liver cells (F) surrounding the cartilage cells (C).   (b) Reaggregation of a mixture of cells from chicken mesonephros and mouse cartilage. Reconstitution of the initial tissues is seen: (M) mesonephric tubules; (C) cartilage.   After Moscona.

Following Moscona's work, many authors have studied the reaggregation of cells from birds and mammals. Trinkaus and Groves (34) were the first to show that cells from different embryonic chicken organs were able to reaggregate and reconstitute the structures from which they were derived. Weiss and Taylor (38) experimented with much older embryonic cells, using organs from 8–14 day chick embryos. Trinkaus and Moscona used embryos at a maximum of 5 days of incubation. Weiss and Taylor cultured aggregates on the chorioallantoic membrane of 8-day chick embryos. They used this method in preference to *in vitro* culture, because under these conditions, the explants became vascularized and differentiation occurred for a longer time than would have been possible *in vitro*. Reaggregation of the metanephros, liver, and skin were studied and these three organs were found to reconstitute themselves and differentiate extremely well.

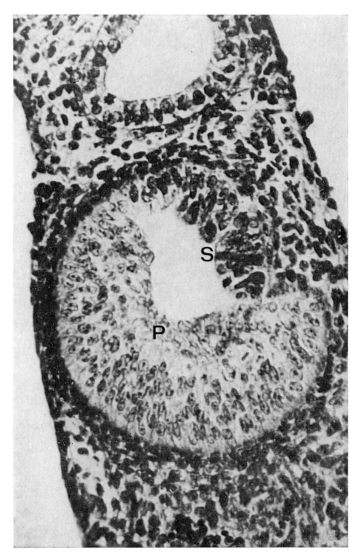

FIG. 12.   Chick embryo lung and mouse embryo lung associated in culture. A chimeric bronchus has formed, composed of chicken cells (P) and mouse cells (S). After Et. Wolff.

In 1960, Abraham (1, 2) showed that testis cells isolated from chick embryos were able to reform their initial morphological structure. He used embryonic cells from late stages, that is, 18 and 19 days of incubation. The organs were dissociated with trypsin using Moscona's technique and the cell suspension was then cultured on a slightly modified version of Wolff and Haffen's medium. The proportion of agar was increased (9 parts being used instead of 6) so that the medium was not liquefied on addition of the cell suspension. Reorganization of the testis was first seen with the formation of a capsule around the explant and proliferation of connective tissue cells. After 3–4 days of culture the epithelial cells formed into condensations and alignments that slowly became organized into testicular tubules (Fig. 13a–e). These experiments again demonstrate the segregation of cells of different types.

III. INTERPRETATIONS OF THE PHENOMENON OF ADHESION

The experiments described above show the ability of dissociated cells to reaggregate themselves and become reorganized according to their specific histological type into positions conforming to the normal. The mechanism by which this reaggregation and selective reassociation occurs must be investigated.

When a study is made of the displacement of cells inside one of these reaggregates, it is seen that the aggregate is not oriented. Similar cells only reassociate when they come into contact with one another as they move through the mass. Reassociation is thus linked with selective adhesion among cells. The cells of a mixed aggregate remain adhering to cells of a similar type, but they continue to move when they come into contact with cells of another type.

Thus it is the adhesion and the selective adhesion among cells that recent experiments have been designed to investigate. Only the main aspects of this work will be indicated.

Weiss (35, 36) compared adhesion between cells with similar enzyme-substrate or antigen-antibody reactions. Spiegel's work on sponges (26) and Gregg's work on the myxomycetes (13) were successful in using specific antibodies to modify reaggregation and seems to verify the hypothesis.

In further work (1958) Weiss returned to his original idea. Spiegel and Gregg's experiments were not sufficient proof, since they only showed that the molecules on the cellular surface that are implicated in adhesion have antigenic properties. Weiss himself had previously tried unsuccessfully to interfere with selective reaggregation by using organospecific antisera.

Taking into account Moscona's results, Weiss suggested another factor involved in the specificity. This was that adhesion between cells occurred

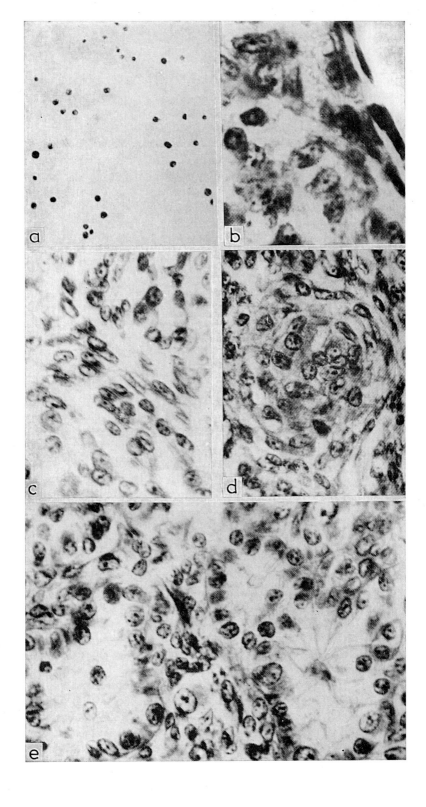

by means of an intermediary exudate. Homologous cells would synthesize homologous exudates that would be likely to mix together and form a communal envelope around the cells. Nonhomologous exudates would not become mixed (37).

Moscona has worked on this idea of an exudate as a factor in cellular reaggregation and reassociation and some of his experiments tried to demonstrate the existence and role of such a matrix.

Steinberg undertook a series of experiments to prove that this matrix played no part either in reaggregation or in selective reassociation. The results of these two different experiments and the conclusions derived from them will be discussed.

Moscona began by observing closely the first phases of reaggregation. He studied the reaggregation of embryonic chicken cells that had been previously dissociated by tryptic digestion. Observation of the cell suspension even before true reaggregation had commenced showed the appearance of a colloidal material, probably derived from the cells. According to the culture conditions, this material formed either as a continuous film or as a network of filaments, along which the cells moved, met, and formed aggregates. This material was collected and analyzed and was found to be probably a mucoprotein (22).

This matrix of extracellular material (E.C.M. of the author) played a double role. It acted as a physical substrate, necessary for the cells to move and meet, and on the other hand, since it was a product of the cells themselves, it reflected in its structure and functions the diversity or similarity of the cells present. Thus it acted not only as a physical bond between the cells but also as an integrating network that would transmit many signals toward many responding mechanisms (22).

The dissociated cells had to synthesize the E.C.M. that had been destroyed or removed at dissociation. This renewal process was linked to the level of metabolic activity. Thus, the more active the synthesis of E.C.M., the greater was the adhesion of the cells responsible for this synthesis. Moscona verified this hypothesis by studying the effect of both temperature and synthetic inhibitors on reaggregation.

In the first experiment the cells used were nerve cells from the retina, liver cells, and mesonephros of 7-day chick embryos. The tissues were dissociated, then cultured by the usual method. The cell suspensions were maintained at 38°, 30°, 25°, and 15°C for 24 hours (23).

FIG. 13.   Reaggregation of cells from chick embryo testis.   (a) Testicular cells a few minutes after dissociation.   (b) Formation of a capsule around the explant. (c) Cords of connective tissue cells.   (d) Condensation of epithelial cells surrounded by connective tissue cells.   (e) Reconstitution of typical testicular tubules.   After Abraham.

The degree of cellular adhesion was evaluated by measuring the mean diameter of the aggregates formed. (The more intercellular adhesion took place the larger were the aggregates.) The curve representing the mean aggregate diameter as a function of temperature showed that cellular adhesion diminished with decreasing temperature.

Hence Moscona concluded that cellular adhesion was not simply the result of the joining together of two surfaces but depended also on the synthetic activity of the cells.

It was shown that the colloidal network formed in the first stages of reassociation had the properties of a protein. For this reason Moscona studied the effect on reaggregation of two inhibitors of protein synthesis, puromycin, and actinomycin D. Puromycin acts at the RNA-protein level and actinomycin D acts at the DNA-RNA level (25). This study was carried out on the retinal nerve cells of 10-day chick embryos. Dissociation and culture were carried out using the usual techniques and the inhibitors were added to the culture medium. As in the preceding experiment, intercellular adhesion was measured indirectly by measuring the size of the aggregates formed. Measurements were taken after 1, 2, 4, 6, 12, and 24 hours of culture.

Moscona showed that cells cultured in the presence of puromycin did not reaggregate. The blocking was reversible, since if the cells were then placed in a puromycin-free medium, reaggregation occurred normally. If puromycin was added to the medium after reaggregation had begun, further aggregation was prevented and the cell masses remained at the size already attained. The cells began to aggregate in the presence of actino-mycin D, but after 4 hours of culture, the cell masses did not increase in size. If actinomycin D was added after 6 hours' culture, the effect was not seen for a further 5 hours.

Since actinomycin D blocks RNA synthesis (and hence blocks the RNA-dependent protein synthesis), it might be thought that this delay reflected the lifespan of the RNA present in the cells at the time the inhibitor was added. It might also be thought that this delay represented the speed of reaction between actinomycin D and DNA.

The overall results of these experiments led Moscona to conclude that the adhesion of previously dissociated cells depends on the production of a proteinaceous substance. By slowing down the synthesis of this protein either by lowering the temperature of culture, or by blocking with inhibitors, the cells were prevented from reaggregating.

In 1962, Steinberg (30) refuted Moscona's conclusions starting from Moscona's work. He studied the reaggregation of chick embryo cells using the epidermis from the back of 8-day chick embryos and cells from the cardiac ventricle and retinal pigment cells of 5-day embryos.

Steinberg made use of a cellular property discovered by Moscona. When dissociated cells are maintained in flasks rotating at known speeds the dimensions of the aggregates formed are inversely proportional to the speed of rotation. The mean diameter of an aggregate was constant for a given cell type at a given speed.

Steinberg thought that if the variations in the cellular capacity to reaggregate were a function of temperature and really reflected a process of secretion of adhesive material, it should be possible, by combining the factors of speed of rotation and temperature, to obtain reaggregation at a low temperature. His work was carried out in two phases.

1. The dissociated cells were maintained for 6 hours at 30°C in flasks turning at a rate of 140 revolutions per minute. If Moscona's hypothesis is accepted, extracellular material can be synthesized at this temperature.

2. The suspensions were then maintained for 24 hours at 6.5°C at a speed of rotation of 70 revolutions per minute.

If extracellular material was effectively formed on the surface of the cells during the first phase of culture, the cells should form aggregates in spite of unfavorable temperature. However, aggregates did not form. According to Steinberg, this negative result showed either that no material had been synthesized or that it had been dissolved as it was gradually produced and that this dissolution continued at the low temperature.

The second explanation was rejected by the author, since he said that if it were true, aggregates in the process of formation and subjected to a low temperature would dissociate owing to dissolution of the cement substance. Nothing like this occurred. Aggregates in the process of formation remained coherent at low temperatures.

In consequence, Steinberg could not accept that intercellular adhesion was linked with the synthesis of adhesive material. He did not deny that an extracellular matrix appeared in the course of reassociation, but he would not admit that this material had the significance attributed to it by Moscona.

He repeated the analysis of the matrix (31) and showed that a crude extract of pancreatin would digest the E.C.M. completely. He further showed that it was the DNase fraction of the crude extract that was active.

Study of the physicochemical properties (that is, the UV absorption spectrum, the effect of NaCl, the effect of pH) and histochemical reactions of the E.C.M. led Steinberg to regard it as a strongly hydrated gel of deoxyribonucleoproteins. Its production was not bound with the metabolic activity of the cells, but it was derived from cells damaged during dissociation. For example, if instead of finely cutting the cells before subjecting them to trypsin dissociation, they were finely excised, the amount of E.C.M. formed during reaggregation was greatly reduced. In contrast, reaggregation itself occurred normally.

In the same way, if the cells were incubated in the presence of DNase no E.C.M. was formed but reaggregation occurred normally.

Steinberg thus concluded that the existence of E.C.M. was linked to the processes of dissociation and could not play any part in reaggregation.

In another series of experiments in 1962, Steinberg (27–29) investigated these problems from a different angle concentrating on the phenomenon of selectivity. First he showed that, in contrast to Holtfreter's suggestion, the final position of the cells in a mixed aggregate did not depend on their "centripetal" or "centrifugal" potentialities. In fact, by varying the proportions of the two cell types in the aggregate, so-called "centripetal cells" can be made to occupy a peripheral position. This was shown for example, when he mixed embryonic retinal and heart cells. When the mass contained 23% of cardiac cells and 77% retinal cells, the cardiac cells formed a large mass in the middle. When the proportion of cardiac cells was reduced to 9%, the masses that they formed within the aggregate were more dispersed and eccentric. Lastly, when the proportion of cardiac cells fell to 1%, they often remained isolated near the periphery.

Thus, the position of the cells in the aggregate does not depend on gradients to which they respond negatively or positively according to their type.

In contrast, this phenomenon could be explained by comparing the mixed aggregate to an unstable emulsion and by admitting that the behavior of the cells depends on their degree of cohesion. In an unstable emulsion, the fluid with the lowest surface tension, that is, that in which the intermolecular bonds are the weakest, tends to come to occupy the surface of the system. Conversely, the fluid with the stronger intermolecular bonds forms droplets that are small and numerous initially, but eventually give rise to a single internal mass in relation to the other constituent.

If the reaggregation of a mixture of cells from heart and retina is followed over a period of time, it is seen that at first the cardiac cells disappear progressively from the surface of the aggregate. They then associate in clumps, initially small and numerous, later larger and fewer.

The general appearance of the phenomenon thus resembles the separation of the two phases of an emulsion. The tissue with the weakest intercellular cohesion occupies a superficial position and the tissue with the strongest intercellular cohesion occupies an internal position.

It is not necessary for the cells present to have been previously dissociated. Steinberg showed that when a culture of retinal fragments and precartilage is confronted with a culture of liver and heart cells, the tissue with the lowest intercellular cohesion surrounds the other, as though they had been dissociated previously.

The idea of intercellular cohesion as a factor in segregation was also confirmed by the fact that the final position of a given cell type was not absolutely constant. It was constant only in relation to another given cell type. For example, cardiac cells occupied an internal position in relation to liver cells, but they were peripheral when associated with precartilage cells (32).

The concept of intercellular cohesion permitted Steinberg to explain many aspects of selective reassociation without needing to refer to the intervention of a substance produced by the dissociated cells.

Curtis also thought that the existence of an extracellular matrix was unnecessary. He believed that adhesion was a physicochemical phenomenon derived from the very structure of the cell membrane.

Danielli (7) had shown that the cell membrane is composed of a bimolecular lipid layer, with a monomolecular layer of proteins adsorbed on either side.

Curtis applied to the cell surface the results derived from the study on the rheological behavior of monomolecular protein films. The details of his reasoning will not be given here. Suffice it to say that Curtis regarded the primary adhesion between cells as the result of an equilibrum between forces of electrostatic repulsion (the cells are negatively charged) and van der Waals–London attraction forces. Thus, cohesion depends on the charge of the cells, which itself depends not only on the structure of the cell surface but also on the state of expansion or contraction of the external protein layer (3, 6).

The latter factor was profoundly modified by the processes of dissociation. The speed of reaggregation depended on the speed at which the cell surface returned to a state of equilibrium. Curtis thought that segregation in the interior of a mixed aggregate was due to the fact that the different cells returned to the equilibrium state at different rates.

Thus, if this theory is correct, it should be possible to modify the final position of a cell type in an aggregate, if instead of mixing the different kinds of cells immediately after dissociation one of the types is allowed to begin to reaggregate before the other is added to the culture.

Curtis first verified this with embryonic amphibian cells (4). The three layers of a gastrula of *Xenopus laevis* were dissociated. It has been shown (33) that if dissociated cells from the three layers are mixed immediately after dissociation, they reaggregate and become rearranged so that each tissue occupies the place that it would normally occupy in the embryo.

However, when endodermal cells were allowed to reaggregate for 4 hours before being added to a mixture of freshly dissociated ectodermal and mesodermal cells, the final aggregate formed showed a central mesodermal mass surrounded by a mixture of endodermal and ectodermal cells.

When the endodermal cells were left to aggregate for 6 hours before they were added to the mesoderm-ectoderm mixture, yet another result was obtained. There was a central mesodermal mass, surrounded by an ectodermal layer that was itself surrounded by the endodermal cells.

Curtis carried out the same type of experiment using sponges where the speed of reaggregation is different. Four species were used, *Microciona sanguinea, Halichondria panicea, Suberites ficus,* and *Hymeniacidon perleve;* these were dissociated by chemical means (5).

If cells from two species with similar rates of reaggregation were mixed together a mixed aggregate was obtained. In contrast, if cells from a species with a slow reaggregation rate were mixed with cells from a species with a fast reaggregation rate, there was complete segregation of the two kinds of cells. However, in the latter case, if the cells from the slowest species were allowed to begin their reaggregation before mixing occurred, inter-mediate types of reaggregation were obtained. By varying this time interval, different types of reaggregation could be obtained at will (Fig. 14).

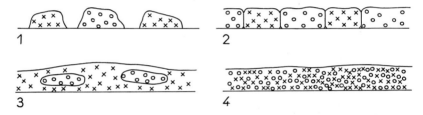

FIG. 14. Diagrammatic representation of four types of segregation in a mixture of cells from two species of sponge. (1) Complete separation of the two cell types. (2) Chain aggregates. (3) Concentric aggregates; one type of cell completely surrounds the other. (4) Perfect mixture of the two cell types. (○) Cells from one species; (×) cells from the other species. After Curtis.

These results could explain reaggregation and selective reassociation without requiring the presence of specific materials secreted by the cells.

However, Moscona (24) and Humphreys (19), working with sponges, demonstrated a diffusible substance that favored reaggregation and acted in a specific fashion. Two species of sponge were used, *Microciona prolifera* and *Haliclona occulata.* The sponges were dissociated chemically or mechanic-ally by washing in artificial sea water lacking calcium and magnesium.

The dissociation fluid was shown to contain a substance that favored reaggregation when added to the medium in which the cell suspension was being cultured. This substance was only active on the cell suspension from which it had been derived. Thus, the compound produced by *Microciona prolifera* did not favor reaggregation of cells from *Haliclona occulata,* and extracts from the dissociation fluid of *Haliclona* were not effective on *Microciona.* If the extract from one of the species was added to a mixture of both cell types, only the cells of that species reaggregated and the other cells remained in suspension.

IV. CONCLUSION

If the dissociated cells from an organ or an organism are cultured, they tend to regroup and reorganize themselves. Experiments have shown that the phenomenon of reorganization results from a sorting out process in the middle of the primary agglomerate, and is due entirely to chance. Similar cells adhere to one another and form a tissue while dissimilar cells merely slide over one another. Homologous cells do not show mutual attraction at a distance. Some workers, such as Townes and Holtfreter, have shown that in an aggregate, cells dissociated from different tissues retain their properties and migrate in such a way that they occupy a position in the aggregate similar to the one that they occupied prior to dissociation (for instance, the epidermal cells tend to form a covering layer).

It has been possible to describe fairly precisely the various stages of reaggregation. The workers who have investigated the phenomenon of reaggregation are not yet in agreement as to its possible explanation. Three principal theories have been put forward.

1. Originated by Weiss and followed up by Moscona, who carried out the experimental work. Adhesion occurs through an intermediary exudate secreted by the cells. The properties of the exudate depend on the synthetic activity of the cells. In addition, Moscona and Humphreys demonstrated the existence of a diffusible substance that has a specific effect on reaggregation.

2. Steinberg did not doubt the presence of an exudate but denied its role in the process of reaggregation. He suggested that segregation of the cells depends on the degree of cohesion that exists between them, and compared the phenomenon with that of the separation of the different phases of an unstable emulsion.

3. Curtis also thought that reaggregation was not due to the effect of a cellular exudate. He thought that adhesion depends only on the electrical charge at the cell surface, this charge being disturbed at the time of dissociation. The different types of cells do not regain their initial charge at the same time. Those that regain their charge most quickly reaggregate first, while those that regain their charge at a later time reaggregate later.

The problem of the mechanisms involved in reaggregation and selective reassociation are far from being solved. The many contradictions seen between the ideas of the different workers reflect the complexity of the problem.

It cannot be denied that purely physical mechanisms do occur in reaggregation, but they are not the only mechanisms. Biological factors also play a large part. In addition, it is certainly artificial to separate the two types of mechanism, which undoubtedly act together.

BIBLIOGRAPHY

1. Abraham M.   Formation de structures tubulaires par des cellules de tissue testiculaire embryonnaire isolées à l'aide de trypsine. *C. r. Acad. Sci.*, 1959, **249**, 2627–2629.
2. Abraham M.   Processus de réorganisation dans les agrégats formés par les cellules des gonades dissociées d'embryon de Poulet. *Arch. Anat. micros. Morphol. exp.*, 1960, **49**, 333–344.
3. Curtis A. S. G.   Cell contacts: Some physical considerations. *The Amer. Natur.*, 1960, **94**, 37–56.
4. Curtis A. S. G.   Timing mechanisms in the specific adhesion of cells. *Exp. Cell Res.*, 1961, suppl. **8**, 107–122.
5. Curtis A. S. G.   Pattern and mechanism in reaggregation of sponges. *Nature*, 1962, **196**, 245–248.
6. Curtis A. S. G.   Cell contact and adhesion. *Biol. Rev.*, 1962, **37**, 82–129.
7. Danielli J. F.   Surface chemistry and cell membranes, 246-265. *In*: Danielli J. F., Pankhurst K. G. A., Riddiford A. C. *Surface phenomena in Chemistry and Biology*. Un vol., Pergamon, édit., London, 1958.
8. Fauré-Frémiet E.   Le mécanisme de la formation des complexes à partir de cellules d'Eponges dissociées. *C. r. Soc. Biol.*, 1925, **93**, 618–620.
9. Fauré-Frémiet E.   Morphogénèse expérimentale chez *Ficulina ficus* L. Arch. *Anat. micr.*, 1932, **28**, 1–80.
10. Fauré-Frémiet E.   Involution expérimentale et tension de structure dans les cultures de *Ficulina ficus* L. *Arch. Anat. micr.*, 1932, **28**, 121–157.
11. Galtsoff P.   The amoeboid movement of dissociated sponge cells. *Biol. Bull.*, 1923, **45**, 153–161.
12. Galtsoff P.   Regeneration after dissociation (an experimental study on sponges). Part I: Behavior of dissociated cells of *Microciona prolifera* under normal and altered conditions; Part II: Histogenesis of *Microciona prolifera*. *J. Exp. Zool.*, 1925, **42**, 183–255.
13. Gregg J. H.   Serological investigations of cell adhesion in the slime molds, *Dictyostelium discoideum*, *Dictyostelium purpureum* and *Polyspondylium violaceum*. *J. Gen. Physiol.*, 1956, **39**, 813–820.
14. Holtfreter J.   Differenzierungspotenzen isolierter Teile der Urodelengastrula. *Arch. Entw. mech.*, 1938, **138**, 522–565.
15. Holtfreter J.   Structure, motility and locomotion in isolated embryonic amphibian cells. *J. Morphol.*, 1946, **79**, 27–62.
16. Holtfreter J.   Observation on the migration, aggregation and phagocytosis of embryonic cells. *J. Morphol.*, 1947, **80**, 25–56.
17. Holtfreter J.   Changes of structure and the kinetics of differentiating embryonic cells. *J. Morphol.*, 1947, **80**, 57–92.
18. Holtfreter J.   Significance of the Cell Membrane in embryonic processes. *Ann. N. Y. Acad. Sc.*, 1948, **49**, 709–760.
19. Humphreys T.   Chemical dissolution and *in vitro* reconstruction of sponge cell

adhesions. I: Isolation and functional demonstration of the Components involved. *Devel. Biol.*, 1963, **8**, 27–48.

20. Moscona A.   Cell suspensions from organ rudiments of chick embryos. *Exp. Cell Res.*, 1952, **3**, 535–539.

21. Moscona A.   The development *in vitro* of chimeric aggregates of dissociated embryonic chick and mouse cells. *Proc. Nat. Acad. Sc. U. S.*, 1957, **43**, 184–194.

22. Moscona A.   Patterns and mechanisms of tissue reconstruction from dissociated Cells, 45-70. *In*: *"Developing Cell Systems and their Control"*. 18th Growth Symposium, 1960.

23. Moscona A.   Effects of temperature on adhesion to glass and histogenetic cohesion of dissociated cells. *Nature*, 1961, **190**, 408–409.

24. Moscona A.   Studies on Cell aggregation: demonstration of material with selective cell binding activity. *Proc. Nat. Acad. Sc.*, 1963, **49**, 742–748.

25. Moscona M. H. and Moscona A.   Inhibition of Adhesiveness and Aggregation of dissociated cells by inhibitors of Protein and RNA synthesis. *Science*, 1963, **142**, 1070–1071.

26. Spiegel M.   The role of specific surface antigens in Cell adhesion. Part I: The reaggregation of sponge cells. Part II: Studies on embryonic amphibian cells. *Biol. Bull.*, 1954, **107**, 130–155.

27. Steinberg M. S.   On the mechanism of tissue Reconstruction by dissociated Cells. I: Population kinetic, differential adhesiveness and the Absence of directed Migration. *Proc. Nat. Acad. Sc.*, 1962, **48**, 1577–1581.

28. Steinberg M. S.   Mechanism of tissue reconstruction by dissociated Cells. II: Time-course of events. *Science*, 1962, **137**, 762–763.

29. Steinberg M. S.   On the mechanism of tissue reconstruction by dissociated Cells. III: Free Energy Relations and the Reorganisation of fused, heteronomic Tissue Fragments. *Proc. Nat. Acad. Sc.*, 1962, **48**, 1769–1776.

30. Steinberg M. S.   The role of temperature in the Control of Aggregation of dissociated embryonic Cells. *Exp. Cell Res.*, 1962, **28**, 1–10.

31. Steinberg M. S.   "ECM": its nature, origin and function in Cell Aggregation. *Exp. Cell Res.*, 1963, **30**, 257–280.

32. Steinberg M. S.   The Problem of Adhesive selectivity in cellular interactions. *In*: "Cellular Membranes in Development". Un vol., Ac. Press, édit., 1964, 321–366.

33. Townes P. L. and Holtfreter J.   Directed Movements and selective Adhesion of embryonic Amphibian Cells. *J. Exp. Zool.*, 1955, **128**, 53–120.

34. Trinkaus J. P. and Groves P. W.   Differenciation in Culture of mixed Aggregates of dissociated Tissue Cells. *Nat. Acad. Sc.*, 1955, **41**, 787–795.

35. Weiss P.   Nerve Patterns: the Mechanics of Growth. *Growth*, 1941, **5** (suppl.), 163–203.

36. Weiss P.   The Problem of specificity in Growth and Development. *Yale J. Biol. and Med.*, 1947, **19**, 235–278.

37. Weiss P.   Cell Contact. *International Review of Cytology*, 1958, **7**, 391–423.

38. Weiss P. and Taylor A. C.   Reconstitution of complete Organs from single-cell Suspensions of Chick Embryos in advanced Stages of Differenciation. *Proc. Nat. Acad. Sc.*, 1960, **46**, 1177–1186.

39. Wilson H. V.   On some Phenomena of Coalescence and Regeneration in Sponges. *J. Exp. Zool.*, 1907, **5**, 245–258.

40. Wolff Et.   Potentialités et affinités des tissus révélés par la culture *in vitro* d'organes en associations hétérogènes et xénoplastiques. *Bull. Soc. Zool. Fr.*, 1954, **79**, 357–368.

ADDENDUM

It is difficult to summarize the results obtained in the last few years on the reaggregation of dissociated animal cells. The apparently simple course of events, in fact, involves phenomena of great complexity, and an interpretation of the experimental findings is not always easy. This explains why, despite the number of recent investigations dealing with this problem, the mechanism of reaggregation is still not fully elucidated and many points remain controersial.

Before discussing the results of this research, mention should be made of the conclusions deduced from previous work.

The reaggregation of dissociated cells takes place, at least broadly speaking, in a consistent manner. During the first stage, the dispersed cells become regrouped at random and form masses in which all the cell types present in the initial suspension are randomly distributed. Then, in the second stage, the masses become reorganized with cells of the same type coming together and forming histological structures such as they would normally form in the intact organism.

Experiments have also shown that the reaggregation and selective regrouping of similar cells are phenomena that depend on linkages established by the cells when they come into contact with one another.

The nature of these linkages is still under discussion, and the theoretical considerations, like the experimental findings, do not lead to any definitive conclusions.

Some authors consider that the intercellular linkages are purely physical in nature and that the physical and chemical characteristics of the cell surfaces involved are sufficient to explain the phenomena; according to others, the linkages responsible for reaggregation and intercellular cohesion depend on a material factor synthesized by the cells in suspension.

These hypotheses have been the starting point for the investigations described here.

This account will consist of three sections, the first dealing with ultrastructural studies on reaggregation, the second with results obtained with substances that interfere with cellular metabolism, and the third with findings on certain factors that stimulate reaggregation.

I. ULTRASTRUCTURAL STUDY OF REAGGREGATION

Lesseps (16) used electron microscopy in an attempt to verify a theory previously proposed by Steinberg (26). This stated that the intercellular linkages are achieved by means of Ca^{2+} ions that unite cell surfaces coming into contact. Lesseps studied the first stages of reaggregation using cells from different organs of the chick embryo.

He found that the first contacts between cells were established by projections with a very small radius of curvature, and that at the point of these first contacts the distance between the membranes of adjacent cells was much smaller than that between two flat resting cell surfaces. Although the radii of curvature and the distances actually measured by Lesseps were greater than the theoretical values, the author considered his observations to be indicative of the action of Ca^{2+} ions during the first stages of reaggregation, thus supporting Steinberg's hypothesis.

Other results, obtained by Millonig and Giudice (22), showed that these conclusions cannot be applied in any general way. Dissociated cells of sea urchin larvae suspended under suitable conditions did not at any time show the slightest projection. From the beginning of reaggregation, the cell surfaces that came into contact remained flat, and the distance between them was such that Ca^{2+} bridges could not have been established.

Finally, Overton (25) recently made some new and interesting observations using special staining techniques. This worker examined the ultrastructure of chick embryo cells, dissociated and in the process of reaggregation, and demonstrated that the intercellular space, hitherto considered as being empty (see main article, Curtis' theory, Ref. 3), in fact contained a fibrillar material that disappeared almost completely after trypsin-induced cell dissociation. The material reappeared progressively during reaggregation, and appreciable quantities could be detected after 6 hours of this process.

Although cautions in drawing conclusions, Overton stressed that the existence of this fibrillar material should be taken into account when considering possible reaggregation mechanisms.

II. REAGGREGATION AND INHIBITION OF METABOLISM

As referred to earlier, Moscona (see main article, Ref. 22) had inferred the existence of a factor synthesized by the dissociated cells and responsible for their reaggregation. His first experiments, designed to confirm the existence of this factor, provided only indirect evidence. When the metabolic level of reaggregating cells was lowered nonspecifically (low-temperature culture) or when the cells were subjected to the action of more specific metabolic inhibitors (puromycin, actinomycin D), a retardation or complete arrest of reaggregation was obtained. Moscona concluded from these results that, because of an inability to synthesize the material responsible for reaggregation, reaggregation had not taken place.

These conclusions were soon criticized on the grounds that neither the metabolic inhibitors nor variations in temperature necessarily act directly on reaggregation; the arrest of reaggregation could have been a secondary effect.

Curtis (1), for instance, believed that temperature influenced reaggregation by modifying the viscosity of the medium in which the cells were suspended. Lowering the temperature might inhibit cell movement and thus reduce the chances of their forming aggregates.

Kemp *et al.* (13) also regarded the inhibition of reaggregation as a secondary phenomenon. Isolated cells are extremely sensitive to temperature variations; when the temperature is lowered they become rounded, and their surface contracts thereby becoming much less adhesive.

The role of inhibitory substances is even more disputed.

Curtis and Greaves (2) showed that if chick embryo cells were maintained in the presence of inhibitors in serum-free medium, they reaggregated normally. The serum, in fact, contained a factor that Curtis was able to isolate and which inhibited reaggregation. This factor was progressively destroyed by the metabolic products of the suspended cells. It is these antiserum factors that are inhibited, rather than the synthesis of a cohesive material, when cell metabolism is repressed.

Giudice (5–7) showed that actinomycin, puromycin, and ethionine inhibited the reaggregation of dissociated sea urchin cells. However, this inhibition was accompanied by a perceptible fall in respiration. The results concerning reaggregation should thus be interpreted with caution.

Kemp *et al.* (13) also studied the effect of puromycin on reaggregation. They found that puromycin added to cell suspensions stopped the reaggregation processes in about an hour, whether it was added to the medium at the start of the experiment or introduced once reaggregation had begun. This suggests that puromycin does not act directly on the synthesis of a possible reaggregation material since, if its action were direct, the addition of puromycin should not affect reaggregation once it has started. Puromycin is believed to inhibit reaggregation by reducing cellular metabolism to a level below which the adhesive mechanisms, whatever they are, are no longer functional.

According to these results, the action of inhibitors on reaggregation is not necessarily direct. However, recent experiments by Glaeser *et al.* (8) indicate otherwise. Glaeser dissociated cells of chick embryo retina using either trypsin or EDTA treatment. He subsequently studied the behavior of these cells when suspended in the presence of various inhibitors, and found that the cells that had been separated by trypsin did not reaggregate. The cells separated by means of EDTA did reaggregate, although more slowly than control cells.

One possible interpretation of this result is as follows: EDTA separates the cells by removing divalent ions from the structure concerned with intercellular contacts but does not attack proteins at the cell surface. Trypsin, on the other hand, acts by destroying these same proteins. Thus, for reaggregation to take place after trypsin treatment, these proteins have to be resynthesized by the cell. This would explain why only the reaggregation of cells dissociated by trypsin is affected by the presence of metabolic inhibitors.

Puromycin and actinomycin are not the only substances capable of influencing reaggregation. Glucosamine in certain concentrations (3, 8) was found to inhibit reaggregation, as did chloramphenicol in some cases (24). The action of certain substances that act on the contractile proteins is most interesting. Jones (10) showed that a tanning agent, p-benzoquinone, inhibited the reaggregation of chick embryo cells. This inhibition was thought to be caused by a contraction of the cell surface due to the tanning agent, the contraction leading to an increase in the charge density of the surface, thus making it less adhesive.

Knight, Jones, and Jones (14) showed that the presence of ATP in a suspension of dissociated embryonic cells had the same inhibitory effect. If the ATP were added to a suspension in which the cells were already partially aggregated, the masses dissociated and the cells dispersed. Last, it should be noted that 2,4-dinitrophenol, which suppresses cellular metabolism by inhibiting ATP formation, also leads to the arrest of reaggregation of dissociated cells (13).

The effects of ATP and the tanning substances led Jones (11) to consider the existence of contractile proteins of the type of actinomyosin at the cell surface. Cellular adhesion would depend on the degree of contraction of these proteins and would reflect an equilibrium between the mechanisms of contraction and relaxation.

The relation between the mechanical properties of the cell surface and reaggregation seems to be confirmed by a recent result of Kemp (12). Neuraminidase, an enzyme that attacks sialic acids, inhibits reaggregation. The sialic groups are present at the surface of many cells and form an integral part of glycoproteins to which they give structural rigidity. They, therefore, certainly have a role to play in the phenomena of intercellular adhesion.

As we have just seen, the results obtained by studying the effects of various substances, inhibitory or otherwise, on the reaggregation of dissociated cells do not permit any definite conclusions to be drawn.

Many other esperiments have been performed to demonstrate the existence of a factor specifically involved in reaggregation. It should be recalled that in 1963 Moscona and then Humphreys had isolated from the supernatant fluid of dissociated sponge cells a factor stimulating reaggregation.

Since then analogous factors have been isolated from other species of sponges and even from chick embryo cells. Some of these factors have been analyzed. Finally, both Lilien and Moscona have recently analyzed the mode of action of this factor, hoping to identify it as the actual factor of reaggregation.

A. Demonstration of Stimulating Factors in Different Species

Kuroda (15) filtered the supernatant fluid from a suspension of chick embryo liver cells and obtained a factor that stimulated the reaggregation of freshly dissociated cells. This factor was active even when the cells were maintained at temperatures that normally do not permit reaggregation. Using Moscona's and Humphreys' preparation methods, MacLennan and Dodd (20) isolated stimulating factors from new species of sponges. Among the 17 species studied, only a single species, *Hymeniacidon perleve*, consistently yielded an active factor. Two or three other species also did so, but inconsistently. The results obtained with the factor from *Hymeniacidon* were less clear-cut than those obtained by Moscona and Humphreys; this factor stimulated not only the reaggregation of cells from *Hymeniacidon* cells but also those of *Ficulina ficus* and *Halichondria panicea*. In a mixed suspension of cells from *Hymeniacidon and Halichondria* the aggregates that formed were strictly monospecific, but addition of the *Hymeniacidon* factor brought about the formation of mixed aggregates. The authors believed that this relative absence of specificity in the activity of the factor reflects a certain taxonomic relationship between the species studied.

B. Analysis of Stimulating Factors

Humphreys (9) used techniques of differential centrifugation to analyze the stimulating factor prepared from cell suspensions of the sponge *Microciona*. He showed that this factor was composed of uniform particles measuring about 200 Å and having a protein and polysaccharide character. According to the author, these particles represent "organelles" responsible for intercellular adhesion.

Margoliash *et al.* (21) obtained similar results. These authors studied not only the factor from *Microciona*, but also one from *Haliclona* (it should be recalled that the stimulating action of these factors is strictly specific, the *Microciona* factor having no effect on the reaggregation of *Haliclona* and, conversely, the *Haliclona* factor being inactive in the reaggregation of *Microciona*). They showed that, in both cases, the factor was a glycoprotein present in particle form. The two preparations studied were qualitatively similar, but they differed quantitatively, especially with regard to their monosaccharide content.

Gasic and Galanti (4) treated the stimulating factor with a large number of enzymes. All the proteolytic enzymes used denatured the factor, but the results with keratinase were of particular interest. This enzyme has the property of reducing disulfide groups. As the stimulating factor lost its activity when treated with keratinase, it would appear that the reaggregation of dissociated sponge cells requires the presence of proteins and intact disulfide groups.

All these results are consistent with those obtained by MacLennan (19). Using immunochemical methods, this author showed that the cell surfaces of many sponges contain glycoproteins that probably play a part in reaggregation phenomena. Qualitatively, the composition of the carbohydrates was the same in all species studied but all the glycoproteins were serologically distinct.

C. Mode of Action of the Stimulating Factors

Lilien and Moscona (18) demonstrated the presence of a factor that stimulated the reaggregation of cells from the chick embryo retina. The factor was isolated from the supernatant fluid of cells maintained in monolayer culture. It stimulated significantly and consistently the reaggregation of freshly dissociated cells but was found to have no effect when tested on cells from the liver, heart, or limb bud. Its action is, therefore, specific.

By various methods, which would take too long to discuss here Lilien (17) showed that the dissociated cells can take up the active factor from the medium, this factor then becoming fixed very probably at the cell surface. He also showed that the fixation was independent of the metabolic level of the cells and could take place at low temperatures. However, utilization of the for actual reaggregation occurred only when the metabolic level of the cells was normal.

The specificity of the factor was realized at the stage of cell fixation. Live cells were shown to be incapable of taking up from the medium a factor prepared from cultured retinal cells.

Moscona (23) studied the stimulating factor obtained from suspensions of sponge cells. Using various techniques under complex experimental conditions, Moscona investigated the mode of the action of the factor and attempted to demonstrate that it represented the actual factor of reaggregation.

In particular, he compared the reaggregation of cells dissociated by a variety of techniques, e.g., mechanical dissociation, dissociation by chemical means (treatment with artificial sea-water lacking Ca^{2+} and Mg^{2+}), and dissociation by enzyme digestion (pronase).

The more the cells were injured by these treatments the later the reaggregation began, the latent period probably corresponding to the time required by the cells to regenerate or synthesize the material required for reaggregation.

When the cells were suspended in a solution containing the stimulating factor the same latent period was observed, but once it had begun the reaggregation proceeded very rapidly. This shows that the stimulating factor can act only if the cells whose surfaces have been injured at the time of dissociation have regenerated a normal surface.

Moscona also studied reaggregation of killed, dissociated cells in the presence of the stimulating factor. These dead cells were incapable of synthesizing their own reaggregation material. The results show that the stimulating factor acts by becoming fixed at the cell surface, and also that the quantity of factor fixed by the killed cells varies according to the dissociating treatment. Cells dissociated mechanically before being fixed in formaldehyde fixed a larger quantity of material than cells dissociated by chemical means. These results thus complement the previous ones. The stimulating factor acts by fixation at the cell surface, and the degree of fixation, which is reflected by the cells capacity to reaggregate, depends on the condition of the cell surface. The more the surface is damaged, the less it is capable of fixing the stimulating factor. At the same time, the more the cells are injured, the longer they take to regenerate a healthy surface, capable of maximum fixation of the stimulating factor.

All these results, only an outline of which has been presented here, led Moscona to consider that the stimulating factor isolated from the supernatant fluid of reaggregating cells undoubtedly represents the actual material of reaggregation.

It is interesting to note that all these experiments, including those of Lilien, stress the importance of cell surface integrity and emphasize the probably fundamental role that it plays in reaggregation phenomena.

In conclusion, all the results described here confirm the complexity of reaggregation phenomena. Cellular integrity and normal functioning appear to be essential. It is also evident that the properties of the cell surface, whether physical or chemical, play a fundamental role. Last, it is possible that the intercellular fibrillar material, whose existence has recently been demonstrated also plays a part.

BIBLIOGRAPHY

1. Curtis A. S. G.   Effect of pH and temperature on cell reaggregation. *Nature*, 1963, **200**, 1235.
2. Curtis A. S. G. and Greaves M. F.   The inhibition of cell aggregation by a pure serum protein. *J. Embryol. Exp. Morphol.*, 1965, **13**, No. 3, 309–327.
3. Garber B.   Inhibition by glucosamine of aggregation of dissociated embryonic cells. *Devel. Biol.*, 1963, **7**, 630.
4. Gasic G. J. and Galanti N. L.   Proteins and disulfide groups in the aggregation of dissociated cells of sea sponges. *Science*, 1966, **151**, 203–205.
5. Giudice G.   Restitution of whole larvae from disaggregated cells of sea-urchin embryos. *Devel. Biol.*, 1962, **5**, 402–411.
6. Giudice G.   Aggregation of cells isolated from vegetalized and animalized sea-urchin embryos. *Experientia*, 1963, **19** (2), 83.
7. Giudice G.   The mechanims of aggregation of embryonic sea-urchin cells. A biochemical approach. *Devel. Biol.*, 1965, **13**, 213–232.

8. Glaeser R. M., Richmond J. E. and Todd P. W. Histotypic self-organization by trypsin dissociated and EDTA dissociated chick embryo cells. *Exp. Cell Res.*, 1968, **52**(1), 71–85.

9. Humphreys T. Cell surface components participating in aggregation: evidence for a new cell particulate. *Exp. Cell Res.*, 1965, **40**, 539–543.

10. Jones B. M. Inhibitory effect of *p*-benzoquinone on the aggregation behaviour of embryo chick fibroblast cells. *Nature*, 1965, **205**, 1280–1282.

11. Jones B. M. A unifying hypothesis of cell adhesion. *Nature*, 1966, **212**, 362–365.

12. Kemp R. B. Effect of the removal of cell surface sialic acids on cell aggregation "*in vitro.*" *Nature*, 1968, **218**, 1255–1256.

13. Kemp R. B., Jones B. M., Cunningham I. and James M. C. M. Quantitative investigation on the effect of puromycin on the aggregation of trypsin and versen dissociated chick fibroblast cells. *J. Cell Sci.*, 1967, **2**, 323, 340.

14. Knight V. A., Jones B. M. and Jones P. C. T. Inhibition of the aggregation of dissociated embryo chick fibroblast cells by adenosine triphosphate. *Nature*, 1966, **210**, 1008–1010.

15. Kuroda Y. Preparation of an aggregation-promoting supernatant from embryonic chick liver cells. *Exp. Cell Res.*, 1968, **49**, 626–638.

16. Lesseps R. J. Cell surface projections: their role in the aggregation of embryonic chick cells as revealed by electron microscopy. *J. Exp. Zool.*, 1963, **153**, 171–182.

17. Lilien J. E. Specific enhancement of cell aggregation "*in vitro.*" *Devel. Biol.*, 1968, **17**, 657–679.

18. Lilien J. E. and Moscona A. A. Cell aggregation: its enhancement by a supernatant from cultures of homologous cells. *Science*, 1967, **157**, 70–72.

19. MacLennan A. P. The sponge cell surface in relation to aggregation specificity. *Biochem. J.*, 1963, **89**, 99.

20. MacLennan A. P. and Dodd R. Y. Promoting activity of extracellular materials on sponge cell reaggregation. *J. Embryol. Exp. Morphol.*, 1967, **17**, 473–481.

21. Margoliash E., Schenk J., Hargie M., Burokass, Richter W., Barlow G. and Moscona A. Characterization of specific cell aggregating materials from sponge cells. *Biochem. Biophys. Res. Commun.*, **20**, 383–389.

22. Millonig G. and Giudice G. Electron microscopic study of the reaggregation of cells dissociated from sea-urchin embryos. *Devel. Biol.*, 1967, **15**, 91–101.

23. Moscona A. A. Cell aggregation: properties of specific cell ligands and their role in the formation of multicellular systems. *Devel. Biol.*, 1968, **18**, 250–278.

24. Nakanishi Y. H., Katao H. and Iwasaki T. Inhibitory effect of chloramphenicol on the histogenetic aggregation of dissociated cells. *Jap. J. Genet.*, 1963, **38**, 257–260.

25. Overton J. A fibrillar intercellular material between reaggregating embryonic chick cells. *J. Cell Biol.*, 1969, **40**, 136–144.

26. Steinberg M. S. On the chemical bonds between animal cells. A mechanism for type specific association. *Amer. Natur.*, 1958, **92**, 65–82.

CHAPTER IX

STUDY OF ORGANOGENESIS
BY DISSOCIATION AND REASSOCIATION
OF EMBRYONIC RUDIMENTS *IN VITRO*

Philippe Sengel

LABORATOIRE D'EMBRYOLOGIE EXPÉRIMENTALE DU COLLÈGE DE FRANCE
PARIS, FRANCE

I. INTRODUCTION

Many vertebrate organs are composed of two tissues having different structures and origins. These are the epithelial tissue and the connective tissue. The epithelial tissue is the distinguishing part and is essential for the functional activity of the organ. The connective tissue gives the organ its physical support and provides nutrition. For example, the skin is composed of a superficial epithelium, the epidermis and a deep connective tissue, the dermis. The epidermis is derived from the ectoderm and the dermis from the mesodermal mesenchyme.

Other organ systems such as the nervous system, the musculature, and the skeleton do not have this double origin, differentiating from a single homogeneous embryonic tissue. The nervous system is derived entirely from ectoderm, and the muscles and skeleton are derived from the mesodermal mesenchyme.

Organ culture of embryonic organs has contributed to the understanding of the formation of these homogeneous and heterogeneous organs. The factors affecting differentiation and the mechanisms of differentiation can be studied. It is possible to isolate a system composed of inductor tissue and effector tissue and to study it under ideal and simple conditions that can be modified at will.

The principal results that have been obtained using organ culture techniques to investigate the field of experimental organogenesis can be summarized in three parts:

1. Morphogenesis of the nervous system and the axial organs. This is the result of primary induction and has been the object of much research,

particularly on amphibians. Some of the fundamental experiments that have been carried out on this subject will be discussed.

2. Formation of the vertebral skeleton, with special reference to the differentiation of cartilage, as induced by the neural tube and the notochord.

3. Interactions between epithelium and mesenchyme that are the origin of heterogeneous organs, where epithelium and mesenchyme unite. Embryonic bird skin and fetal mouse kidney will be discussed in most detail as they are the organs that have been studied most closely.

II. ANALYSIS OF PRIMARY INDUCTION

A. Amphibians

In 1931, Holtfreter (30) described a technique of *in vitro* explantation that made possible the study of differentiation in isolated rudiments from amphibian gastrulas. The so-called "sandwich" technique (Fig. 1) consists

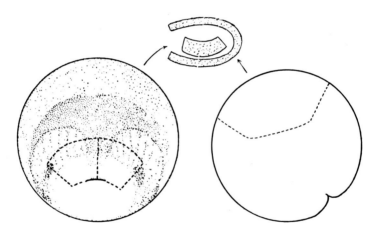

FIG. 1.   The "sandwich" technique. Half of the dorsal lip of the blastopore from a young gastrula is surrounded by a strip of ectoderm taken from the region of the animal pole. After Holtfreter (32).

of wrapping a piece of undifferentiated ectoderm from a young gastrula inside a piece of tissue whose inductive properties are being investigated (31). The inductor and effector tissues are thus brought into close contact with one another. When cultured alone, the ectoderm usually only gave rise to atypical undifferentiated epidermis. However, if a piece of the dorsal lip of the blastopore was included in the sandwich, the ectoderm differentiated and gave rise to the central nervous system.

Holtfreter first used the "sandwich" technique to study the inductor effects of various killed tissues (31). Later (1936) he carried out his famous experiments and explanted heterologous "sandwiches" (32). In these experiments, a piece of the dorsal lip of the blastopore from *Triton alpestris* was associated with a strip of ectoderm from *Bombinator pachypus* (Fig. 2) and a piece of the dorsal lip of the blastopore from *Bombinator* was associated with a strip of epidermis from *Triton* (Fig. 3). The tissues of these two species are easy to distinguish histologically (Figs. 4 and 5). These heterologous

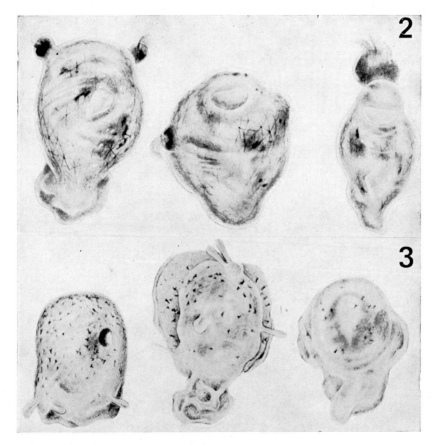

FIG. 2. Dorsal lip of the blastopore of *Triton* surrounded by ectoderm from *Bombinator*. Macroscopic appearance of three explants with secretory adhesive papillas and pigment cells, 10 days after explantation. Approx. × 30. After Holtfreter (32).

FIG. 3. Dorsal lip of the blastopore from *Bombinator* surrounded by ectoderm from *Triton*. Macroscopic appearance of three explants showing balancers and pigment cells 10 days after explantation. Approx. × 30. After Holtfreter (32).

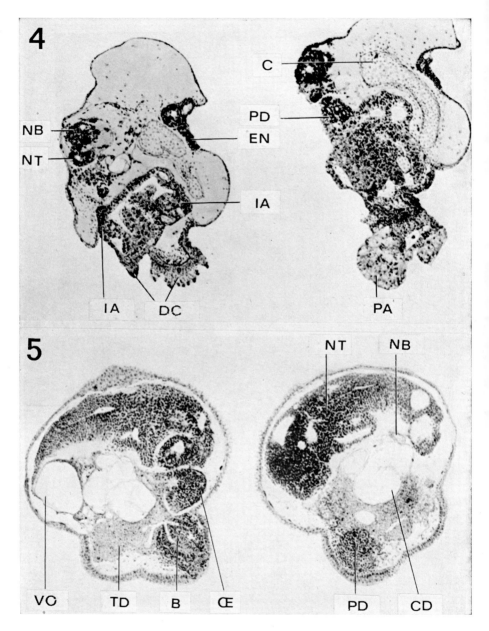

FIG. 4. Transverse sections of an explant derived from the dorsal lip of the blastopore of *Triton* and *Bombinator* ectoderm after 10 days of culture. Tissue derived from *Triton* (large nuclei) has developed into notochord, nerve cells (NT), foregut (IA) and dental papillae (PD). The *Triton* tissue has induced, in the *Bombinator* ectoderm, neural tissue

associations made it possible to determine the potentialities of each of these tissues when they were brought into contact with one another. The blastopore lip usually differentiated into notochord, muscles, and sometimes a small rudiment of the central nervous system. The ectodermal strip gave rise to various tissues, in particular the central nervous system and the sense organs (Figs. 2–5). The epidermis always differentiated true to type, whether the combination was homologous or heterologous. Thus, even under the influence of the blastopore lip from *Bombinator*, *Triton* ectoderm produced balancers and dentinous tooth rudiments (Urodele characteristics). In the same way, *Bombinator* ectoderm in contact with the *Triton* inductor formed adhesive glandular papillae and horny tooth rudiments (Anuran characteristics).

These experiments demonstrate that primary induction has no specific characteristic. The specificity is in the competent ectoderm. They also show that primary induction is not connected with morphogenetic movements, but rather with the transmission of a morphogenic agent from the inductor to the effector tissue.

The transmission of this substance has been the subject of many experiments (8–10, 31, 33). Saxen (46) has demonstrated it using another technique of explantation *in vitro*. This involved placing a filter between the inductor and the ventral ectoderm (Fig. 6). A piece of the ventral ectoderm of a young

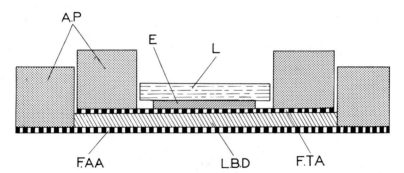

FIG. 6.   Arrangement of filters used in Saxen's experiments (46). A.P., Plexiglass rings; E, ectoderm; F.AA., Millipore filter of type AA; F.TA., Millipore filter of type TA; L, coverslip; L.B.D., dorsal lip of the blastopore acting as an inductor. After Saxen (46).

(NB), horny teeth (DC), nasal epithelium (EN), cartilage (C), and an adhesive papilla (PA). Approx. × 50. After Holtfreter (32).

FIG. 5.   Transverse sections from an explant derived from the dorsal lip of the blastopore of *Bombinator* and *Triton* ectoderm after 10 days of culture. Tissue derived from *Bombinator* has formed a notochord (CD), a little neural tissue (NB), and parts of the digestive tract (TD). It has induced in the *Triton* ectoderm considerable neural material (NT) with an eye (OE), buccal cavity (B) with dental papillae (PD), and an otic vesicle (VO). Approx. × 50. After Holtfreter (32).

gastrula of *Taricha torosa* or *Triturus vulgaris* was explanted with a piece
of blastopore lip from one or other species. The tissues were placed on opposite sides of a Millipore filter type TA* (20 μ thick, mean pore diameter 0.8 μ).
The apparatus used prevented the passage of any cells or physiological
saline around the edges of the filter. The two tissues could only communicate
through the filter pores. The ectoderm was removed 6–24 hours after explantation, then cultured alone for 9 days. Out of a total of 78 experiments,
37 pieces of ectoderm showed typical neural differentiation (Fig. 7). Pieces

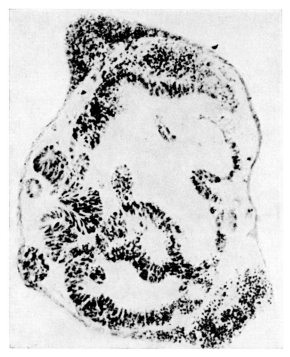

FIG. 7. Explant of *Triton* ectoderm that had previously been placed for 6 hours on a
Millipore filter with a dorsal lip of the blastopore on the opposite surface. The explant
was then cultured alone for 9 days. Anterior neural formations have differentiated and
also an eye with a lens. After Saxen (46).

of ectoderm placed in contact with the filter but no inductor were used as
controls and these formed no recognizable structures.

The inducing agent can thus pass across the filter. Cellular contact between
the inductor and the effector is not necessary. Exposure to this filtrable
agent for 6 hours is sufficient to produce neural differentiation.

* Millipore Filter Corporation, Bedford, Massachusetts.

B. Birds

Similar experiments to those described above were carried out by Waddington (58–60) using chick embryo blastoderm; the results obtained demonstrated the role of the endoderm and the primitive streak in the differentiation of the axial structures.

The blastoderms were taken at the beginning of the primitive streak formation. The epiblast was separated from the underlying endoderm. The anteroposterior axis of the epiblast was then rotated through 180° in relation to the anteroposterior axis of the endoderm. In this way, the anterior part of the epiblast was in contact with the posterior part of the endoderm and vice versa. The reconstituted blastoderm was then cultured *in vitro* using a previously described technique.

This operation generally had a marked effect on the subsequent development of the epiblast. Sometimes the turning of the endoderm inhibited the growth of the normal primitive streak and sometimes it induced the formation of a new primitive streak, oriented in the opposite direction to the original one. In some cases the new primitive streak induced by the endoderm did not persist and disappeared in the course of later development. In other cases the two primitive streaks persisted and gave rise to double monsters. In yet other cases only the secondarily induced primitive streak differentiated, while the original one regressed.

These experiments show that the endoderm is able to induce the formation of a primitive streak in the epiblast. The orientation of the primitive streak is determined by the position of the anteroposterior axis of the endoderm. Waddington thought it unlikely that the endoderm would induce differentiation in a determined tissue. It seemed, rather, that it is the beginning of the morphogenetic movements that results in the formation of the primitive streak.

In 1933, Waddington and Schmidt (61) tested the inductor activity of the primitive streak itself. Pieces of primitive streak from chicken or duck blastoderms were implanted into the area pellucida of blastoderms from both species cultured *in vitro*. The graft differentiated and gave rise to an embryonic axis composed of a neural plate, notochord, and somites. In addition, the host epiblast was induced to differentiate a secondary axis, characterized by a neural plate, the anterior part of the intestine, and mesodermal structures. Pieces of the posterior part of the primitive streak (without Hensen's node) of the heat process and of the rhomboid sinus had the same inductor capacity as the anterior part of the primitive streak. [See also the details of recent experiments on this subject by Hara (29).]

Recently, Butros (11) carried out the same type of experiment using the blastoderm of chick embryos and reached the same conclusions as the previous authors. Blastoderms were incubated for 22 hours and were then cut into two pieces, a prenodal part with Hensen's node and a postnodal part. The postnodal part was used as the effector tissue and various tissues were associated with it in order to determine their inductor capacities. The combination of the inductor tissue and the postnodal portion was cultured *in vitro*.

The prenodal axial structures induced neural, notochordal, and somite differentiation in the postnodal parts. Pieces of the dorsal notochord implanted in the postnodal part induced differentiation of nephrotomes and ducts. Pieces of the neural folds resulted in the differentiation of neural folds, notochord, and mesenchyme.

Thus the primitive streak and its axial derivatives play the same role in birds as does the primary organizer in amphibians. Experiments with combined chick and duck tissues show that this inductor action is not species specific.

It can be concluded from these experiments that primary induction in amphibians is due to the transmission of a diffusible material able to pass through a filter which can act within 6–24 hours on appropriate ectoderm. The morphogenetic movements that accompany axial differentiation are not necessary for the histological differentiation of the nervous system. In birds, the endoderm exerts an oriented inductor effect on the epiblast which results in the formation of the primitive streak. The primitive streak and its axial derivatives can induce differentiation of the neural plate and the axial mesodermal structures.

III. ANALYSIS OF THE INDUCTION OF VERTEBRAL CARTILAGE

Since the work of Watterson (62), Strudel (55, 56), and Holtzer and Detwiler (35) it has been known that the neural tube and the notochord are the inductors of vertebral cartilage (34). *In vitro* culture techniques have allowed a detailed study of this morphogenetic effect and have resulted in the partial characterization of a compound of low molecular weight responsible for the differentiation of somitic mesenchyme into cartilage cells.

Grobstein and Parker (28) cultured, on a plasma clot, somites taken from 9-day fetal mice (fewer than 25 somites). The somites were explanted in groups of 8 and cultured for 4 to 7 days, on a medium composed of 2 parts of horse serum, 2 parts of Tyrode's solution, and 1 part of chick embryo extract. They remained mesenchymal and did not form cartilage (Fig. 8). When a piece of the neural tube from an embryo of the same age was added, it induced differentiation of cartilaginous nodules in the middle of the somitic mesenchyme (Fig. 9).

Grobstein and Holtzer (27) showed subsequently that only the basal plate of the neural tube, that is, the ventral portion, was active. The alar plates were inactive. Moreover, the inductor capacity of the neural tube decreased with increasing age of the donor embryo. The neural tube of a 12–13 day embryo had a poor inductor action, whilst that of a 15-day embryo had lost all inductor ability. It was also established that direct contact between the neural tube and somites was unnecessary for induction to occur. A piece of neural tube was cultured at some distance from the

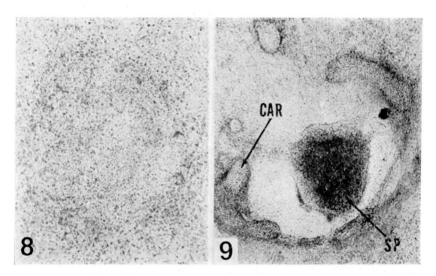

FIG. 8.   Somites from a 9-day mouse embryo after 6 days of culture ($\times$ 26). After Grobstein and Parker (28).

FIG. 9.   Somites from a 9-day mouse embryo after 6 days of culture in the presence of mouse embryo neural tube (SP). Nodules of cartilage have formed (CAR). Compare with Fig. 8 ($\times$ 26). After Grobstein and Parker (28).

somites and was able to induce the formation of cartilaginous nodules in them (Fig. 10). The brain and the otic vesicle also possessed the same inductor effect as the spinal medulla. In contrast, other tissues such as costal cartilage or liver of 15-day mouse embryo and adult mouse liver, kidney, or spleen had no morphogenic effect on somitic mesenchyme. In addition, heating of the neural tube destroyed its inductor effect.

Lash, Holtzer, and Holtzer (38) used chick embryos to study the specificity of the inductor action of the neural tube and the notochord, the differences between the morphogenic effects of these two inductors, and lastly the transmission of the inductor agent across a filter. The conclusion was that only the ventral part of the neural tube and the notochord of the 3-day embryo can induce cartilage formation; all other chick embryo organs tested were found to be inactive. The organs used were either living or killed by alcohol, freezing, or formalin. Glass, wood, and cauterization were also ineffective.

There was a striking difference between the inductor effect of the notochord and that of the neural tube. When placed in contact with a piece of somitic

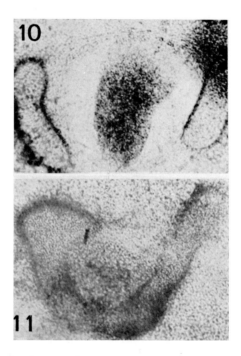

Fig. 10. Association between the neural tube and six somites from a 9-day mouse embryo cultured for 6 days. Nodules of cartilage have been induced at a distance from the neural tube. × 40. After Grobstein and Holtzer (27).

Fig. 11. Differentiation of cartilage in the somitic mesenchyme of a mouse embryo, cultured on a Millipore filter with 11-day mouse embryo neural tube on the opposite surface. The cartilage has surrounded the area above the neural tube, but has not impinged on it. After Grobstein (21).

mesoderm, the notochord always induced the formation of a *single* cartilaginous mass contiguous with the notochordal sheath. Under the same conditions, the neural tube often induced the formation of several small cartilaginous nodules at a distance of up to 2.5 mm from the inductor (Fig. 10). It was also noted that the notochord lost its activity when the notochordal sheath was removed. The sheath itself was able to induce morphogenesis, but could not transmit the induction across a tissue barrier, such as a piece of muscle. The neural tube could exert its effect across a barrier of muscle fibers.

Thus, the morphogenic effects of the neural tube and notochord are different. The neural tube acts by transmission of a diffusible agent, whereas the notochord requires direct cellular contact between the inductor and the effector cells.

These results were confirmed and demonstrated by placing a Millipore filter (Type TA, 20 μ thick, mean pore diamter 0.8 μ) between the inductor organs and the somites (Fig. 11). The notochord, even with the sheath present, could not induce cartilage formation across the filter. The inductor agent from the neural tube could cross the filter and induce the formation of a cartilaginous nodule in the center of the mesenchyme on the other side of the filter. It was also shown that the morphogenic agent did not diffuse in the culture medium, since it was not transmitted unless the two explants were exactly superimposed on either side of the filter. A piece of neural tube four times the normal size had no inductor effect when placed at the edge of the filter with somitic mesoderm in the middle.

Lash, Holtzer, and Whitehouse (39) demonstrated that it was the synthesis of chondroitin sulfate that was dependent on the neural tube or the notochord. This substance is an essential constituent of cartilage. The experiments were carried out using ^{35}S-labeled Na_2SO_4. Only somites cultured in association with the neural tube or the notochord were shown to incorporate actively labeled sulfur into chondroitin sulfate. Somites cultured alone did not incorporate labeled sulfur.

Cartilage synthesis is not linked with the maintenance of histological structure in the somites. In fact, cells that have reaggregated following dissociation of somites by trypsin are able to respond in the same way as normal somites. They react to the morphogenetic effects of the neural tube and the notochord (54).

Lastly, Lash and co-workers (40) and Strudel (57) showed that the morphogenic factor contained in the neural tube could be extracted, and would act in aqueous solution on somites cultured *in vitro*. Hommes *et al.* (36) succeeded in isolating the factor in a nucleotide fraction of neural tube extract obtained using perchloric acid in the cold. The factor possessed the same chondrogenic properties as the intact neural tube, but it has not yet been identified.

The T malformation in mice was studied by Bennett (6) using *in vitro* culture to associate neural tube and somites. Mice carrying the T/T mutation develop normally up to the 4-somite stage. Subsequently, the posterior part of the body does not differentiate any further. There is no more notochord, the somites are rudimentary, and the neural tube is abnormal. To find out if the mutation affected the neural tube or the somite mesenchyme, Bennett cultured somites from normal $+/+$ or mutant T/T embryos in association with neural tube from normal or mutant embryos. The results were quite clear. None of the T/T somites differentiated any cartilage, whether they were associated with a normal or mutant neural tube. All $+/+$ somites formed cartilage, whatever the origin of the associated neural tube. The mutation thus affects the somites, which are unable to respond to the inductor action of the neural tube. The neural tube of the mutants functions normally as an inductor of skeletal differentiation in the vertebral skeleton.

Benoit (1) worked on the induction of cartilage in the internal ear of the chick embryo. When taken at an early stage ($3\frac{1}{2}$ days of incubation), isolated, and cultured, otic mesenchyme remained undifferentiated and did not form cartilage *in vitro*. However, when reassociated with the inductor otocyst, the mesenchyme did differentiate into cartilage. By carrying out associations of varying duration, Benoit showed that contact (either direct or across the vitelline membrane) was necessary for at least 48 hours before chondrification of the otic mesenchyme was obtained.

Both the neural tube and the notochord have been found to exert an inductor effect on the somitic mesoderm. When associated *in vitro* with undifferentiated somites, each of these organs can induce differentiation of vertebral cartilage. The use of organ culture techniques has demonstrated that the neural tube can act at a distance and that the morphogenic agent derived from it can pass a filter interposed between the inductor and the somites. It has also been shown that the notochord cannot induce the formation of cartilage except by direct contact with the effector cells. The inductor activity of the notochord lies within its surrounding sheath. Lastly, the inductor agent of the nervous system can be extracted and has been shown to act in aqueous solution. It is probably a small nucleotide molecule.

IV. ANALYSIS OF THE MORPHOGENIC INTERACTIONS BETWEEN EPITHELIUM AND MESENCHYME IN THE RUDIMENTS OF HETEROGENEOUS ORGANS

Many organs are derived from the union between, and intimate combination of, the epithelium and mesenchyme. At a precise moment during the development of the organs, and in a specific part of the embryo, the rudiments of the two constituents come close to one another. Direct contact may be established and intimate interpenetration may occur. A short time after this union has occurred, one of the two components, and often both of them, differentiates to give form and structure to the organ.

These preferential regions of contact and combination are naturally of interest to the embryologist, who can investigate them in order to demonstrate the mechanisms of organogenesis.

Two kinds of organs have been investigated. These are the skin of bird embryos and certain glandular organs such as the salivary gland and the kidney of mouse embryos.

An analysis of the morphogenic interactions responsible for differentiation in these organs can be carried out only if the two constituents of the organ rudiment can be completely separated. An almost perfect separation is usually obtained using 1–3% trypsin solution in physiological saline lacking Ca^{++} and Mg^{++} ions (Figs. 12, 32A, 33A, 35A). Different workers have used the trypsin digestion technique in different ways, but all the methods are derived from the technique initially described by Moscona (45). Zwilling (68) and others have successfully used Versene (disodium salt of EDTA) at a concentration of 0.1%.

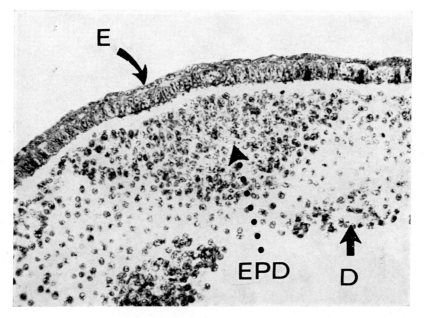

FIG. 12. Separation of the dermis and epidermis of the dorsal skin of 7½-day chick embryo using a 1% trypsin solution. The epidermis is completely released from the dermis and there are no mechanical ties. Cleavage is perfect, even in the region of a young, stage 2 feather germ. D, dermis; E, epidermis; EPD, lenticular mass of dermal cells forming the dermal part of the feather germ. × 420. After Sengel (49).

A. The Skin of Bird Embryos

Three aspects of skin differentiation were studied. These were the development of the skin derivatives, keratinization, and the formation of the uropygial gland. For each of these morphogenetic processes, it was possible to define the role of both the dermal and the epidermal components of the skin. Experimental associations were carried out between pieces of dermis and epidermis that had been previously separated.

1. DIFFERENTIATION OF THE SKIN DERIVATIVES

The principal cutaneous derivatives in birds are the feathers and scales. The feathers cover almost all of the body and are derived in the embryo from small cylindrical papillae, the feather germs. The scales cover the feet of almost all birds and are derived from flattened papillae, the scale germs. The rudiments of both are composed of an epidermal sheath around a mesodermal core.

In order to study what it is that determines the differentiation of these derivatives, a study was made of the mechanisms of interaction between the dermis and the epidermis during the differentiation of embryonic feathers and scales. Fragments of dermis and epidermis of different ages were isolated by treatment with 1% trypsin solution and then associated together in culture (47–50). Wolff and Haffen's method (67) for organ culture was used, and their standard medium was employed.

It is possible to distinguish three stages during the early differentiation of feather germs from the dorsal skin surface. At stage 0 (5–6 days of incubation) the skin is smooth, the epidermis flat, and the dermis homogeneous and undifferentiated. At stage 1 ($6\frac{1}{2}$–7 days of incubation), the dermis shows small lenticular condensations of cells that are the feather rudiments (these form where feathers are present in the chicken) and the epidermis is still flat. At stage 2 ($7\frac{1}{2}$–8 days of incubation) the epidermis above the feather rudiments thickens, and becomes dome-shaped. Thus, there is a formation of the epidermal sheath of the feather germ filled with dermal cells.

a. Differentiation of Ectoderm into Epidermis. Between 5 and 6 days of incubation, the plain ectoderm differentiated into a typical epidermis composed of a basal layer of prismatic cells and a periderm of flattened

iEc/D$_1$

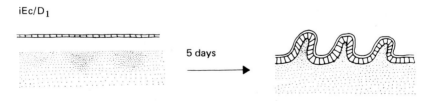

5 days

FIG. 13. *In vitro* development of an association between inverted 5-day ectoderm (iEc) and stage 1 dermis (D$_1$) from a chick embryo: iEc/D$_1$. Differentiation of feather germs has occurred and the epidermis shows the normal polarity of its two layers of cells. After Sengel (49).

cells. Association between stage 1 dermis and 5-day ectoderm demonstrated the histogenetic effect of the dermis (Fig. 13). If 5-day ectoderm or stage 0 epidermis was placed on the piece of dermis with the peridermal surface against the dermis, a remodeling of the epidermis occurred, so that its internal-external polarity was reversed. Thus the peridermis was again on the surface at the end of culture (Fig. 14). This polarity of the skin becomes stabilized by the 7th day of incubation and could not afterward be reversed.

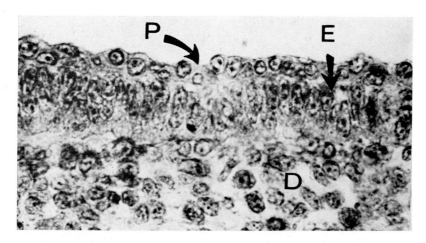

FIG. 14. Histological appearance of the epidermis from an association between stage 0 inverted epidermis and stage 1 dermis (iE_0/D_1) from a chick embryo after 5 days of culture. D, Dermis; E, basal layer of the epidermis; P, peridermis. × 1050. After Sengel (49).

b. Formation of the Feather Germ. The feather germ is the result of inductor interaction between the dermal and epidermal components of the feather rudiment. If a piece of stage 1 dermis and a piece of 0 epidermis are associated in culture on the standard medium, the explant becomes covered with feather germs within 5 days (Fig. 15). This differentiation affirms the

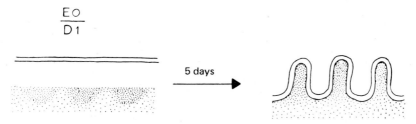

FIG. 15. *In vitro* development of an association between stage 0 epidermis (E_0) and stage a dermis (D_1) from chick embryo: E_0/D_1. Differentiation of feather germs has occurred. After Sengel (49).

inductor role of the dermis in the formation of the epidermal sheath. After stage 2, the dermis loses its inductor activity. The opposite association, that is, between stage 2 epidermis and stage 0 dermis, revealed the former's inductor effect on the latter (Fig. 16). Under the influence of the epidermis,

$$\frac{E\ 2}{D\ 0}$$

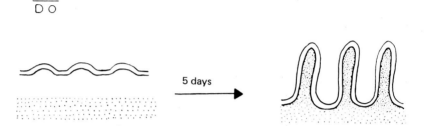

FIG. 16. *In vitro* development of an association between stage 2 epidermis (E_2) and stage 0 dermis (D_0) from a chick embryo: E_2/D_0. Differentiation of feather germs has occurred. After Sengel (49).

the dermal cells colonized the epidermal sheath of the feather germs. This secondary morphogenetic effect was also demonstrated by placing stage 2 epidermis in contact with the deep surface of the dermis from a piece of stage 1 skin (Fig. 17). The epidermal graft induced the differentiation of supplementary feather germs on the deep surface of the dermis (Fig. 18). Lastly, the morphogenic effect of the epidermis was shown by associating feather-producing stage 2 epidermis with dermis from the uropygial region of the duck (17). This area is normally destined to form the uropygial gland. The epidermis induced the formation of feather germs and caused the uropygial dermal cells to deviate from their normal fate, inducing them to form the mesodermal core of the feather germs.

The dermis is thus the primary inductor for the outgrowth of the feather germs. After having been subjected to the first inductor impulse exerted by

$$E_2/iP_1$$

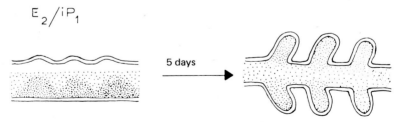

FIG. 17. *In vitro* development of an association between stage 2 epidermis (E) and inverted stage 1 skin (iP_1): E_2iP_1. Differentiation of feather germs has occurred on both sides of the explant (see Fig. 18). After Sengel (49).

the dermis, the differentiated epidermis plays a principal part in the construction of the feather germ.

   c. Orientation of the Feather Germ.   The feather germs in the dorsal region have a definite orientation in relation to the whole embryo. From

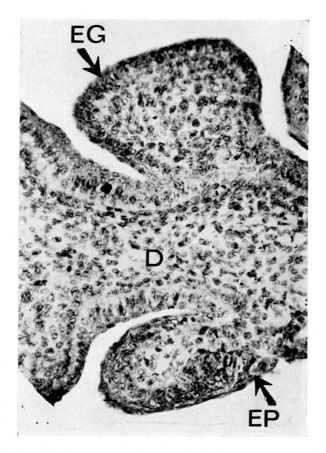

FIG. 18.   Histological appearance of an association between stage 2 epidermis and inverted stage 1 skin (E_2iP_1, see Fig. 17) of a chick embryo after 5 days of culture. D, Dermis of the inverted skin; EG, grafted epidermis; EP, epidermis belonging to the dermis of the inverted skin. $\times$ 450. After Sengel (49).

the beginning of their outgrowth, they are inclined toward the tail of the embryo. Associations of dermis and epidermis were cultured in which the epidermis was rotated through 90° or 180° in relation to the cephalocaudal axis of the dermis, and these showed that the epidermis alone was responsible for the orientation of the feather germs (Fig. 19). The feather germs always inclined toward the caudal edge of the piece of epidermis, whatever the orientation of the dermis.

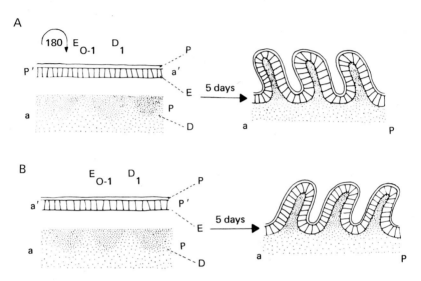

FIG. 19. (A) *In vitro* development of an association between stage 1 dermis (D_1) and stage 0 or 1 epidermis from a chick embryo. The cephalocaudal axis of the epidermis has been rotated through 180° in relation to that of the dermis (180 E_{0-1}): 180 E_{0-1}/D_1.

(B) *In vitro* development of a control association where the epidermis has not been turned: E_{0-1}/D_1. D, dermis; E, basal layer of epidermis; P, peridermis; a—P, cephalocaudal axis of the dermis; a′—P′, cephalocaudal axis of the epidermis. After Sengel (49).

d. Regional Differentiation of the Skin. To investigate why some parts of the skin are covered with feathers, while others such as the feet are covered with scales, and to investigate which tissue is responsible for the difference,

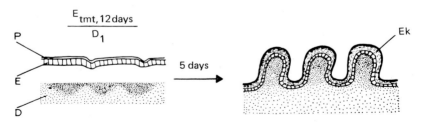

FIG. 20. *In vitro* development of an association between tarsometatarsal epidermis from a 12-day embryo ($E_{tmt\ 12j}$) and stage 1 dorsal dermis (D_1): $E_{tmt\ 12j}/D_1$. Differentiation of feather germs has occurred and keratinization has appeared early. D, dermis; E, basal layer of epidermis; Ek, epidermis in the process of keratinization; P, peridermis. After Sengel (49).

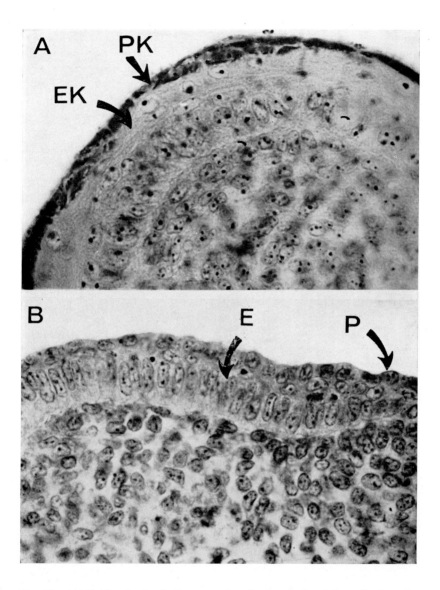

Fig. 21.   (A) Epidermis of a feather germ that developed after 5 days of culture from an association between 12-day tarsometatarsal epidermis and stage 1 dorsal dermis (see Fig. 20). Note the flattened cells of the superficial layers (EK) of the true epidermis and the keratohyalin granules in the peridermis (PK)   (B) In comparison, epidermis of a feather germ derived from stage 1 dorsal skin of a chick embryo cultured for 5 days. The true epidermis (E) is composed of two layers and the peridermis (P) shows only one layer with no keratohyalin granules. × 1050. After Sengel (48).

associations were cultured combining dermis and epidermis from the back
(feather-producing) and the tarsometatarsal region (scale-producing). These
demonstrated the role of the dermis in the regional differentiation of the skin
and the dual potentiality of the skin of bird embryos. Association of stage 1
dorsal dermis with 12-day tarsometatarsal epidermis resulted in an explant
covered with feather germs (Fig. 20). These feather germs differed from
normal feather germs in the early keratinization of the epidermis (Fig. 21).
Under the influence of the dorsal dermis, epidermis from the foot developed
anatomically according to the nature of the dermis. However, the histological
differentiation of the epidermis conformed to its origin. An opposite association between 13-day tarsometatarsal dermis and stage 1 dorsal epidermis
resulted in typical scales (Fig. 22). Under the influence of dermis from the

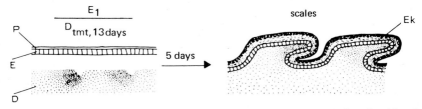

FIG. 22. *In vitro* development of an association between stage 1 dorsal epidermis
(E_1) and 13-day tarsometatarsal dermis ($D_{tmt\ 13j}$): $E_1/D_{tmt\ 13j}$. Differentiation of typical
scales has occurred. D, Dermis; E, basal layer of the epidermis; Ek, epidermis in the
process of keratinization; P, peridermis. After Sengel (49).

foot, keratinization of the dorsal epidermis was as rapid and was of the
same type as that in normal scales (Fig. 23).

Thus, the dermis determines the regional quality of cutaneous differentiation. Whatever the origin of the epidermis, the dorsal dermis induces feather
germs and the tarsometatarsal dermis induces scales.

To summarize, the mechanism of differentiation of the skin can be described
as follows (Fig. 24).

First phase. The dermis induces differentiation of typical epidermis from
simple ectoderm.

Second phase. Under the influence of a factor whose nature has not
yet been defined but which may come from the group of axial organs
(neural tube, notochord, myotomes, or sclerotomes), the dermis of the
dorsal skin forms feather rudiments.

Third phase. The dermal feather rudiments exert a brief inductor effect
on the overlying epidermis which results in the primary outgrowth of the
epidermis. At the same time, the anatomical origin of the dermis determines

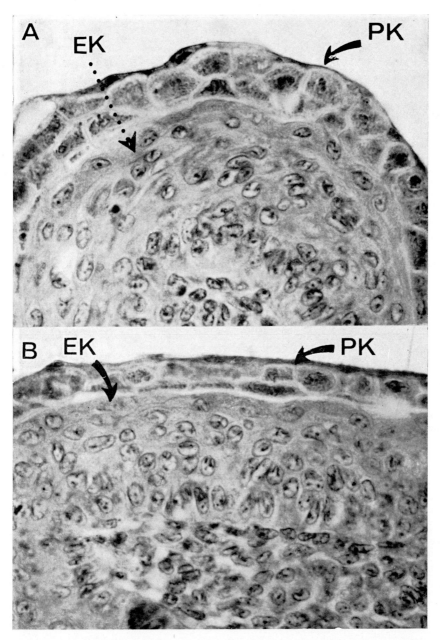

Fig. 23. (A) Development of a scale, developed after 5 days of culture of an association between stage 1 dorsal epidermis and 13-day tarsometatarsal dermis. Note the thickness of the true epidermis with superficial layers (EK) that are flattened and in the process of keratinization. The cells of the three peridermal layers are markedly hypertrophied and are filled with eosinophile granules. (B) In comparison, the epidermis of a scale from a 13-day embryo and cultured for 5 days. Note the same histological features as in Fig. 23A. × 1050. After Sengel (48).

the regional cutaneous differentiation of the epidermis into feathers or scales.

Fourth phase. The epidermis, in its turn, induces the dermal cells to colonize the epidermal sheath and fixes the orientation of the feather germs according to its cephalocaudal polarity.

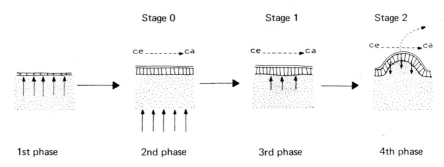

FIG. 24. Diagrammatic representation of four successive inductions (indicated by parallel arrows) resulting in the formation of the feather germ in the chick embryo. The straight broken arrows represent the cephalocaudal orientation (ce-ca) of the epidermis, which determines the orientation of the feather germ (curved arrow). After Sengel (49).

e. Dermal-Epidermal Relationships in the Skin of "Scaleless" Chick Embryos. Abbot used carriers of this mutation selected from the Poultry Husbandry Department of the University of California. Homozygotes are characterized by the absence of scales and by a deficient plumage that covers only part of the body. In particular, the dorsal skin of the thoracic and the anterior lumbar region is completely bare.

The morphogenetic potentialities of the dermis and epidermis of the dorsal and tarsometatarsal skin of these mutants were studied to see if the mutation affected the whole skin or only one of its two constituents (51). Heterogeneous combinations of dermis and epidermis taken from normal and scaleless embryos were cultured *in vitro*. The dorsal skin explants were taken from 6–7½ day embryos, and explants from the tarsometatarsal area were taken from 10–11 day embryos.

Explants containing scaleless epidermis did not differentiate, whether combined with normal or scaleless dermis. Dorsal explants containing normal epidermis formed feather germs, even when combined with scaleless dermis. In explants from the tarsometatarsal region, most of the combinations of normal epidermis and scaleless dermis formed recognizable scales. Thus, in the skin of scaleless embryos the mutation affects only the epidermis. This epidermis cannot respond to the morphogenic effect of the dermis, either normal or scaleless, with which it is associated in culture. Scaleless dermis functions normally and exerts the same differentiating effect as does normal dermis when associated with normal epidermis.

These experiments concentrated essentially on the morphological differentiation of two skin structures, that is, feathers and scales. Other experiments have been carried out to investigate the determination of the histological differentiation of the epidermis, which results in the formation of the cornified layers.

2. KERATINIZATION

After 5 days of incubation, the skin of the chick embryo has not yet become characterized. The dermis is not yet separated from the underlying mesenchyme and the epidermis is still flat and composed of two layers of cells. These are a basal layer of cubical cells and a superficial periderm composed of scanty, very flattened, fusiform cells. At this stage the dorsal epidermis has not been irreversibly determined. Its normal fate would be to become keratinized during the later development which forms the cornified layers of the skin. It can be diverted from its normal differentiation by association in culture with mesenchyme from another region (42, 43).

Epidermis cultured using Fell's techniques keratinized completely within 10 days, with all the cells changing into cornified layers and then dying. When the epidermis was reassociated with mesenchyme from the limb bud, it differentiated normally and only the superficial layers became keratinized. In contact with mesenchyme from the gizzard, the epidermis was transformed into a secretory epithelium and sometimes became ciliated. With mesenchyme from the proventriculus and during the first 7 days of culture the epidermis first differentiated mucous cells, as it did with gizzard mesenchyme. Later, however, keratinization recommenced. When associated with heart mesenchyme, the epidermis behaved differently according to whether it was in contact with myoblasts or fibroblasts. With myoblasts, the epidermis took on the appearance of a thin, squamous layer, whereas with fibroblasts it formed a very thick layer of keratin.

These experiments demonstrate clearly the determining role of the mesenchyme during differentiation of the cutaneous epithelium. This role has been studied closely by Wessells (64, 65) using the tarsometatarsal skin of the chick embryo. Pieces of skin were taken from the anterior part of the foot (tarsometatarsus) of 11-day chick embryos. The dermis was separated from the epidermis using a trypsin-pancreatin solution (1.5–3%). The explants were cultured on a synthetic medium for 5 days. The medium used was a modification of Waymouth's medium 752/1 (63) (for its composition see Chapter 2).

Wessells' results were as follows. The whole skin differentiated normally *in vitro*, with many mitotic figures seen in the basal cells. Kerato-hyalin granules appeared in the peridermis, tonofibrils formed in the subperidermal layer, and the superficial layers became keratinized. Epidermis cultured alone did not undergo this differentiation. The palisade arrangement of the basal cells became rapidly disorganized and the explant became necrotic within 2–3 days. Dermis cultured alone survived longer, and accumulated much intercellular fibrous material which was seen to be birefringent and PAS positive, and could be destroyed by collagenase. This material was distributed uniformly throughout the dermal mass. When the dermis was cultured in contact with a piece of epidermis, the fibrous material only differentiated at a distance from the epidermis, as though the latter inhibited its formation in the immediate vicinity. Epidermis reassociated with dermis differentiated normally, in the same way as normal undissociated skin. Thus the dermis seems to be indispensable for normal differentiation of the epidermis. This morphogenic effect of the dermis disappears at a later stage. When associated with 18-day dermis, 11-day epidermis survived in good condition but did not differentiate. The same occurred when 11-day epidermis was associated with 11-day muscle. Only 11-day dermis seemed able to support the normal histogenesis of the epidermis.

Cellular contact between the dermis and the epidermis is not necessary for the transmission of the dermal morphogenic agent. A Millipore filter could be placed between the two components in culture, without hindering either normal keratinization of the skin, or the maintenance of alignment of the basal cells (Figs. 25 and 26). Wessells tested four types of filter of varying thickness and porosity: (type TH, 25 μ, pores 0.45 μ; type TV, 25 μ, pores 0.1 μ; type HA, 150 μ, pores 0.45 μ; type VC, 150 μ, pores 0.1 μ). Only the VC filter, which was the thickest and had the finest pores, prevented the passage of the morphogenic agent. Epidermis cultured on this filter did not differentiate.

The dermis affects the survival and the histological differentiation of the tarsometatarsal epidermis by means of a morphogenic factor that can be transmitted at a distance and is diffusible in the intercellular spaces. The epidermis seems to exert an inhibitory or localizing influence on the buildup and deposition of intercellular fibers in the dermis.

The dermis also acts on the mitotic activity of the epidermis. Wessells (66) studied this action of the dermis by using historadioautographic techniques after the incorporation of tritiated thymidine. Epidermis cultured alone rapidly lost its ability to incorporate thymidine. After 10 hours of culture, the level of thymidine incorporation was almost zero (Figs. 27 and 28). When replaced in contact with a piece of dermis, the epidermis gradually began to incorporate thymidine. The level of incorporation became normal again after 38 hours of culture (Figs. 29 and 30). If the epidermis was cultured in contact with a piece of cartilage or in a medium enriched with horse serum, the thymidine incorporation was poor. However, the histological development of the basal cells was precocious and well advanced, so that many of

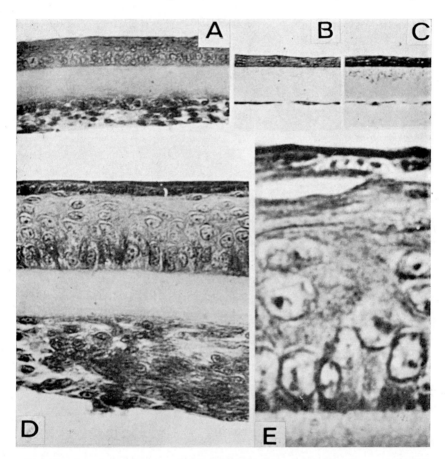

Fig. 25.   Association between dermis and tarsometatarsal epidermis on either side of a Millipore filter. Tissue taken from an 11-day chick embryo.   (A) Dermis and epidermis on either side of a Millipore filter (type TH) after 3 days of culture. Note the palisade arrangement of the basal cells of the epithelium. Unna, × 400.   (B, C) Histological appearance with bright field illumination (B) and phase contrast (C) of the lateral zones of the same filter as shown in Fig. 25A. The epidermal cells are flattened and have not retained their palisade arrangement because so few dermal cells are present on the opposite side of the filter. Unna, × 400.   (D) Differentiation of the epidermis up to the 14-day stage on a type TH filter after 5 days of culture. Unna, × 600.   (E) Histological appearance of epidermis cultured on a type TH filter in association with a piece of dermis. Note the basal palisade arrangement in the epidermis. Phase contrast, × 2160.   After Wessells (65).

27

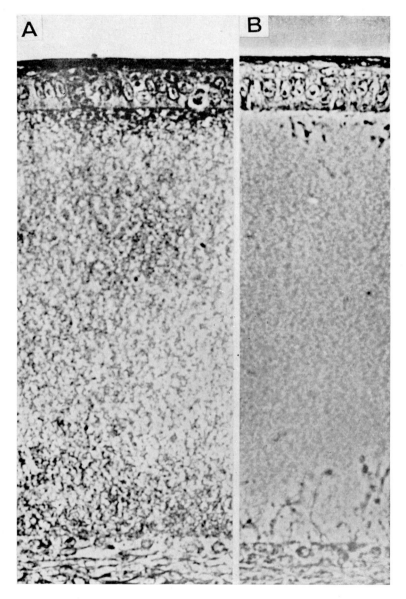

FIG. 26. Association of dermis and tarsometatarsal epidermis from an 11-day chick embryo, with a thick Millipore filter between the explants (150 μ). (A) Bright field. (B) Phase contrast. Note the orientation of the basal layer and the presence of a mitotic figure in the epidermis. The depth and frequency of penetration of cytoplasmic processes into the filter are very variable, but a large area of the central part has not been invaded. Approx. × 740. After Wessells (65).

the cells became keratinized and only a few remained as undifferentiated basal cells.

These last experiments show that the dermis acts on the basal epidermal cells and maintains their ability to multiply actively. Contrary to what might be thought at first, the essential role of the dermis is not to induce differentiation of the basal cells, but rather to prevent them from developing

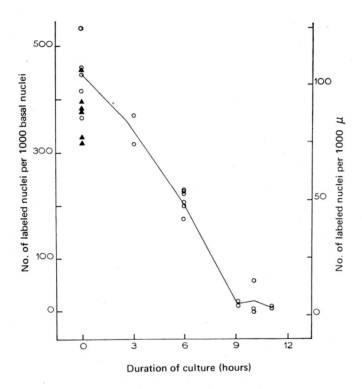

FIG. 27.   Tarsometatarsal skin of an 11-day chick embryo. Incorporation of tritiated thymidine by the intact skin (A) and by the epidermis cultured alone (O) as a function of the duration of culture. After Wessells (66).

in an anarchic fashion toward keratinization. In this way the normal stratification of the epidermal layers is preserved. In the absence of this regulating factor, all the epidermal cells complete their differentiation only if they survive long enough. This was true when the epidermis was cultured alone on a suitable medium, or in contact with other tissues such as cartilage.

Recently, Dodson (15) has carried out some interesting experiments regarding the role of the dermis in the histological differentiation of the epidermis. The dermis was taken from the tarsometatarsal region of a 12-day chick embryo. After various chemical or physical treatments, the dermis was recombined with epidermis from the same region and of the same age, and was then cultured *in vitro* (Fig. 31).

Dermal cells that had been dissociated by trypsin, freed of intercellular material, reassociated, and when placed in contact with epidermis were

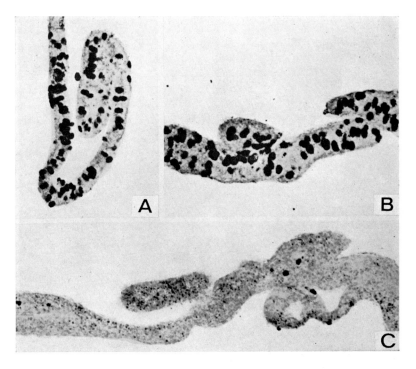

FIG. 28. Radioautographs of tarsometatarsal epidermis from 11-day chick embryos, cultured for (A) 0, (B) 6, and (C) 10 hours. Between 6 and 10 hours of culture, the level of tritiated thymidine incorporation decreases rapidly. Hematoxylin, 8 days' exposure. After Wessells (66).

able to maintain epidermal stratification. A PAS-positive basal membrane was reconstituted after 3 hours of culture and the intercellular material then reformed. The epidermis continued its normal differentiation as it would when in contact with dermis that had not been subjected to trypsin treatment.

Repeated freezing of the dermis did not modify the development of epidermis with which it was associated. When in contact with this dead tissue, the epidermis showed normal keratinization and the basal cells retained their normal palisade arrangement. Dermis that had been killed by heat treatment had no effect on the epidermis. Epidermis associated with this heat-killed dermis behaved as though it was in culture alone, with the basal cells losing their palisade arrangement, mitosis ceasing, and the cells becoming unhealthy.

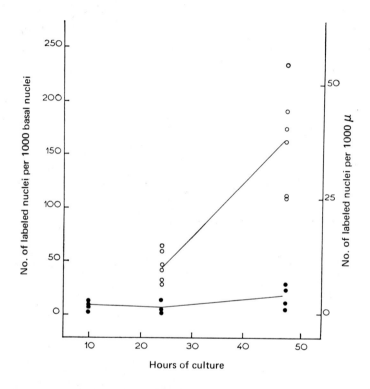

FIG. 29.   Incorporation of tritiated thymidine by the tarsometatarsal epidermis of an 11-day chick embryo. The explant was precultured alone for 10 hours before reassociation with the dermis. o, Epidermis alone; O, epidermis reassociated with the dermis. After Wessells (66).

Dodson also showed that the dermis could be replaced by a gel of collagen without any arrest in the differentiation of the epidermis (Fig. 31D).

These important results show that at least a major part of the activity of the dermis is not connected with the metabolic activity of its cells, but rather with the existence of physicochemical factors independent of the life of the tissue.

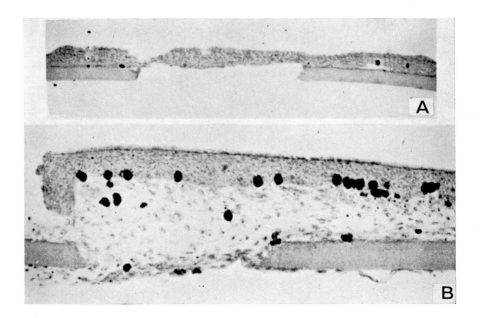

Fig. 30. (A) Radioautograph of an 11-day chick embryo epidermis cultured alone
for 10 hours on a Millipore filter (control for explant in Fig. 30B). There are very few
labeled nuclei. Hematoxylin, 16 days' exposure.   (B) Radioautograph of a recombination
of dermis and epidermis that had been precultured alone for 10 hours. Tritiated thymidine
was added 38 hours after reassociation with the dermis. Marked incorporation of thymidine
took place.   Hematoxylin, 8 days' exposure. After Wessells (66).

3. Differentiation of the Uropygial Gland

The uropygial gland is the only cutaneous gland in birds, and is situated
in the dorsal skin of the tail. It is formed by two ectodermal invaginations
that acquire glandular properties as they become buried in the dermal
mesenchyme. Gomot (17, 18) has studied the interactions occurring between
the ectoderm and the mesoderm during differentiation of this gland in duck
embryos. Explants of dorsocaudal skin were taken from 8–13 day embryos
and were cultured on Wolff and Haffen's standard medium (67).

When explanted *in vitro* before the beginning of the ectodermal invagination (between 8 and 10 days of incubation), the dorsocaudal skin followed
its normal differentiation. The epidermis became invaginated and gave rise
to an obviously normal gland. The reactions of the uropygial dermis and
epidermis were studied when these were associated in culture with pieces
of feather-producing or neutral dermis and epidermis, that is, cells that will
normally give rise to feathers or else form no skin derivatives.

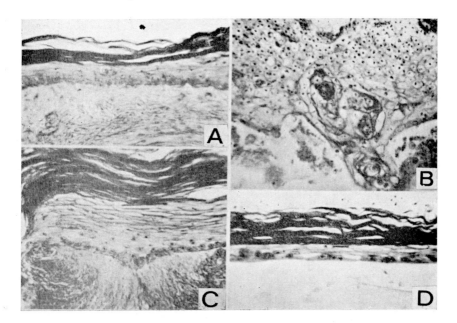

FIG. 31. Differentiation of the tarsometatarsal epidermis of a 12-day chick embryo cultured on various living and inanimate supports. (A) After 10 days of culture in association with living untreated dermis. Normal differentiation. Azan, × 225. (B) After 2 days of culture alone on a rayon (cellulose acetate) support. Disintegration and necrosis. Azan, × 225. (C) After culture for 10 days in contact with dermis killed by freezing. Differentiation of keratin and maintenance of the normal stratification. Azan, × 225. (D) After 10 days of culture on a collagen gel support. Normal keratinization and maintenance of the basal cells. Azan, × 225. After Dodson (15).

Association between 9–10 day uropygial dermis and feather-producing skin (stage 0–1) resulted in normal differentiation with the formation of typical glandular invaginations. The uropygial dermis is thus the inductor of the glandular invaginations. Undifferentiated feather-producing epidermis was still able to respond to this inductor effect and formed a glandular epithelium. A little later, at 12 days, the uropygial dermis had lost this morphogenic activity and was no longer able to induce invaginations in stage 0 or stage 1 feather-producing epidermis. The differentiation of invaginating uropygial epidermis (11–13 days) was studied in association with dermis from the neck of the "bare neck" strain. Such an association did not differentiate normally. A few epidermal folds formed in the region of the early invaginations, but these did not penetrate the dermis.

Thus the dermis plays an essential part in the origin of the uropygial gland. One of its principal activities is of a mechanical nature, since it is able to induce invaginations as easily in foreign epidermis (trout fry or frog tadpole, for instance) as in a dead membrane (epidermis or amniotic membrane fixed in absolute alcohol). Obviously these diverse combinations do not develop for very long. After 2 days of culture, the dermal cells have crossed the membrane that covered them and have progressively invaded the invaginations. However, this does not detract from the finding that the dermis exerts a strong modeling effect during the formation of the uropygial gland.

Finally, Gomot (18) placed the feather-producing inductor (dermal and epidermal) in competition with the uropygial inductor (dermal). It has already been shown that a combination between stage 2 featherproducing epidermis and 10-day uropygial dermis results in the production of many feather germs to the detriment of the gland. The association of $11\frac{1}{2}$-day uropygial epidermis with stage 1 differentiated feather-producing dermis also resulted in the exclusive production of feather germs.

Thus, the differentiation of the plumage takes precedence over that of the uropygial gland under these experimental conditions. In all cases, the feather inductor, either dermal or epidermal, dominates the uropygial inductor.

B. Organs with Cells Arranged in Tubules or Cords

With the exception of the stomach, which is derived directly from localized differentiation of the endoderm, all the organs to be discussed have the following features in common. They arise from a simple or hollow epithelial bud that becomes embedded in a feltwork of mesenchymal cells. Ramifications grow out from this bud, which finally has the appearance of a tube or cell cord, extensively arborized in the middle of the surrounding mesenchyme.

The differentiation of the submaxillary salivary gland and the kidney (metanephros) of mouse embryos has been studied extensively by Grobstein and his school (5, 19–24, 26, 27). Other embryonic organs have also been examined, for example, mouse thymus (3, 4), lung (1, 2), and pancreas (16, 25) and chicken lung (13, 14), metanephros (12), and liver (41). The principal results are summarized below.

1. Salivary Gland (19)

All the experiments of Grobstein and his co-workers were carried out using crossbred mice from BALB/C females and C3H males. The rudiments of the submaxillary gland were taken on the 13th day of gestation. The explants were cultured on a plasma clot in a liquid medium. The epithelial rudiment was isolated from the capsular mesenchyme by means of trypsin and was found to be unable to differentiate *in vitro* when cultured alone. If put back into contact with salivary mesenchyme, it formed many glandular ramifications (Fig. 32A,B). Thus, the mesenchyme is necessary for epithelial differentiation. It was necessary to discover if the morphogenic effect of the mesenchyme was specific, or whether other types of mesenchyme could induce arborization of the epithelial tubules. Epithelial rudiments of the salivary gland were cultured in contact with mesenchyme derived from the

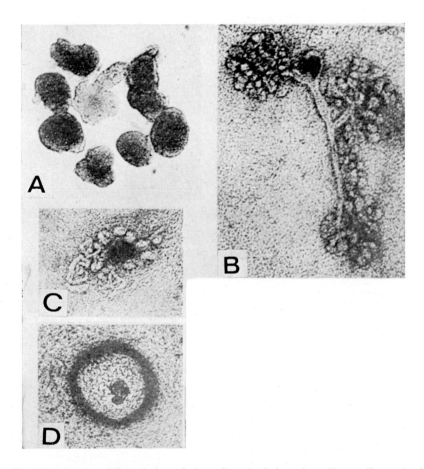

FIG. 32. *In vitro* differentiation of the rudiment of the submaxillary salivary gland from a 13-day fetal mouse. (A) Epithelial rudiment of the salivary gland after trypsin separation, surrounded by pieces of mesenchyme and at the time of explantation. (B) Differentiation of salivary epithelium reassociated with its own mesenchyme after 5 days of culture. (C)Association between salivary epithelium and metanephric mesenchyme from an 11-day embryo after 4 days of culture. The epithelium is not differentiated but convoluted tubules have developed in the renal mesenchyme. (D) Association between salivary epithelium and 11-day pulmonary mesenchyme. The epithelium has formed only an undifferentiated cyst after 4 days of culture. × 40. After Grobstein (19).

metanephros (Fig. 32C), the lung (Fig. 32D), the maxilla (Fig. 33A,B,C), the wall of the coelom, and the limb bud of 8–13 day mouse embryos and the limb bud of 4-day chick embryos. The epithelium did not ramify in any of these combinations. It spread out or formed a cyst and remained undifferentiated. Of all of the mesenchyme tested, only mesenchyme derived from the salivary gland possessed the specific inductor effect that resulted in

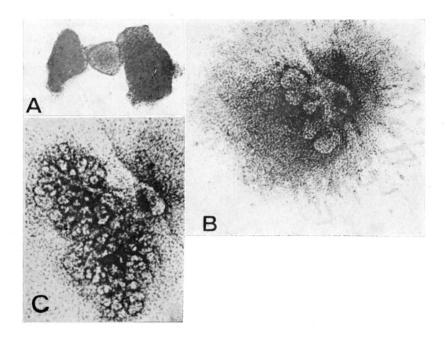

FIG. 33. Association of salivary gland epithelium from one 13-day mouse embryo with its own mesenchyme and with nonsalivary maxillary mesenchyme. (A) At the time of explantation. (B) After 40 hours of culture, the epithelium has differentiated beside the salivary mesenchyme (left) but has remained inactive beside the foreign mesenchyme (right). (C) After 5 days of culture. After Grobstein (21).

differentiation of terminal glandular epithelium. This capacity was associated with the metabolic activity of the mesenchyme cells, as salivary mesenchyme that had been killed by heating or freezing was ineffective.

The differentiation of the epithelium of the submaxillary salivary gland thus depends on the presence of living salivary mesenchyme. It will be shown that for other organs, the relations between the epithelium and the mesenchyme are not so closely limited.

2. KIDNEY (5, 20–24, 26, 37)

In the metanephros, composed of ureteral epithelium and enveloping metanephric mesenchyme, the two components give rise to tubular differentiation. The convoluted secretory tubules develop in the mesenchyme from mesenchymal cells and the collecting tubules form from the ureteral epithelium. During development the two types of tubules become continuous (Fig. 34). The situation in the kidney is more complex than in the salivary gland. The mechanisms of the two types of epithelial differentiation must be elucidated simultaneously. Grobstein (19) used crossed combinations of epithelium and mesenchyme from the kidneys and the salivary glands in culture to investigate the mechanisms.

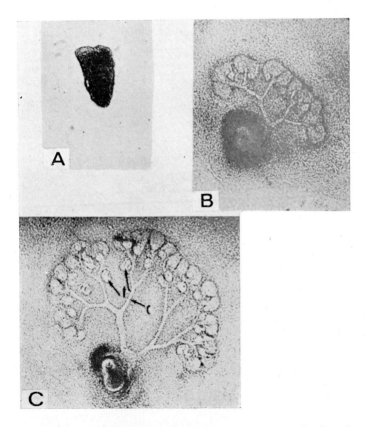

FIG. 34.   Whole renal rudiment from an 11-day mouse embryo at the time of explantation (A) and after 4 (B), and 9 (C) days of culture. C, Collecting ducts derived from the ureteral bud; t, convoluted secretory tubules appearing in the renal mesenchyme. × 27. After Grobstein (20).

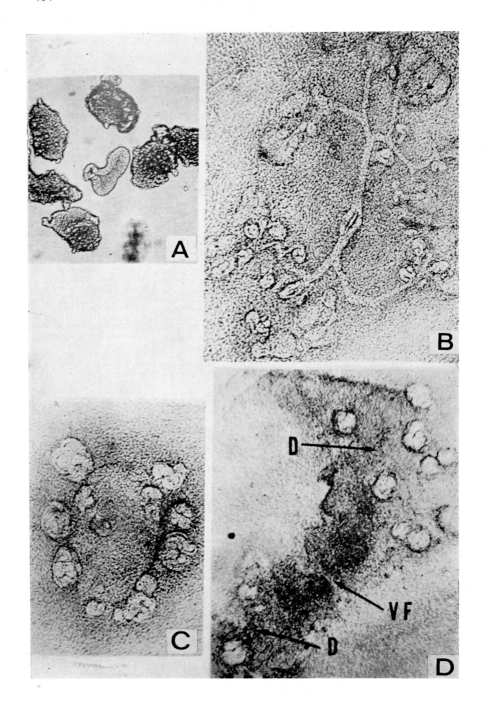

The metanephric rudiments were taken at 11 days of gestation, and those from the salivary gland at 13 days as before. After separation using trypsin followed by culture alone, neither the epithelium nor the mesenchyme of the two rudiments differentiated. The results of the various combinations were as follows:

1. Reassociation of the epithelium and the metanephric mesenchyme resulted in differentiation of the two rudiments and both secretory and collecting tubules were formed (Fig. 35A,B).

2. Association of salivary epithelium and metanephric mesenchyme produced no differentiation of the salivary epithelium (as noted above, the development of this epithelium depended strictly on the presence of salivary mesenchyme). Secretory tubules were seen to develop in the renal mesenchyme (Fig. 32C).

3. The opposite association between renal epithelium and salivary mesenchyme did not result in any morphogenesis.

Thus, the renal epithelium is as narrowly dependent on the presence of its own mesenchyme for differentiation as is the salivary epithelium. Differentiation of the *secretory* tubules in the metanephric mesenchyme can be induced not only by its own ureteral epithelium, but also by foreign epithelium, such as salivary epithelium.

Grobstein (20) then showed that the formation of secretory tubules in the metanephric mesenchyme could be induced by various other living or dead organs from mice or chickens. This was especially true of the neural tube of mouse or chick embryos (Fig. 35C). It was shown that the morphogenic activity of the neural tube lay in the dorsal part of the medulla, with the ventral part having no effect on the metanephric mesenchyme (Figs. 35D and 36). This activity diminished with increasing age of the donor embryos from which the neural tubes were taken and disappeared at birth.

The inductor-effector system constituted by the association of neural tube and metanephric mesenchyme was later used in more advanced investigations

---

FIG. 35. (A) Epithelial renal rudiment from an 11-day mouse embryo, by trypsin and explanted with pieces of renal mesenchyme. × 45. (B) After 6 days of culture, the reassociation has differentiated to form collecting tubules from the ureteral epithelium and secretory tubules from the mesenchyme. These tubules later fuse together. × 45. (C) Association between neural tube (dorsal part) and renal mesenchyme of an 11-day mouse embryo. Secretory convoluted tubules have differentiated in the renal mesenchyme and are closely related to the surface of the neural tube. × 54. (D) Association between a complete section of neural tube (opened and rolled flat) and renal mesenchyme, after 3 days of culture. Note the differentiation of convoluted tubules near the dorsal parts of the neural tube (D) and not near the ventral part which is recognizable by the medial-ventral fissure (VF). × 54. After Grobstein (20).

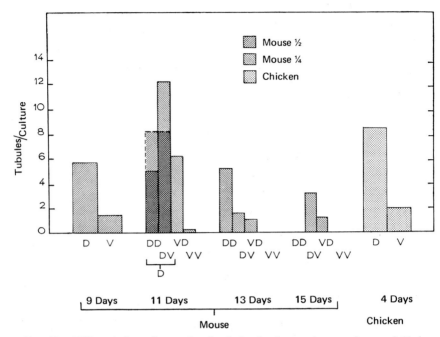

Fɪɢ. 36.   Differentiation of convoluted tubules in the renal mesenchyme of 11-day mouse embryos cultured in the presence of pieces of neural tube from various sources. The ordinate shows the mean number of tubules per culture and the abscissa the various pieces of neural tube that were tested: D, Dorsal half; V, ventral half; DD and DV, respectively dorsal and ventral quarters taken from the dorsal half; VD and VV, respectively dorsal and ventral quarters taken from the ventral half. After Grobstein (20).

by Grobstein and his associates (22, 23, 26). Neural tube and metanephric mesenchyme were associated together in culture and the two tissues were separated by a barrier of varying porosity, such as a Millipore filter or cellophane (Figs. 37 and 38).

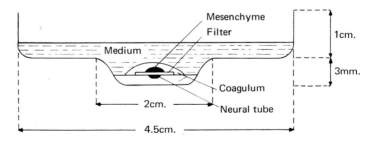

Fɪɢ. 37.   Method of culture using a Millipore filter placed between the renal mesenchyme and the neural tube. After Grobstein (22).

The use of Millipore filters of varying thickness and porosity made it possible to demonstrate that cellular contact between the tissues was unnecessary for the passage of the inductor agent. This agent easily passed filters 20 μ thick and with a mean pore diameter of 0.8 or 0.45 μ (Fig. 39A). The number of secretory tubules induced was always greater with a more porous filter.

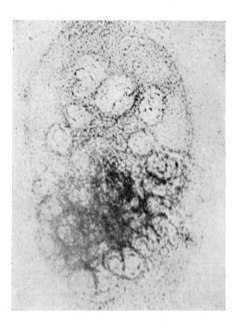

FIG. 38.   Differentiation of convoluted tubules in renal mesenchyme from an 11-day mouse embryo cultured on one side of a Millipore filter; 11-day mouse embryo neural tube on the other side of the filter. Note that the distribution of the tubules coincides well with the contour of the neural tube. After Grobstein (21).

Electron microscopic examination of the filters at the end of the experiments showed the presence of abundant cytoplasmic prolongations in the most porous filters (0.8 μ). These prolongations were less numerous in filters of moderate porosity (0.45 μ). With an even finer filter (mean pore diameter 0.1 μ) there was practically no penetration by cytoplasmic elements. Even so, the inductor activity was still transmitted across this filter, as long as the thickness did not exceed 20 μ. The inductor agent was thus carried across the filter by some extracytoplasmic and diffusible substance.

It was necessary to determine across what distance this inductor effect could be exerted. Several 20 μ thick filters with a mean pore diameter of 0.4 or 0.8 μ were superimposed (Fig. 39B), and it was shown that the mesen-

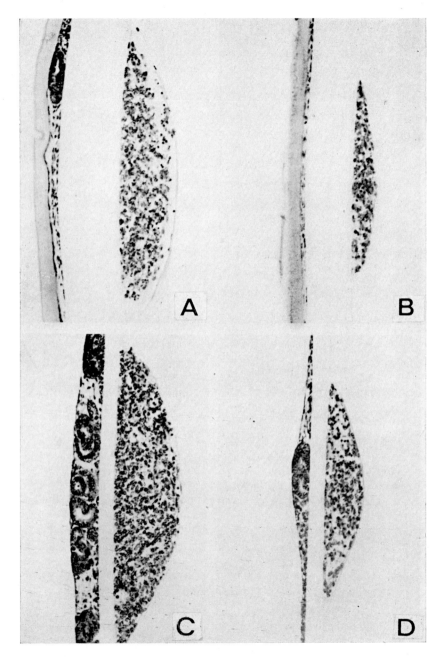

FIG. 39. Induction of convoluted tubules in renal mesenchyme from 11-day mouse embryos. (A, C) Inductor effect of an explant of neural tube of "standard" volum

chyme could no longer differentiate when four filters were placed between it and the neural tube. The morphogenic agent could travel no further than 80 μ. A layer of cellophane, 20 μ thick, placed between two Millipore filters 20 μ thick, was found to be impermeable to the inductor agent (Fig. 40A). If a hole 0.1–0.2 mm in diameter was made in the cellophane, differentiation of tubules did occur in a restricted zone immediately overlying the hole in the cellophane (Fig. 40B). The number of tubules induced across a hole 0.1 mm in diameter was never greater than one, whereas when the hole was 0.2 mm in diameter the mean number of tubules induced was five. In consequence, while the morphogenic agent was held up by the fine pores of the cellophane (0.045 μ ?), it was able to traverse the 20 μ distance through the physiological saline filling the hole. Moreover, the metanephric mesenchyme showed a response to induction proportional to the amount of incoming morphogenic material (Fig. 39C,D).

Later experiments (24, 37) proved irrefutably that there is a transfer of substances from the inductor tissue to the effector tissue. Before being explanted on one side of the Millipore filter, the neural tube was incubated for 2 hours, either in a solution containing 17 tritiated amino acids, or simply in a solution of tritiated leucine. In a first series of experiments, a count was made of the silver grains seen by historadioautography after culture periods of 1, 3, 6, and 24 hours. After 24 hours the radioactivity was 7–16 times higher in the part of the filter in contact with the mesenchyme than it was in a control part of the filter removed from the mesenchyme. In the mesenchyme itself, the radioactivity was almost equal to or slightly higher ($\times$ 1.5) than that in the part of the filter supporting the mesenchyme. This shows that the morphogenic agent (and the substances that accompany it) crosses the filter only in the region between the two explants and that there is no diffusion either laterally in the filter, or into the fluid bathing the tissue. Lastly, it demonstrates the storage of the morphogenic agent in the effector tissue.

The following results were derived from a second series of experiments.

1. Labeled compounds were carried from the inductor tissue to the induced tissue in two forms, one of which could be demonstrated in the filter by histological fixatives. The other could not be demonstrated in this way.

---

across a Millipore filter (C) and across three filters (A). Note the small number of tubules induced across three layers of filter.   (B, D) Inductor effect of an explant of neural tube with a volume reduced to one quarter of the "standard" volume used normally across one (D) and three (B) filter thicknesses. No tubules were induced in the latter case. After Grobstein (37).

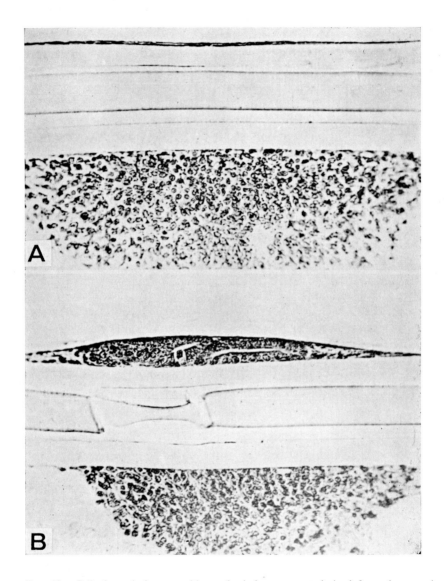

Fig. 40. Cellophane is impermeable to the inductor agent derived from the neural tube of mouse embryo. (A) Association of neural tube and renal mesenchyme of the mouse embryo. Two Millipore filters are separated by a piece of cellophane and are placed between the two explants. After 72 hours of culture, there has been no differentiation of the mesenchyme. (B) A similar experiment, but carried out after making a hole in the cellophane. After 72 hours of culture tubules differentiated in the mesenchyme in the zone immediately over the hole in the cellophane (37).

2. The radioautographic distribution of the first of these forms (that which can be fixed in the filter) was closely related to ease of transmission of the inductor agent. This was proved in the following way:

(a) A piece of labeled neural tube was placed on a Millipore filter 150 μ thick. At the end of culture, radioactive material could be shown up to a maximum distance of 100 μ into the center of the filter. The region of the filter in contact with the mesenchyme was not radioactive, but the mesenchyme itself showed radioactivity (moreover, it was at least 150 μ away from the neural tube). Thus, besides the radioactive material fixable in the filter, there was a second radioactive substance that could not be fixed, that had crossed the filter, and had reached the mesenchyme and accumulated there. This second material did not induce tubule formation (the inductor activity could not be transmitted further than 80 μ; see above).

(b) If a layer of cellophane was interposed between two Millipore filters 20 μ thick (Fig. 41), the mesenchyme did not differentiate but became radioactive owing to accumulation of the nonfixable material crossing

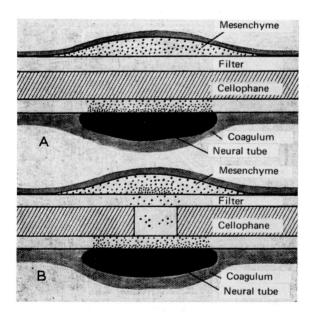

Fig. 41. Diagrammatic representation of culture radioautography in which cellophane was placed between the neural tube and the renal mesenchyme. (A) Note that there are no traces in the filter apposed to the mesenchyme, but there is uniform distribution of grains in the mesenchyme. (B) Note the presence of traces in the filter apposed to the mesenchyme. These are situated directly above the hole in the cellophane. Note also the increased density of grains in the mesenchyme above the hole. After Grobstein (37).

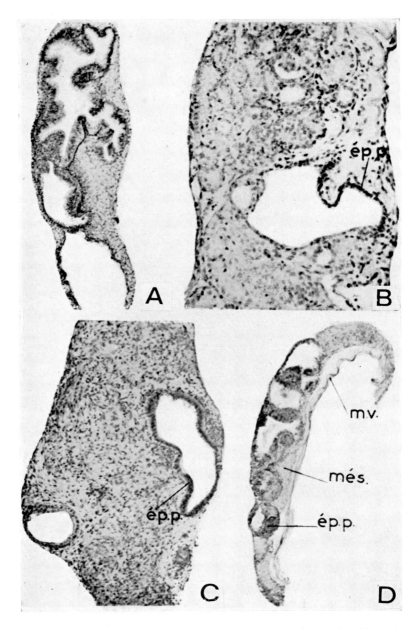

FIG. 42. Associations between pulmonary epithelium (ép. p) from 5-day chick embryos with chick embryo mesenchyme from various regions, after 5 days of culture. (A) Reassociation with 5-day pulmonary mesenchyme. Differentiation and branching of the pulmonary epithelium has occurred. × 135. (B) Association with 5-day mesonephros.

the filter. No radioactivity was shown in the filter that was in contact with the mesenchyme, while that in contact with the neural tube was heavily labeled. Thus, cellophane was permeable to the nonfixable labeled material that possessed no inductor activity. It was only necessary to make a small hole in the cellophane for tubules to develop in the mesenchyme. At the same time, radioactivity appeared in the filter adjacent to the mesenchyme, and was greatly increased in the mesenchyme immediately over the hole in the cellophane, where the tubules had formed.

It is thus well established that two substances come from the neural tube, cross the filter, and collect in the mesenchyme. One of these substances has small molecules that can cross the cellophane but it has no effect on the differentiation of the secretory tubules in the metanephric mesenchyme. The other substance is probably composed of macromolecules that can be fixed by histological methods and that cannot pass cellophane or travel further than 100 μ from the neural tube. However, this substance contains the inductor factor responsible for the differentiation of the secretory tubules.

3. OTHER ORGANS

Similar mechanisms probably occur in the morphogenesis of many other organs where studies have been made. These experiments were not so advanced as those of Grobstein and his school, but it was suggested that analogous morphogenic interactions occur between the epithelium and the mesenchyme of these organs. The essential details of these experiments will be given below.

The thymus gland from a $12\frac{1}{2}$-day mouse embryo is composed of an epithelial bud surrounded by a small mass of mesenchyme cells. When it was taken at this stage and cultured *in vitro*, the thymus differentiated by characteristic lobulation of its epithelium (3). Epithelium cultured alone did not form lobules. When reassociated with thymus mesenchyme, or with mesenchyme from 12-day embryo lung, 13-day submaxillary gland, or 11-day kidney, the epithelium developed the characteristic lobulation. Mesenchyme from the limb bud of a 12-day embryo or a newly born animal had only a weak effect on thymus epithelium. Twelve-day embryonic neural tube or 12-day pulmonary epithelium had no effect. The same results were obtained when a Millipore filter was placed between the mesenchyme and the

---

The epithelium has remained undifferentiated and there are no branches. × 340. (C) Association with 3-day somitic mesenchyme. The epithelium has not differentiated. × 216. (D) Association with metanephric mesenchyme from a 5-day embryo. Good differentiation of the pulmonary epithelium; més., Mesenchyme; m.v., vitelline membrane (which serves as a support to the culture). (× 124). After Dameron (13).

epithelium. By using crossed associations between the epithelium and the mesenchyme from mouse and chicken, Auerbach demonstrated that the epithelium was the source of the lymphocytes and that the mesenchyme gave rise to the connective stroma of the gland (4).

The formation of bronchial branches from the pulmonary epithelium was studied by Dameron (13, 14) in the chick embryo and by Alescio and Cassini (1, 2) in the mouse embryo. In the chicken, the pulmonary mesenchyme could be replaced by metanephric mesenchyme from a 5-day embryo and the bronchial branches differentiated almost as well as they did in the pulmonary mesenchyme (Fig. 42A,D). In contrast, mesenchyme from the mesonephros (Fig. 42B), the somites (Fig. 42C), or the chorioallantoic membrane of the 3–5 day embryo did not induce differentiation of the bronchial epithelium.

In the mouse, the apical mesenchyme of the lung is the inductor of bronchial budding (1, 2). Grafted in the place of a piece of tracheal mesenchyme (noninductor of bronchial budding), the apical pulmonary mesenchyme induced a supplementary bronchial bud in the tracheal epithelium (Fig. 43). The mesenchyme of the submaxillary gland had no effect on the tracheal epithelium.

When cultured alone *in vitro*, the two rudiments of the metanephros of the chick embryo of $5\frac{1}{2}$ days' incubation did not differentiate. They underwent normal morphogenesis when the two rudiments were reunited (12).

The pancreatic epithelium of 11-day mouse embryos differentiated into glandular lobules (with the appearance of zymogen granules) when they were cultured in direct association with embryonic mesenchyme from various sources, such as pancreas, lung, and stomach of 11-day embryos and salivary gland or coelomic wall from 13-day embryos (16, 25). Across a Millipore filter, the morphogenic effects were more variable. With salivary mesenchyme the lobulation was good but, curiously, was less good with its own pancreatic mesenchyme. There was no morphogenesis with the renal mesenchyme.

The chicken stomach is divided into two parts, the proventriculus, which is essentially glandular, and the gizzard, which is chiefly masticatory. Sigot (52, 53) demonstrated the morphogenic role of the mesenchyme of the two parts of the stomach on the lining epithelium of the digestive tract. The experiments were carried out on rudiments from 5-day embryos. Associated with its own mesenchyme, the epithelium of the proventriculus differentiated in a characteristic fashion, forming many glandular invaginations into the mesenchyme (Fig. 44). Associated with gizzard mesenchyme the proventricular epithelium did not form any glandular rudiments, but always assumed the appearance of gizzard epithelium (Fig. 44). After 6 days of culture, glycogen granules characteristic of the gizzard could be seen in the epithelium. These were not seen in the epithelium of the proventriculus

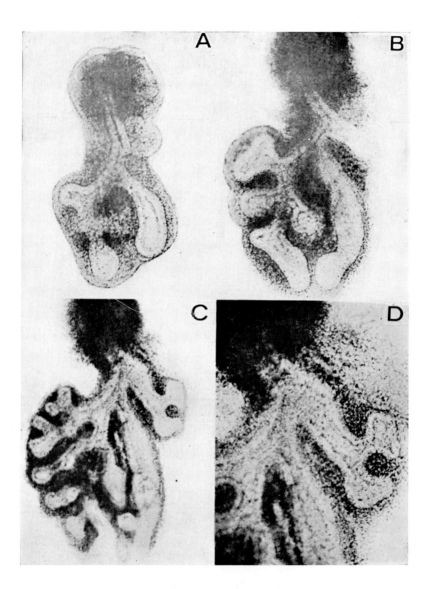

Fig. 43.   Culture of the lung rudiment of an 11-day mouse embryo. A piece of bronchial mesenchyme has been taken from the distal end of the rudiment and then grafted in contact with the left-hand wall (on the right in the photograph) of the trachea.   (A) After 6 hours of culture, an extra lung bud has begun to grow out from the trachea at the site of the graft. × 50.   (B) After 1 day of culture the extra bud has grown longer. × 50.   (C, D) After 3 days of culture, the extra bud has produced two secondary branches in which a lumen can be seen. C (× 50); D (× 65). After Alescio and Cassini (2).

(Fig. 45). Thus, in contact with gizzard mesenchyme, the normally glandular proventricular epithelium is transformed into typical gizzard epithelium.

Marin and Sigot (44) have made an interesting observation regarding the mechanism of the transmission of this inductor effect of the mesenchyme. Pieces of mesenchyme from the gizzard or proventriculus of 5-day embryos were cultured using Wolff and Haffen's method (67). The fragments were covered with a glass coverslip for 7 days and were then removed. An organic

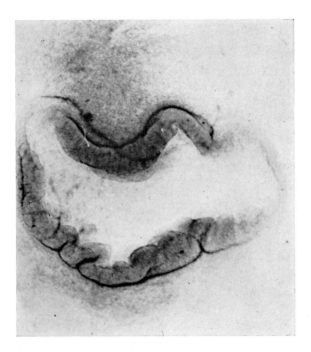

FIG. 44. Association of epithelium from the proventriculus of a 5-day chick embryo with mesenchyme from proventriculus (left) and gizzard (right). After 6 days of culture in contact with its own mesenchyme, the epithelium of the proventriculus has developed many glandular invaginations (unpublished observation, Sigot).

deposit was seen to remain on the coverslip. The inductor effect of this deposit was then tested on 5-day proventricular epithelium. After a short period of culture the epithelium adhered strongly to the coverslips that had been covered with mesenchyme. The epithelium did not adhere to clean coverslips used as controls. After 5–6 days the coverslips were removed and the epithelium was cultured alone for a further 24 hours. Histological examination showed that the differentiation of the epithelium depended on the origin of the organic material with which it had been cultured. The deposit left by proventricular mesenchyme oriented epidermal differentiation toward the formation of glandular folds. On a clean coverslip with no deposit, or in contact with the deposit left by the gizzard mesenchyme, the proventricular epithelium differentiated into gizzard epithelium and the cells accumulated glycogen. Thus, differentiation into epithelium of the gizzard type corresponds to autodifferentiation of proventricular epithelium in the absence of the inductor stimulus.

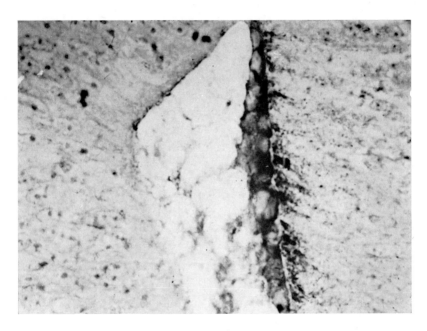

FIG. 45. Histological appearance of an association between epithelium from the proventriculus with mesenchyme from proventriculus (left) and gizzard (right). Note the glycogen granules and the abundant mucus that indicates the differentiation of proventricular epithelium into gizzard epithelium. PAS ($\times$ 1070). After Sigot (53).

Le Douarin (41) showed that organogen of the liver in chick embryos also resulted from an interaction between hepatic mesenchyme and an endodermal epithelial bud. An obstacle (such as shell membrane) placed transversely in the presumptive region of the liver in a 13-somite embryo made it possible to obtain development of hepatic mesenchyme completely free from epithelial cords. The effect of this hepatic mesenchyme, and other mesenchyme, on the proliferation of the hepatic bud was tested *in vitro*. Hepatic mesenchyme stimulated epithelial arborization and induced the differentiation of hepatic cells, which were characterized by their glycogen content (Fig. 46). Association with pulmonary mesenchyme also resulted in the differentiation of hepatic cells, but epithelial proliferation was slower. Somitic mesenchyme had no effect on hepatic epithelium.

During their embryonic development, these heterogeneous organs are the site of important inductor reactions between their mesenchymal and epithelial constituents. Generally, it is the mesenchymal component that is the primary inductor for epithelial differentiation. In some cases, as in the

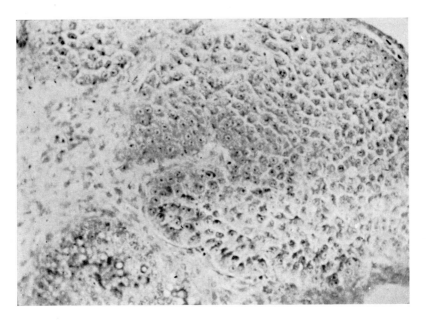

FIG. 46. Association between the hepatic bud and hepatic mesenchyme from a 5-day chick embryo after 3 days of culture. Differentiation of hepatic cell cords from the endodermal epithelium. Note the presence of glycogen in the epithelial cells. PAS ($\times$ 400). After Le Douarin (41).

salivary gland of the mouse embryo, the epithelium has strictly specific needs and must be associated with its own mesenchyme before it can differentiate. In other cases, mouse embryo thymus or pancreas, for instance, it seems that any mesenchyme, either simple or specialized, can give the epithelium the necessary stimulus for development. It has been shown that in several organs the inductor effect can be transmitted across a filter placed between the inductor and the effector.

The induction can be exerted in the absence of inductor cells or tissues, either by accumulation of the inductor substance in a filter or by intermediary compounds left on the glass surface by the inductor tissue. Finally, it is interesting to comment that in the case of the skin, the dermis (which plays an important part in the survival, stratification, and ordered keratinization of the epidermis) can be replaced by an inanimate collagen gel.

V. CONCLUSIONS

In vitro explantation has produced some interesting results, and a number of simple facts emerge. From these facts can be derived certain general rules regarding the morphogenesis of many organs.

In many cases, the inductor effect appears to be a simple one, with no organ or species specificity. The effector tissue carries the specific characteristics of its future differentiation. This is true of primary induction, at least so far as specificity in the zoological sense of the word is concerned—for example, ectodermal differentiations such as balancers and adhesive papillae and dentinous or horny teeth. This is also true as regards differentiation of the secretory tubules of the metanephrogenic mesenchymes. In genetic malformations it is the competent tissue that is damaged by the mutation, the inductor functioning normally.

Morphogenic interactions avoid this rule, particularly where the nature of the inductor tissue determines the nature of the differentiation of the effector tissue. The determination of cutaneous epithelial differentiation is an example. According to the origin of the mesenchyme with which it is associated the epithelium gives rise to feather, scales, keratin, and ciliated and glandular mucus cells.

The method of organ culture has made it possible to obtain much useful information, regarding the development of feather germs, for example. One rudiment acts on a second which in turn acts on a third tissue. The latter, in return, exerts a morphogenic effect on the second. Such chains of induction are of a fairly general character, having also been discovered in other embryonic organs such as the limb bud.

Most of the inductor effects that have been studied until now have been linked with the transmission of an agent able to diffuse into the intercellular spaces. These substances seem to be of moderate molecular weight, small enough to pass through the 0.1 μ pores of a Millipore filter, but too large to pass through the pores of cellophane. Where induction occurs due to such an agent being transmissible across distance, direct cellular contact between the two tissues is not necessary. However, not all forms of induction are of this type. Induction of cartilage formation by the sheath of the notochord can only occur where the cells are in direct contact.

Lastly, it is remarkable to note that in some system it is possible to replace the living inductor tissue with dead tissue or even with an inanimate collagen gel, without hindering the normal development of the competent tissue in the process. Such results open up promising avenues toward the study of the physicochemical conditions occurring in the differentiation of organs.

BIBLIOGRAPHY

1. Alescio T. and Cassini A. L'interazione epitelio-mesenchimale nell'organogenesi del polmone embrionale di topo coltivato *in vitro*. *Z. Anat. Entw.-gesch.*, 1962, **123**, 369–396.

2. Alescio T. and Cassini A. Induction *in vitro* of tracheal buds by pulmonary mesenchyme grafted on tracheal epithelium. *J. exp. Zool.*, 1962, **150**, 83–94.

3. Auerbach R. Morphogenetic interactions in the development of the mouse thymus gland. *Devel. Biol.*, 1960, **2**, 271–284.

4. Auerbach R. Experimental analysis of the origin of cell types in the development of the mouse thymus. *Devel. Biol.*, 1961, **3**, 336–354.

5. Auerbach R. and Grobstein C. Inductive interaction of embryonic tissues after dissociation and reaggregation. *Exp. Cell Res.*, 1958, **15**, 384–397.

6. Bennett D. *In vitro* study of cartilage induction in T/T mice. *Nature*, 1958, **181**, 1286.

7. Benoit J. A. A. Action inductrice de durée variable sur le mésenchyme otique de l'embryon de Poulet en culture *in vitro*. *C. r. Acad. Sci.*, 1964, **258**, 334–336.

8. Brachet J. Quelques observations sur le mode d'action de l'organisateur chez les Amphibiens. *Experientia*, 1950, **6**, 56–57.

9. Brachet J. and Hugon de Scœux F. Remarques sur le mode d'action de l'organisateur chez les Amphibiens. *Commun. 3ᵉ Journée cyto-embryol. belgo-néerland.*, 1949, 56–60.

10. Brahma S. K. Experiments on the diffusibility of the Amphibian evocator. *J. Embryol. exp. Morphol.*, 1958, **6**, 418–423.

11. Butros J. Studies on the inductive action of the early chick axis on isolated post-nodal fragments. *J. exp. Zool.*, 1962, **149**, 1–20.

12. Calame S. Le rôle des composants épithélial et mésenchymateux du métanéphros d'après les résultats de la culture *in vitro*. *Arch. Anat. micr. Morphol. exp.*, 1961, **50**, 299–308.

13. Dameron F. L'influence de divers mésenchymes sur la différenciation de l'épithélium pulmonaire de l'embryon de Poulet en culture *in vitro*. *J. Embryol. exp. Morphol.*, 1961, **9**, 628–633.

14. Dameron F. Rôle du mésenchyme dans la différenciation de l'ébauche épithéliale du poumon embryonnaire de Poulet en culture *in vitro*. *Pathol.-Biol.*, 1962, **10**, 811–816.

15. Dodson J. W. On the nature of tissue interactions in embryonic skin. *Exp. Cell Res.*, 1963, **31**, 233–235.

16. Golosow N. and Grobstein C. Epithelio-mesenchymal interactions in pancreatic morphogenesis. *Devel. Biol.*, 1962, **4**, 242–255.

17. Gomot L. Interaction ectoderme-mésoderme dans la formation des invaginations uropygiennes des Oiseaux. *J. Embryol. exp. Morphol.*, 1958, **6**, 162–170.

18. Gomot L. Contribution à l'étude du développement embryonnaire de la glande uropygienne chez le Canard. *Arch. Anat. micr. Morphol. exp.*, 1959, **48**, 63–141.

19. Grobstein C. Epithelio-mesenchymal specificity in the morphogenesis of mouse submandibular rudiments *in vitro*. *J. exp. Zool.*, 1953, **124**, 383–413.

20. Grobstein C. Inductive interaction in the development of mouse metanephros. *J. exp. Zool.*, 1955, **130**, 319–339.

21. Grobstein C.   Tissue interaction in the morphogenesis of mouse embryonic rudiments *in vitro*. In: *Aspects of Synthesis and Order in Growth* (D. Rudnick, ed.), Princeton U. Press, 1955.

22. Grobstein C.   Transfilter induction of tubules in mouse metanephrogenic mesenchyme. *Exp. Cell Res.*, 1956, **10**, 424–440.

23. Grobstein C.   Some transmission characteristics of the tubule inducing influence on mouse metanephrogenic mesenchyme. *Exp. Cell Res.*, 1957, **13**, 575–587.

24. Grobstein C.   Autoradiography of the interzone between tissues in inductive interaction. *J. exp. Zool.*, 1959, **142**, 203–213.

25. Grobstein C.   Interactive processes in cytodifferentiation. *J. cell. comp. Physiol.*, 1962, **60** (suppl. 1), 35–48.

26. Grobstein C. and Dalton A. J.   Kidney tubule induction in mouse metanephrogenic mesenchyme without cytoplasmic contact. *J. exp. Zool.*, 1957, **135**, 57–73.

27. Grobstein C. and Holtzer H.   *In vitro* studies of cartilage induction in mouse somite mesoderm. *J. exp. Zool.*, 1955, **128**, 333–357.

28. Grobstein C. and Parker G.   *In vitro* induction of cartilage in mouse somite mesoderm by embryonic spinal cord. *Proc. Soc. exp. Biol. Med.*, 1954, **85**, 477–481.

29. Hara K.   Regional neural differentiation induced by prechordal and presumptive chordal mesoderm in the chick embryo. *Drukkerij Libertas N. V.*, Utrecht, 1961, 1–44.

30. Holtfreter J.   Ueber die Aufzucht isolierter Teile des Amphibienkeimes. II: Züchtung von Keimen und Keimteilen in Salzlösung. *Roux' Arch. Entw.-mech. Organ.*, 1931, **124**, 404–466.

31. Holtfreter J.   Nachweis der Induktionsfähigkeit abgetöteter Keimteile. Isolations- und Transplantationsversuche. *Roux' Arch. Entw.-mech. Organ.*, 1933, **128**, 584–633.

32. Holtfreter J.   Regionale Induktionen in xenoplastisch zusammengesetzten Explantaten. *Roux' Arch. Entw.-mech. Organ.*, 1936, **134**, 466–550.

33. Holtfreter J.   Studies on the diffusibility, toxicity and pathogenic properties of "inductive" agents derived from dead tissues. *Exp. Cell Res.*, 1955, **3**, 188–209.

34. Holtzer H.   The development of axial structures in regeneration and embryogenesis. In "*Regeneration in Vertebrates*" (C. Thornton, ed.), 1959, 15–33, U. Chicago Press.

35. Holtzer H. and Detwiler S. R.   An experimental analysis of the development of the spinal column. III: Induction of skeletogenous cells. *J. exp. Zool.*, 1953, **123**, 335–369.

36. Hommes F. A., Leeuwen G. van and Zilliken F.   Induction of cell differentiation. II: The isolation of a chondrogenic factor from embryonic chick spinal cords and notochords. *Biochim. biophys. Acta*, 1962, **56**, 320–325.

37. Koch W. E. and Grobstein C.   Transmission of radioisotopically labeled material during embryonic induction *in vitro*. *Devel. Biol.*, 1963, **7**, 303–323.

38. Lash J. W., Holtzer S. and Holtzer H.   An experimental analysis of the development of the spinal column. VI: Aspects of cartilage induction. *Exp. Cell Res.*, 1957, **13**, 292–303.

39. Lash J. W., Holtzer H. and Whitehouse M. W.   *In vitro* studies on chondrogenesis: the uptake of radioactive sulfate during cartilage induction. *Devel. Biol.*, 1960, **2**, 76–89.

40. Lash J. W., Hommes F. A. and Zilliken F.   Induction of cell differentiation. I: The *in vitro* induction of vertebral cartilage with a low-molecular-weight tissue component. *Biochim. biophys. Acta*, 1962, **56**, 313–319.

41. Le Douarin N.   Isolement expérimental du mésenchyme propre du foie et rôle morphogène de la composante mésodermique dans l'organogenèse hépatique. *J. Embryol. exp. Morphol.*, 1964, **12**, 141–160.

42. McLoughlin C. B. The importance of mesenchymal factors in the differentiation of chick epidermis. II: Modification of epidermal differentiation by contact with different types of mesenchyme. *J. Embryol. exp. Morphol.*, 1961, **9**, 385–409.

43. McLoughlin C. B. Metaplasia of epidermis transplanted on to different types of mesenchyme in the chick. *Coll. internat. C.N.R.S.*, No. 101, Nogent-sur-Marne, 29 août-3 septembre 1960, 1961, 145–154.

44. Marin L. and Sigot M. Évolution d'une ébauche épithéliale au contact d'une surface ayant porté un mésenchyme inducteur. *C. r. Acad. Sci.*, 1963, **257**, 3475–3477.

45. Moscona A. Cell suspensions from organ rudiments of chick embryos. *Exp. Cell Res.*, 1952, **3**, 535–539.

46. Saxén L. Transfilter neural induction of Amphibian ectoderm. *Devel. Biol.*, 1961, **3**, 140–152.

47. Sengel P. Analyse expérimentale du développement *in vitro* des germes plumaires de l'embryon de Poulet. *Experientia*, 1957, **13**, 177–182.

48. Sengel P. Déterminisme de la différenciation régionale des phanères de l'embryon de Poulet. *Bull. Soc. zool. Fr.*, 1958, **83**, 82–86.

49. Sengel P. Recherches expérimentales sur la différenciation des germes plumaires et du pigment de la peau de l'embryon de Poulet en culture *in vitro*. *Ann. Sci. nat., Zool.*, 1958, **20**, 431–514.

50. Sengel P. La différenciation de la peau et des germes plumaires de l'embryon de Poulet en culture *in vitro*. *Année biol.*, 1958, **34**, 29–52.

51. Sengel P. and Abbott U. K. *In vitro* studies with the scaleless mutant: interaction during feather and scale differentiation. *J. Hered.*, 1963, **54**, 255–262.

52. Sigot M. Sur le rôle du mésenchyme dans la différenciation des glandes du proventricule chez le Poulet. *C. r. Acad. Sci.*, 1962, **254**, 2439–2441.

53. Sigot M. Induction de la formation de glycogène dans l'épithélium du proventricule par le mésenchyme de gésier chez l'embryon de Poulet. *C. r. Acad. Sci.*, 1963, **256**, 4970–4971.

54. Stockdale F., Holtzer H. and Lash J. W. An experimental analysis of the development of the spinal column. VII: Response of dissociated somite cells. *Acta Embryol. Morphol. exp.*, 1961, **4**, 40–46.

55. Strudel G. Conséquences de l'excision de tronçons du tube nerveux sur la morphogenèse de l'embryon de Poulet et sur la différenciation de ses organes: contribution à la genèse de l'orthosympathique. *Ann. Sci. nat., Zool.*, 1953, **15**, 251–329.

56. Strudel G. L'action morphogène du tube nerveux et de la chorde sur la différenciation des vertèbres et des muscles vertébraux chez l'embryon de Poulet. *Arch. Anat. micr. Morphol. exp.*, 1955, **44**, 209–235.

57. Strudel G. Autodifférenciation et induction de cartilage à partir de mésenchyme somitique de Poulet cultivé *in vitro*. *J. Embryol. exp. Morphol.*, 1963, **11**, 399–412.

58. Waddington C. H. Experiments on the development of chick and duck embryos cultivated *in vitro*. *Phil. Trans. roy. Soc.*, B, 1932, **221**, 179–230.

59. Waddington C. H. Induction by the endoderm in Birds. *Roux' Arch. Entw.-mech. Organ.*, 1933, **128**, 502–521.

60. Waddington C. H. Induction by the primitive streak and its derivatives in the chick. *J. exp. Biol.*, 1933, **10**, 38–46.

61. Waddington C. H. and Schmidt G. A. Induction by heteroplastic grafts of the primitive streak in birds. *Roux' Arch. Entw.-mech. Organ.*, 1933, **128**, 522–563.

62. Watterson R. L. Neural tube extirpation in *Fundulus heteroclitus* and resultant neural arch defects. *Biol. Bull.*, 1952, **103**, 310.

63. Waymouth C. Rapid proliferation of sublines of NCTC clone 929 (strain L) mouse

cell in a simple chemically defined medium (MB 752/1). *J. nat. Canc. Inst.*, 1959, **22**, 1003–1015.

64. Wessells N. K.   An analysis of chick epidermal differentiation *in situ* and *in vitro* in chemically defined media. *Devel. Biol.*, 1961, **3**, 355–389.

65. Wessells N. K.   Tissue interaction during skin histodifferentiation. *Devel. Biol.*, 1962, **4**, 87–107.

66. Wessells N. K.   Effects of extraepithelial factors on the incorporation of thymidine by embryonic epidermis. *Exp. Cell Res.*, 1963, **30**, 36–55.

67. Wolff Et. and Haffen K.   Sur une méthode de culture d'organes embryonnaires *in vitro*. *Texas Rep. Biol. Med.*, 1952, **10**, 463–472.

68. Zwilling E.   Ectoderm-mesoderm relationship in the development of the chick limb bud. *J. exp. Zool.*, 1955, **128**, 423–442.

ADDENDUM

Since 1962 there has been an increase in the amount of research dealing with morphogenetic interactions during embryonic development. The existence and importance of inductions between two or more components of a differentiating organ are now established beyond doubt. In view of the diversity of organs whose development has been studied, it can be stated with almost complete certainty that the formation of all embryonic organs results from such interactions, during which substances and stimuli, still of a hypothetical nature, are transmitted from one tissue to another.

It would be tedious to report in detail the numerous results obtained using not only *in vitro*, but also other techniques of manipulation *in situ* or explantation *in vivo*. Most of the recent experiments have, in fact, only confirmed, when necessary, the fundamental role and the universality of organogenetic inductions.

From Table A-I the reader can form some idea—simplified but nonetheless sufficiently varied—of the morphogenetic interactions which have been demonstrated since 1964 by the use of *in vitro* organ culture techniques.

The new concept that arises from recent research is that of the existence of several inductions, succeeding one another in time and acting on the same tissue, for example, an epithelium. The first induction, which occurs at an early stage, is usually of brief duration, is determining and specific, and originates from a tissue near the epithelium. The subsequent inductions, which replace the first, often exercise a less specific morphogenetic action. They may continue for some time and even become permanent. Under the influence of the first induction, the epithelium is rendered competent; it is determined, and from then on contains all the information necessary for its subsequent differentiation. For differentiation to be accomplished, a second induction is necessary; all this does is to set in motion a morphogenetic process already written into the still latent epithelium. Successive inductions of this type have been specifically demonstrated (see Table A-I) in the differentiation of hepatic entoderm (31, 36), lens (46), pancreas (60), adenohypophysis (12, 13, 41), and pharyngeal entoderm (38, 39).

To illustrate the process of stepwise inductions, we shall take as an example mouse pancreas, which has been fully studied by Wessells and Cohen (60). This organ, whose main differentiation takes place between 8 days (11 pairs of somites) and 10 days of gestation (31 pairs of somites), is formed from a dorsal evagination of the gut entoderm; a surrounding layer of dense mesenchyme becomes associated with this at the 26-somite stage. The midgut,

435

TABLE A-I

DISSOCIATION AND REASSOCIATION OF ORGAN RUDIMENTS[a]

Effector tissue	Tissue whose inductive activity is being tested	Results (0 = absence of differentiation and morphogenesis)	References
Ectodermal Effectors			
Chick tarsometatarsal epidermis (11–12 d)	Peritumoral adult human epidermis, living or killed by freezing	Maintenance and normal histogenesis of the epidermis	(48)
Chick tarsometatarsal epidermis (11–12 d)	Adult human dermis, normal, inflammatory or cicatricial, or peritumoral dermis treated with collagenase or trypsin, or heat-killed	0	
Chick tarsometatarsal epidermis (11 d)	Mouse dorsal dermis (15–16 d)	Normal histogenesis of the chick type (keratinization more intense than in chick–chick combinations)	(45) (see text)
Chick tarsometatarsal epidermis (11 d)	—	0 (degeneration of epidermis)	
Mouse dorsal epidermis (15–16 d)	Chick dorsal or tarsometatarsal dermis (11 d)	Normal histogenesis of the mouse type	
Mouse dorsal epidermis (15–16 d)	—	0 (degeneration of epidermis)	
Mouse muzzle epidermis (11–13 d)	Dermis of muzzle (11–13 d) or of back (14 d)	Hair follicles of the vibrissal type	(27) (see text)
Mouse dorsal epidermis (11–13 d)	Dorsal dermis	Hair follicles of the coat type	

[a] Experiments on the dissociation and reassociation of organ rudiments carried out since 1964 using *in vitro* culture (N.B.: some associations carried out *in ovo* are also mentioned when they complement the results obtained *in vitro*). Unless otherwise indicated, the tissue whose inductive activity is being tested (Column 2) belongs to the same species and is of the same age as the effector tissue (Column 1) with which it is associated. The stage of the embryonic rudiments is given in days (d) of incubation or gestation, or as the number of pairs of somites (s). The experiments of Dodson (8, 9) on differentiation of tarsometatarsal epidermis, those of Flaxman *et al.* (14) on histogenesis of the reptilian epidermis, those concerning chondrogenesis of the somitic mesenchyme (1, 15, 23, 29, 30), and those studying the role of extracellular substances (18–20, 25, 25a, 44, 50, 59, 61) do not figure in the table but are reported in detail in the text.

TABLE A-I *(continued)*

Effector tissue	Tissue whose inductive activity is being tested	Results (0 = absence of differentiation and morphogenesis)	References
Mouse dorsal epidermis (11–13 d)	Dermis of muzzle (14 d)	0 (or abortive follicles)	
Mouse epidermal cells (dissociated and reaggregated) (13–14 d)	Chick skin cells (dissociated and reaggregated) (8 d)	Construction of barbar crests in which mouse cells participate; construction of hair follicles from mouse cells only; early keratinization of chick epidermal cells	(16)
Mouse epidermal cells (dissociated and reaggregated) (13–14 d)	Chick skin cells (dissociated and reaggregated) (8 d)	Inhibition of feather germs	
Chick skin cells (dissociated and reaggregated) (8 d)	Mouse dermal cells (dissociated and reaggregated (14–15 d)	Inhibition of feather germs	
Rabbit mammary epidermis (12 d)	Anterior ventral nonspecific cutaneous mesenchyme	0	(47)
Rabbit mammary epidermis (13–14 d)	Anterior ventral nonspecific cutaneous mesenchyme (13–14 d)	Primary mammary buds	
Anterior ventral nonspecific epidermis (12–14 d)	Mammary mesenchyme	Primary mammary buds	
Chick dorsal epidermis (7–8 d)	Duck dorsal dermis (8–9 d)	Neoptile feather of general ducklike appearance with chick-type barbules	(7)
Duck dorsal epidermis (8–9 d)	Chick dorsal dermis (7–8 d)	Neoptile feather of general chicklike appearance with barbules and barbicels of duck type (cultures on chorioallantoic membrane)	
Chick dorsal epidermis (7–8 d)	Subepidermal mesenchyme from the medioventral apteric zone (10–15 d)	0	(53)

TABLE A-I *(continued)*

Effector tissue	Tissue whose inductive activity is being tested	Results (0 = absence of differentiation and morphogenesis)	References
Chick epidermis from the medioventral apteric zone (10–13 d)	Dorsal dermis (7 d)	Normal or nearly normal feather germs	
Chick epidermis from the medioventral apteric zone (14–16 d)	Dorsal dermis (7 d)	Feather germs, less developed as the epidermis is older (cultured on chorioallantoic membrane)	
Mouse dental epithelium (16 d)	Dental mesenchyme	Absence of morphogenesis but cytodifferentiation of adamantoblasts and odontoblasts (F)[b]	(26)
Mouse molar dental epithelium (14–16 d)	Dental mesenchyme of incisor	Tooth resembling an incisor	(28)
Mouse molar dental epithelium of incisor	Dental mesenchyme of molar	Tooth resembling a molar	
Mouse lens presumptive epithelium (20–23 s, 9 d)	Optic cup (10 d)	Lens	(46)
Mouse lens presumptive epithelium (20–23 s, 9 d)	Periocular mesenchyme (10 d), splenic or salivary mesenchyme (13 d), or salivery mesenchyme (13 d) + optic cup (10 d)	Thick-walled vesicle, not lenslike	
Mouse lens presumptive epithelium (24–25 s, 9 d)	Salivary mesenchyme (13 d) + optic cup (10 d)	Lens	
Lens placode (27–30 s, 10 d)	Ocular or pulmonary mesenchyme (11 d), salivary or splenic mesenchyme (13 d), or neural tube	Lens vesicle without lens fibers	
Lens placode (27–30 s, 10 d)	Optic cup (10 d)	Lens (F)[b]	
Anterior lens epithelium of mouse (13 d)	Retina and salivary mesenchyme	Reconstitution of a complete lens	

[b] The inductive factor can traverse a Millipore filter (25 μ thick; 0.45 μ pore diameter) interposed between the two components of the association.

TABLE A-I *(continued)*

Effector tissue	Tissue whose inductive activity is being tested	Results (0 = absence of differentiation and morphogenesis)	References
Anterior lens epithelium of mouse (13 d)	Neural tube and salivary mesenchyme	Nonlens type vesicle	
Rathke's and Sessel's pouches of chick (17–24 s)	Encephalic floor and postocular mesenchyme	Adenohypophysis	(12)
Rathke's and Sessel's pouches of chick (17–24 s)	Hypophyseal or postocular mesenchyme, or hypophyseal mesenchyme + notochord, or postocular mesenchyme + roof of mesencephalon	0	
Rathke's and Sessel's pouches of chick (3 d)	—	0	
Rathke's and Sessel's pouches of chick (3 d)	Lateral or somitic cephalic mesenchyme	Adenohypophysis	(41)
Rathke's pouch of mouse (11 d)	Postocular cephalic mesenchyme	Adenohypophysis	(13)
Endodermal Effectors			
Pharyngeal endoderm of chick (7–27 s) or quail (15–35 s)	Chick somatopleural mesoderm (or splanchnopleural mesoderm *in ovo*)	Various typical digestive or glandular organs (gizzard, ventriculus liver, pancreas)	(38, 39)
Pharyngeal endoderm of chick (7–27 s) or quail (15–35 s)	Chick axial mesoderm or limb bud mesoderm *(in ovo)*	0	
Chick pharyngeal endoderm (3rd and 4th branchial slits) (15–30 s)	Somatopleural mesoderm	Thyroid and thymus	(34)
Chick pharyngeal endoderm (3rd and 4th branchial slits) (15–30 s)	—	0	
Chick pharyngeal endoderm (3rd and 4th branchial slits) (20–35 s)	Proventriculus mesenchyme (6–7 d), or metanephric mesenchyme (6 d)	Normal thyroid	(43)

TABLE A-I *(continued)*

Effector tissue	Tissue whose inductive activity is being tested	Results (0 = absence of differentiation and morphogenesis)	References
Chick pharyngeal endoderm (3rd and 4th branchial slits) (20–35 s)	Gizzard mesenchyme (6–7 d)	Thyroid little developed	
Chick pharyngeal endoderm (3rd and 4th branchial slits) (20–35 s)	Gizzard mesenchyme + gastric endoderm	Inhibition of thyroid differentiation	
Dissociated and reaggregated cells of chick thyroid (8 and 16 d)	—	0	(21. 22)
Dissociated and reaggregated cells of chick thyroid (8 and 16 d)	Dissociated and reaggregated cells of thyroid mesenchyme (16 d)	Numerous typical thyroid follicles (F^b for 16-day rudiments)	
Dissociated and reaggregated cells of chick thyroid (8 and 16 d)	Dissociated and reaggregated cells of mesentery or heart fibroblasts		
Dissociated and reaggregated cells of chick thyroid (8 d)	Thyroid mesenchyme (8 d)	0 (necrosis)	
Dissociated and reaggregated cells of chick thyroid (16 d)	Thyroid mesenchyme (8 d)	Epithelial cords, rare follicles (stage 8 d)	
Dissociated and reaggregated cells of chick thyroid (16 d)	Perichondral cells	Rare follicles	
Mouse esophageal, gastric, intestinal, or tracheal epithelium (12–19 d)	Various mesenchymes	Epithelial differentiation according to origin	(55)
Rabbit gastric epithelium (16 d)	—	0 (degeneration)	(6)
Rabbit gastric epithelium (16 d)	Gastric mesenchyme	Normal differentiation	
Rabbit gastric epithelium (16 d)	Chick esophageal, tracheal, or crop mesenchyme (9 d)	Subtypical differentiation	
Rabbit gastric epithelium (16 d)	Hepatic mesenchyme, or gizzard mesenchyme of chick (9 d)	0	

TABLE A-I *(continued)*

Effector tissue	Tissue whose inductive activity is being tested	Results (0 = absence of differentiation and morphogenesis)	References
Chick prehepatic endoderm (head process stage)	Mesoderm of cardiac area + hepatic mesenchyme (15 s)	Hepatocytes	(31)
Chick prehepatic endoderm (head process stage)	Hepatic mesenchyme (15 s)	0	
Chick hepatic endoderm (20–22 s)	Various mouse mesenchymes from hypomere: hepatic (3–13 s), pulmonary (5 d), mesenteric (15–23 s), parietal coelomic (27–30 s), or metanephric (12 d)	Typical hepatocytes (synthesizing glycogen)	(24, 32, 36, 40, 42)
Chick hepatic endoderm (20–22 s)	Various mesenchymes from epimere or mesomere: of limb (3 d), cephalic (10–20 s), somitic (3 d), mesonephric (17–20 s), metanephric ($5\frac{1}{2}$ d)	0 or atypical hepatocytes (not synthesizing glycogen)	(33, 35, 37, 40, 42)
Chick pulmonary epithelium (5 d)	Pulmonary, proventriculus, gizzard, intestinal, hepatic mesenchyme (5–6 d), cutaneous (5–6 d), mesenchyme, metanephric mesenchyme, or mouse pulmonary mesenchyme (11 d), or lung (postnatal, 2–6 d)	Ramification and differentiation of epithelium (the morphogenetic factors cross the vitelline membrane but not a Millipore filter or a cellophane membrane)	(2–4)
Chick pulmonary epithelium (5 d)	Mesonephric (3–6 d), cephalic, allantoic, somitic (2–3 d), or no tissue associated	0	
Chick pulmonary epithelium (3 d)	Pulmonary mesenchyme (5 d)	Ramification and differentiation of epithelium	(5)
Chick pulmonary epithelium (5 d)	Pulmonary mesenchyme (3 d)	0	

TABLE A-I *(continued)*

Effector tissue	Tissue whose inductive activity is being tested	Results (0 = absence of differentiation and morphogenesis)	References
Chick epithelium, pre-cultured for 48 hours in association then cultured alone	Pulmonary mesen-chyme (5 d)	0 (interposition of vitel-line membrane)	
Chick epithelium, pre-cultured alone for 48 hours then in associa-tion	Pulmonary mesen-chyme (5 d)	0 (loss of competence)	
Mouse pulmonary epithelium (12 d)	Pulmonary mesen-chyme	Arborization and dif-ferentiation of epithe-lium $(F)^b$	(56)
Mouse pulmonary epithelium (11–12 d)	Chick pulmonary mesenchyme (5 d)	Monopodial and di-chotomous arboriza-tion intermediate be-tween avian and mammalian type $(F)^b$	
Mouse pulmonary epithelium (11 d)	Salivary mesenchyme (13 d)	0 (cysts with smooth musculature)	
Mouse pulmonary epithelium (12 d)	Salivary mesenchyme (13 d)	Little arborization $(F)^b$	
Mouse pancreatic epi-thelium (0–5 s)	Own intestinal meso-derm	0	(60) (see text)
Mouse pancreatic epi-thelium (6–8 s)	Own intestinal meso-derm	A few acini in some cases	
Mouse pancreatic epi-thelium (9–15 s)	Own intestinal meso-derm	Exocrine pancreatic acini	
Mouse pancreatic epi-thelium (0–2 s)	Pancreatic mesen-chyme (11 d)	0	
Mouse pancreatic epi-thelium (3–6 s)	Pancreatic mesen-chyme (11 d)	Few acini in some cases	
Mouse pancreatic epi-thelium (7–19 s)	Pancreatic mesen-chyme (11 d)	Exocrine pancreatic acini	
Mouse pancreatic epi-thelium (2–13 s)	Salivary mesenchyme (13 d)	0	
Mouse pancreatic epi-thelium (14–20 s)	Salivary mesenchyme (13 d)	Exocrine pancreatic acini	
Mouse pancreatic epi-thelium (0–30 s)	— (with chick embryo extract 20%)	0	(17)
Mouse pancreatic epi-thelium (30–32 s)	— (with chick embryo extract 20%)	Exocrine pancreatic acini (F^b for all expe-riments)	

TABLE A-I *(continued)*

Effector tissue	Tissue whose inductive activity is being tested	Results (0 = absence of differentiation and morphogenesis)	References
Mouse pancreatic epithelium (11 d)	—	0	
Mouse pancreatic epithelium (11 d)	Pancreatic, salivary, renal, pulmonary, gastric, splenic, or nonspecific mesenchyme	Exocrine pancreatic acini (F)[b]	
Mesodermal Effectors			
Chick precardiac mesoderm (5 s)	—	0	(49)
Chick precardiac mesoderm (5 s)	Endoderm of precardiac area	Tubular heart	
Chick precardiac mesoderm (5 s)	Ectoderm of precardiac area	Tubular heart (less endocardium in some cases)	
Chick pulmonary mesenchyme (5 d)	Mouse pulmonary or intestinal epithelium (12 d)	Smooth musculature, vascularization, connective tissue	(56)
Chick pulmonary mesenchyme (5 d)	Mouse renal epithelium (12 d)	Vascularization (little), connective tissue	
Chick pulmonary mesenchyme (5 d)	Mouse salivary epithelium (13 d) or notochord (12 d)	0	
Chick pulmonary mesenchyme (5 d) or mouse pulmonary mesenchyme (12 d)	Mouse pulmonary epithelium (12 d)	The smooth musculature does not develop if a Millipore filter is interposed	

in association with its own mesoderm, acquires the capacity to form exocrine pancreas *in vitro* at about the 8-somite stage. At 10 somites the pancreatic rudiment is identifiable, and at 15 somites it is determined and capable of forming pancreatic acini when in "transfilter" association with (nonspecific) salivary mesenchyme from a 13-day-old mouse embryo. Later on, after the 30-somite stage, the salivary mesenchyme is no longer necessary and may be effectively replaced by a higher concentration (20% instead of 3%) of chick embryo extract in the culture medium.

Thus, during development, the pancreatic epithelium goes through three phases. During the first it is incapable of undergoing glandular differentiation *in vitro*, even if it remains associated with its own mesenchyme; during the second it is capable of differentiation either in combination with pancreatic mesenchyme, or with a foreign mesenchyme (salivary); last, during the third phase it differentiates even in the absence of living mesodermal cells. The origin of the determining factors that make the pancreatic epithelium capable of differentiating in the absence of its own mesenchyme is still unknown.

The numerous results summarized above, although of vital significance, tell us very little about the precise mechanisms of organogenesis. However, there are other investigations, which provide new data on the way in which tissue rudiments act on one another and on the nature of the substances transmitted between single rudiments. These investigations deal with vertebral chondrogenesis, with differentiation of the skin and exoskeleton, and with the role of various extracellular substances, such as collagen and the mucopolysaccharides, in the formation of salivary gland, pancreas, and other organs.

I. FACTORS INVOLVED IN VERTEBRAL CHONDROGENESIS

We have seen that differentiation of cartilage from the somites depends on inductive factors which come from the ventral neural tube and the notochord. Remarkable differences were found between the inductive actions of these organs (30). The notochord brings about the formation of a single cartilaginous nodule in direct contact with the sheath, while the cartilage induced by the neural tube always differentiates at a certain distance from the inductor and usually in the form of small distinct nodules. The inductive agent coming from the neural tube is capable of traversing a Millipore filter, while the notochord seems to require direct contact with the somitic cells to transmit its chondrogenetic influence.

New experiments (1, 15, 29), however, have shown that these earlier conclusions were erroneous. The inductive agent coming from the notochord has been shown to be capable of traversing a Millipore filter, and the morphological response of the somitic mesenchyme to either of the inductive tissues can be modified by the culture conditions. The principal results are as follows:

Tissues whose inductive activity has been tested (1) are first, the notochord from 9-day-old mouse embryos or from chick embryos at stages 12–18, 21–24, and 27–37$\frac{1}{2}$ of Hamburger and Hamilton, and second, costal, humeral, or tracheal cartilage of 12- to 15-day-old mouse embryos and costal or tibial cartilage of 5$\frac{1}{2}$- to 15$\frac{1}{2}$-day-old chick embryos. The effector somitic mesoderm was taken from 9-day-old mouse embryos or from chick embryos at stages 12 to 18 of Hamburger and Hamilton. A Millipore filter (25 μ thick, porosity 0.45 μ) was interposed between the inductor and the somitic mesenchyme in some of the experiments. The associated tissues were cultured in a liquid medium containing Eagle's solution, horse serum (10%), and chick embryo extract (3%). The results showed that chondrogenetic activity is a property associated with the stage of histogenetic differentiation of the inductive tissue. As regards the notochord, only the cells in the course of vacuolization and hypertrophy were inductive. A notochordal tissue, which at the time of the explantation had not reached this characteristic stage in its differentiation, or which did not attain this stage during culture, remained without effect on the somitic mesenchyme. Similarly, with respect to the cartilage, only that portion of the tissue containing cells in the process of hypertrophy produced an inductive effect. The small flattened cells that had not reached the stage of chondrification or cells which had completed the process of hypertrophy either did not yet possess or had lost their chondrogenetic activity. In "transfilter" associations, where the cartilage contained cells at various stages of chondrogenesis, cartilaginous nodules formed in the somitic mesenchyme solely in relation to zones of inductive tissue where cells in the process of hypertrophy were found. It thus seems that the inductive activity of cartilage is restricted to the phase during which its cells are synthesizing and excreting the components of the ground substance.

It has been confirmed (1), that in general, only a single cartilaginous nodule is formed in somitic mesenchyme cultured in combination with notochord or cartilage, this nodule being characteristically localized in direct contact with either the notochord (in associations without an interposed filter) or with the filter. The histology of these nodules was entirely typical for the inductions obtained by notochord or cartilage, in comparison with the cartilage masses produced by neural tube induction. In the presence of inductive notochord or cartilage the induced nodule was only surrounded by a perichondrium in those regions farthest from the filter. In the proximal portion of the nodule the induced cartilaginous cells were in direct contact with the filter and oriented themselves perpendicularly to its surface ("partial" nodule). In contrast, with a neural tube as the inductor, the induced nodules always formed at a certain distance from the filter and were completely surrounded by a perichondrium ("entire" nodule).

This difference in the response of the somitic mesenchyme to inductions arising on the one hand from the notochord or cartilage and on the other from the neural tube seems to indicate that the inductions are not of the same type. In point of fact, either of the responses can be obtained with either of the inductive tissues by varying the culture conditions (15). If the inductive effect of the neural tube is reduced by interposing two or three filters, each $25\,\mu$ thick, then the number of nodules induced decreases with increasing distance separating the two explants. However, no "partial" nodules were obtained in this way. In turn, intensification of inductive factors achieved by culturing somitic mesenchyme as a "sandwich" between two filters, each bearing a fragment of neural tube, produced the expected effect. From a total of 26 nodules formed in 5 cultures, 11 were of the "partial" type. Conversely, attenuation of the notochordal inductive action by interposing more than one filter, by reducing the usual size of notochord explants by about half, or by culture of the notochordal tissue for 2 days prior to the association led to the differentiation of a certain proportion of whole nodules that formed at some distance from the filter. These results show that the chondrogenetic inductive substances that emanate from the neural tube or from the notochord are not significantly different in nature. It is, therefore, reasonable to suppose that two influences can be distinguished in the differentiation of a cartilaginous nodule: first, there is the inductive agent of cytodifferentiation that initiates synthesis of the components of the cartilaginous matrix, and second, there are the factors, still of unknown nature and origin, which determine the precise location of differentiation.

Holtzer (23) considered that other factors play a part in the induction of chondrogenesis. The concept according to which the inductor produces, releases, and transmits a specific macromolecule carrying information to an undifferentiated cell, does not seem to apply to the differentiation of cartilage. In fact, neither the notochord not the neural tube is capable of inducing cartilage in any mesenchyme cells other than those of the somites, which must have reached a certain stage of development (3 days in the chick). From this it is clear that the inductors can act effectively only on competent cells, already conditioned (at a latent stage) by their earlier development to respond to the inductive action. It was also found that 3-day-old somites removed prior to undergoing the inductive action of the notochord and the neural tube regularly formed large masses of cartilage when cultured on the chorioallantoic membrane, while not producing any *in vitro*. Conversely, if 4-day-old somites (already induced) were placed in *in vitro* organ culture, they differentiated cartilage in the absence of the inductor tissue but did not form any in cell culture.

It is thus clear that, although neural tube and notochordal induction is still undoubtedly a morphogenetic factor, it is probably neither essential nor sufficient to bring about chondrification of the somitic cells. Before becoming capable of chondrification, the somitic cells have to go through a phase of intense multiplication between Days 3 and 5 of incubation. The necessity for this preliminary mitotic activity is demonstrated by culture of clones from isolated somitic cells, removed at 3 and 5 days of incubation.

Cells isolated at 5 days first formed clones, about 20% of which were made up of chondrogenetic cells. Thus, 20% of explanted cells were already determined to form cartilage at the time they were placed in suspension. If they were first allowed to multiply rapidly for 7–10 days in cell culture, the proportion of chondrogenetic clones reached 60%. Cells isolated at 3 days were incapable of forming clones unless previously cultured. Only after 3 weeks of cell culture and three subcultures, were they capable of giving rise to a reasonable proportion (about 30%) of chondrogenetic clones.

Thus there seems to be a latent period, during which the future cartilaginous cells must divide a certain number of times before they acquire the capacity to synthesize the cartilaginous matrix. For 3-day somitic cells *in situ*, this period is 2–3 days. When cultured in association with the inductor tissue, it is 3–5 days. It is approximately 2–3 weeks in cloning experiments. On the contrary, differentiated cartilaginous cells isolated *in vitro* reconstituted a metachromatic capsule in less than 12 hours.

Experiments on mitotic inhibition have shown that this phase of preliminary cell multiplication is a necessary prerequisite for chondrification. Associations of 3-day-old somites and notochord were cultured for 10 days. At times varying from 0 to 9 days after the beginning of culture, they were subjected for 4 hours to the action of a mitotic inhibitor ($10^{-6}M$ colchicine, $10^{-6}M$ Colcemid, or $10^{-3}M$ fluorodeoxyuridine) and then replaced on fresh medium without the inhibitor. These substances, which block mitosis either by disruption of the achromatic spindle or by inhibition of DNA synthesis (fluorodeoxyuridine), inhibited chondrogenesis only if they were applied during the first 3–4 days of culture. After this period, when the necessary latent period was over, mitotic blocking agents had no effect on the differentiation of cartilage.

II. MECHANISMS OF DIFFERENTIATION OF SKIN AND EPIDERMAL APPENDAGES

The investigations described previously demonstrate amply the importance of tissue interactions during histogenesis of skin and epidermal structures in birds. Recent studies have provided various interesting details on the role of the dermis and the basal cell layer in maintenance of the epidermis (8, 9).

Tarsometatarsal epidermis from 12-day-old chick embryos, separated from the dermis by treatment with versene (0.02–0.04%) and then isolated *in vitro*, was incapable of re-forming its basal layer (the latter had remained fixed to the dermis after versene treatment). It was unable to maintain its normal histological differentiation and rapidly underwent necrosis. On the contrary, if it was cultured on a dermal layer, either intact or previously dissociated by trypsin, the epidermis reconstituted its basal layer after 14 hours of explantation, and then continued to keratinize normally in the same way as intact control skin cultures. Various nonliving substrates have been used in order to define the morphogenetic role of the dermis. Dermis previously killed by heat, a Millipore filter, gelatin, agar agar, fibrin, or alginate did not enable the epidermis to reconstitute its basal layer. Under these conditions, it disintegrated and died. On the other hand, if cultured on dermis previously killed by freezing, or on a reconstituted collagen gel, the epidermis did construct a new basal layer. The germinative layer was maintained in a state capable of cellular proliferation, and the superficial layers keratinized in an orderly fashion. It is interesting to note that dermis killed by freezing and then subjected to the action of trypsin (which destroys a large part of the ground substance but leaves the collagen intact) lost its morphogenetic properties. According to Dodson (8), at least two factors are necessary for normal histogenesis of the epidermis. These are collagen and a solid substrate presenting the basal cells of the epidermis with a smooth and continuous surface. It should be noted that chick embryo tarsometatarsal epidermis, when isolated *in vitro*, could maintain its germinative basal layer and produced virtually normal stratification, as long as the mucopolysaccharide material exuded on trypsin treatment by the subepidermal mesenchyme remained in contact with the basal membrane (44).

Thus, in birds, the isolated epidermis is incapable of surviving for very long *in vitro;* however, its degeneration is fairly gradual. It can be cultured alone for 24 or even 30 hours and then reassociated with living dermis, without its capacities for histodifferentiation being perceptibly decreased (9). When contact is reestablished with dermal cells (even those without a basal layer, such as cells from deep in the dermis), it reconstitutes a PAS-positive basal layer in about 10 hours. The cells of the germinative basal layer, which became considerably flattened during the period of isolation, resumed their characteristic cuboidal appearance and began to divide. After 2 days a complete epidermis containing all the strata had regenerated. If cultured alone for 48 hours, however, the epidermis was incapable of recovering its histogenetic powers.

In addition, Dodson (9) has demonstrated that epidermal secretory mucoid metaplasia induced by the administration of an excess of vitamin A (10, 11) could be obtained in isolated epidermis cultured on a reconstituted collagen gel. Vitamin A thus acts directly on epidermal protein syntheses in the absence of dermal cells.

Investigations analogous to those demonstrating the existence of morphogenetic interactions in the skin of birds have recently been carried out in mammals to see if the development of hair proceeds by inductive mechanisms comparable to those which lead to feather formation. Kollar's (27) experiments have provided some information on this question. Fragments of dorsal skin (which produces coat hairs) and muzzle skin (which produces vibrissae) were removed from mouse embryos of 11- to 14-days' gestation. The dermis was separated from the epidermis by the usual technique of trypsin dissociation. Various homotopic or heterotopic combinations were cultured *in vitro*. As in the skin of chicks, neither the isolated epidermis nor the isolated dermis could survive for very long in culture, or carry out any sort of differentiation. The homotopic recombinations formed typical hair follicles, either of coat hair or vibrissae, depending on their origin. Of the heterotopic recombinations, only those in which muzzle epidermis of 11-, 12-, or 13-day gestation was associated with 14-day dorsal dermis gave rise to well-developed follicles that were of the "vibrissal" type. The converse association, i.e., 13-day dorsal epidermis with 14-day muzzle dermis, at best only gave rise to a few abortive hair follicles. It is concluded from this that 11-day-old muzzle epidermis is already determined to form vibrissae, and already contains the information necessary for this typical regional differentiation. Fourteen-day-old dorsal dermis did not impose a dorsal coat regional character on the muzzle epidermis, but supplied the growth and differentiation factors necessary for follicle construction. Last, 14-day-old muzzle dermis had little effect on the dorsal epidermis; the inductive action is nonspecific and probably of brief duration. Experiments carried out at earlier stages may well clarify the roles of both the dermis and epidermis in regional determination of hair-producing areas.

It has, however, been established that in both mammals and birds, the dermis or one of its constituents (e.g., collagen) is essential first, for maintaining the germinative basal layer and the orderly histogenesis of cell-layer formation, and second for the construction of epidermal cutaneous differentiations.

Reptilian skin behaves quite differently as has been shown by experiments with three species of lizards (*Anolis carolinensis, Gecko gecko,* and *Iguana iguana*) (14). These experiments were carried out using the skin of adult animals and therefore no direct comparison can be made with the results obtained on avian and mammalian embryos. Even so, the skin is the one organ that retains in the adult the distinctive embryonic characteristics of the germinative basal layer that is capable of giving rise to the differentiated cells of the upper layers at all times.

In contrast to the skin of homeothermic amniotes, in which the epidermis undergoes a slow continuous sloughing off of cells, the epidermis of reptiles molts periodically; shedding part of the horny superficial layers (exuviation). The structure of the epidermis is highly complex, consisting of many layers of keratinized cells, each characterized by a specific conformation. Shortly before molting, two generations of horny cells become superimposed. The external generation is ready for shedding and is entirely composed of dead cells, containing no less than six different layers (from the outisde inward: epidermis, β-layer, mesos, α-layer, lacuna layer, and clear layer). The internal generation consists of three to four layers, the deepest being in the process of differentiation and resting on the germinative basal layer.

When explanted *in vitro* 1 day after shedding, the skin rapidly reconstituted its superficial layers and in this way a new external generation was formed.

After 16 days, the skin reached the stage characteristic of the next shedding. After 49 days *in vitro*, superimposition of three complete external generations was observed (each containing its six typical layers), together with an internal generation of three layers in the process of formation. True molting, i.e., the elimination of the external generations, cannot take place in culture; explaining why successively differentiated generations accumulated on the explant. The maintenance of intense proliferation by the basal layer and the typical heterogenesis of cells arising from it (although more rapid than under normal *in situ* conditions) demonstrate the excellence of the culture conditions used by the authors.

Skin dissociation experiments have given very interesting results. Trypsin treatment has been used to separate the supragerminative layers in process of keratinization from the germinative basal layer that remains attached to the dermis. On the other hand, versene (EDTA) separates the skin into dermis and epidermis. If the "germinative basal layer-dermis" portion is isolated *in vitro* it has been shown to develop in an atypical manner. The basal layer became flattened and gave rise to only a single superficial squamous cell type, not so far identified with any of the normally keratinized layers. Control skin explants, trypsinized but not dissociated, have shown that this abnormal histogenesis is not due to a deleterious action of the enzyme. On the other other hand, when epidermis was cultured alone on a Millipore filter, there was typical construction of various keratinized layers of the external generation and of part of the internal generation in 10 days.

From these results it appears that the epidermis of the adult reptile skin possesses a surprising degree of autonomy with respect to the dermis; the latter is unnecessary for normal histogenesis of the epidermis. However, the integrity of the epidermis is essential for maintaining its capacities for differentiation. According to the authors' hypothesis, the horny superficial layers or those in the process of keratinization, may exercise, through a feedback mechanism, an inductive morphogenetic action on the germinative basal layer.

Returning to the birds, the histogenetic regulatory action exercised by the dermis on the epidermis seems to be nonspecific in character and it can be exercised in xenoplastic combinations of dermis and epidermis from chick and mouse (45). Tarsometatarsal epidermis of the chick (11 days of incubation) and dorsal epidermis of the mouse (15–16 days of gestation) responded to the influence of foreign dermis by keratinizing normally in the way appropriate to each species.

The course of events is quite different in the dermal–epidermal interactions that lead to feather formation. The dermis in this instance transmits specific information (7). Duck dermis associated with chick epidermis (see Table A-I) brought about the formation of neoptile feathers whose general morphology was of the duck type, although the fine structure of the barbular cells retained a chick character. The converse combination gave rise to feathers of chicklike appearance, but the barbular cells demonstrated their duck origin by the formation of barbicellar spines.

This capacity of avian dermis to organize the spatial arrangement of epidermal cells is also manifested in heterospecific combinations between birds and mammals. Cultures were carried out on the chorioallantoic membrane, in which cells of 13- or 14-day-old mouse embryo skin (or epidermis) were mixed, as a suspension of dissociated cells with cells of 8-day-old chick embryo skin (16). It was shown that mouse epidermal cells could participate in the formation of barbar crests of chimeric feather germs. However, since the chick dermal and epidermal cells were not separated from each other in all these experiments, it cannot be concluded that the organization of mouse epidermal cells into barbar crests came about through dermal induction. It is possible that the chick epidermal cells, which are normally capable of forming barbar crests through the morphogenetic action of the dermis, led the mouse epidermal cells to behave similarly.

The most important conclusion to be drawn from these recent results is that the avian dermis (and also, perhaps, that of the mammal) can exercise at least two types of inductive action on the epidermis. The first type, non-specific in nature, and perhaps primarily trophic, is characterized by a continuous influence that permits maintenance of the germinative basal layer and orderly keratinization of the epidermis. The second type, which doubtless includes multiple inductions specific for each stage in differentiation of the epidermal outgrowths (52), consists of the transmission of qualitative morphogenetic information, which leads to the formation of the epidermal structures whose regional and specific character conforms to the origin of the dermis.

III. ROLE OF COLLAGEN AND OTHER EXTRACELLULAR SUBSTANCES IN EPITHELIAL DIFFERENTIATION

We have seen earlier that the pancreatic epithelium of mouse embryos taken at 11 days of gestation (more than 30 pairs of somites) is capable of forming glandular acini *in vitro* in the absence of mesenchyme, provided that a medium enriched with chick embryo extract is used (10 or 20% instead of 3%). Rutter, Wessells, and Grobstein (50) have shown that the active substances can be found in the sediments when the embryonic extract is centrifuged at, 1,000, 10,000, and 100,000g. After centrifugation at 100,000g the supernate as well as the filtrate was inactive. Adult liver microsomal and mitochondrial fractions, salmon sperm DNA, yeast RNA, calf skin tropocollagen, and a collagen gel reconstituted from rat tail tendon were also inactive (59). The activity of the sediment from embryonic extract (100,000g) was not altered either by ribonuclease or deoxyribonuclease, but it was destroyed by incubation in trypsin for 60 minutes. The active factor is thus very probably protein in nature.

The results obtained so far indicate the importance of collagen and mucoproteins, at least in the organogenesis of certain organs such as mouse embryo salivary gland (25, 25a).

The two components of the gland from 13-day-old embryos were previously separated by trypsin-pangestin and then cultured with a Millipore filter between them (Fig. 37, p. 428). The capacities of this combination for differentiation have been described earlier (p. 422 ff). One or other of the components was labeled with ^{3}H-proline (25). If the mesenchyme were labeled, the radioactivity accumulated in a fibrous material deposited at the filter-epithelium interface under the epithelial basal membrane. If the epithelium were labeled, no such accumulation was observed. In addition, in the first case, digestion with collagenase caused disappearance of the labeling associated with the fibers. Hyaluronidase did not have this effect. The same results were obtained if the mesenchyme was labeled with ^{3}H-glycine, but not if it was labeled with ^{3}H-leucine. It is, therefore, very probable that the fibrous material synthesized between the epithelium and the filter is collagen, and that the mesenchyme provides at least part of the precursors necessary for this synthesis. This idea has recently been confirmed by biochemical analyses [Bernfield, cited by Grobstein (19)]. Estimations were made of the proline and hydroxyproline contents of the material synthesized by the mesenchyme and epithelium. Only the association of proline-labeled mesenchyme with non-labeled epithelium produced radioactive substances with a high proportion of hydroxyl-containing proteins, i.e., collagen. It is also interesting to note that if the salivary mesenchyme was replaced by ordinary maxillary mesenchyme (which has no morphogenetic influence on the salivary epithelium), no radioactive material accumulated at the filter-epithelium interface.

The next question that arises is whether the epithelium plays a role in the synthesis of these collagen fibers. Kallman and Grobstein (25a) have suggested that the epithelium provides a polymerizing factor, possibly mucopolysaccharidic in nature, which would provide the collagen precursors with the necessary framework for fiber synthesis. The study of ^{3}H-glucosamine incorporation into the same organogenetic system as before (salivary epithelium-salivary mesenchyme) has provided convincing arguments in favor of this hypothesis.

After 24 hours of culture, and using combination in which the epithelium, but not the mesenchyme, was labeled, radioactive material accumulated at the periphery of the epithelial explant, outside the cells. In opposite combinations, in which only the mesenchyme was labeled, no accumulation was produced. The kinetics of incorporation, studied by serial fixations of the labeled epithelium after 2, 4, 6, and 24 hours of culture, indicate that glucosamine is first incorporated into a fixable substance within the peripheral epithelial cells and is subsequently transferred to the exterior of the cells.

Enzymatic digestion experiments using hyaluronidase and trypsin–pancreatin, which inhibit periepithelial labeling, and collagenase, which has no effect, have shown that the material synthesized from glucosamine is a true mucopolysaccharide. The mesenchyme seemed to have a negligible role in this synthesis. When cultured alone or in association with noninductive maxillary mesenchyme, the salivary epithelium showed the same glucosamine-incorporating activity and the same level of excretion of mucopolysaccharide material. Since entire salivary rudiments do not incorporate glucosamine, the authors concluded that the preliminary treatment with trypsin–pancreatin was the factor that initiated the epithelial synthetic activity. Enzymatic digestion doubtless degrades an extracellular component that the cells rapidly reconstitute in culture (in less than 6 hours) before beginning histogenesis.

To sum up, the results obtained in experiments on the salivary gland show that the epithelium produces a glucosamine-incorporating substance at the exact point where collagen is to be synthesized, i.e., at the interface between the two tissues. However, it must be seen if the collagen fibers that form over the epithelial basal membrane play any part in morphogenesis.

Experiments in which the collagen has been experimentally degraded by collagenase indicate that it does so, at least as regards the salivary gland (20), the lung, and the ureteral bud (61). Epithelial rudiments pretreated for 20–120 minutes with a collagenase solution (0.3–1 mg/ml) and then explanted in transfilter culture in association with their own mesenchyme temporarily lost the capacity for normal morphogenesis. The salivary epithelium formed a rounded vesicle with no trace of lobule formation: the pulmonary epithelium flattened and spread out on the surface of the filter without forming bronchial ramifications; the ureteral epithelium lost its characteristic form. However, proliferation of epithelial cells was not inhibited. Thus, the collagenase did not interfere with growth-stimulating substances coming from the mesenchyme (in the absence of mesenchyme, the epithelial cells did not divide), but selectively blocked morphogenesis, i.e., the acquisition of the organ's characteristic form. Observations made with the electron microscope, during lobule formation in the glandular epithelium, have shown that collagen was deposited locally, in the epithelial indentations which progressively separate the epithelial outgrowths from one another. Collagen acted as a stabilizing agent on epithelial proliferation at the base of the lobules. The distal end of the lobule, however, remained free of collagen and retained the ability for growth and ramification until stabilized by collagen gradually laid down from the base of the digitations.

Mesenchymal synthesis of collagen precursors was also found to be dependent on exogenous stimulating factors coming from the epithelium. It was unimportant whether the factors were of salivary or pancreatic origin. In the absence of epithelium, the salivary mesenchyme produced little or no collagen [Bergfield, cited by Grobstein (19)]. A reciprocal inductive action on the mesenchyme by the epithelium is thus demonstrated. We have seen other examples of this in feather germ formation [Sengel (51)] and in the differentiation of smooth muscle and blood vessels in the pulmonary mesenchyme (see Table A-I).

The glandular acini in mouse pacreas do not seem to be formed by the same mechanisms as collagenase has been found to have no effect on differentiation of the pancreatic epithelium (61). It was also found that reconstituted collagen was not a suitable support for the morphogenesis of this epithelium (59). In fact, electron microscopy showed [Kallman, unpublished work, cited by Wessells and Cohen (59)] that collagen was not laid down around the pancreatic acini during their differentiation, contrary, for example, to the observations on the salivary gland.

IV. CONCLUSIONS

The recent results briefly reported here or summarized in Table A-I appear to point to some new concepts. In contrast to the findings of previous experiments, these concepts can now be formulated with some precision.

The universality of tissue interactions during organogenesis is impressive. The embryonic organs studied so far all show morphogenetic exchanges between their component parts, whether the latter transmit specific information or a less-specific inductive stimulus.

In organs composed of an epithelium and a mesenchyme, the latter, as far as is known at present, appears to be the *primum movens* of organogenesis, but its action on the epithelium is not a simple one. It appears to exert at least three different effects; i.e., determination, stimulation of cellular proliferation, and differentiation itself. Only the combination of these three effects leads to the characteristic morphogenesis of the organ.

Conversely, it is possible that the epithelium is the initial repository of genetic information, and that it first influences the mesenchyme, thus conferring on it its morphogenetic properties and specificity of action. Recent results (54) indicate that this is what happens in the differentiation of epidermal structures and limbs in both chick and duck embryos. The autopodial ectoderm of the wing bud contains "feather" information which is expressed even when it participates in the tormation of a foot when combined with foot mesoderm. A foot formed in this way always bears feathers as well as scales.

Our present views regarding organogenetic mechanisms may have to be revised. Although it is currently thought that the mesenchyme exerts the initial inductive action, it is possible that the epithelial components of organs may after all prove to be the initiators of differentiation.

BIBLIOGRAPHY

1. Cooper G. W.   Induction of somite chondrogenesis by cartilage and notochord: a correlation between inductive activity and specific stages of cytodifferentiation. *Devel. Biol.*, 1965, **12**, 185–212.

2. Dameron F.   Relations épithélio-mésenchymales dans l'organogenèse du poumon embryonnaire de poulet en culture *in vitro. C. r. Soc. Biol.*, 1965, **159**, 96–98.

3. Dameron F.   Étude de la morphogenèse de la bronche de l'embryon de poulet associé à différents mésenchymes en culture *in vitro. C. r. Acad. Sci.*, 1966, **262**, 1642–1645.

4. Dameron F.   Étude expérimentale de l'organogenèse du poumon: nature et spécifité des interactions épithélio-mésenchymateuses. *J. Embryol. exp. Morphol.*, 1968, **20**, 151–167.

5. Dameron F.   Étude expérimentale de l'organogenèse du poumon chez l'embryon de poulet: I. Mise en évidence et chronologie des interactions épithélio-mésenchyma-teuses. *Ann. Embryol. Morphol.*, 1968, **1**, 373–393.

6. David D.   L'influence de divers mésenchymes sur la différenciation de l'épithélium gastrique du foetus de lapin, en culture *in vitro. C. r. Acad. Sci.*, 1967, **264**, 1062–1065.

7. Dhouailly D.   Analyse des facteurs de la différenciation spécifique de la plume néoptile chez le canard et le poulet. *J. Embryol. exp. Morphol.*, 1967, **18**, 389–400.

8. Dodson J. W.   The differentiation of epidermis. I. The interrelationship of epidermis and dermis in embryonic skin. *J. Embryol. exp. Morphol.*, 1967, **17**, 83–105.

9. Dodson J. W.   The differentiation of epidermis. II. Alternative pathways of differen-tiation of embryonic chick epidermis in organ culture. *J. Embryol. exp. Morphol.*, 1967, **17**, 107–117.

10. Fell H. B.   The effect of excess vitamin A on cultures of embryonic chicken skin explanted at different stages of differentiation. *Proc. Roy. Soc. London, B*, **146**, 242–256.

11. Fell H. B. and Mellanby E.   Metaplasia produced in cultures of chick ectoderm by high vitamin A. *J. Physiol., London*, 1953, **119**, 470–488.

12. Ferrand R.   Influence inductrice exercée par le plancher encéphalique sur l'ébauche adénohypophysaire aux jeunes stades du développement de l'embryon de poulet. *C. r. Acad. Sci.*, 1969, **268**, 550–553.

13. Ferrand R. and Nanot J.   Différenciation de la poche de Rathke isolée de l'ébauche nerveuse de l'hypophyse et associée à un mésenchyme hétérologue chez la souris. *C. r. Soc. Biol.*, 1968, **162**, 983–986.

14. Flaxman B. A., Maderson P. F. A., Szabo G. and Roth S. I.   Control of cell differen-tiation in lizard epidermis *in vitro. Devel. Biol.*, 1968, **18**, 354–374.

15. Flower M. and Grobstein C.   Interconvertibility of induced morphogenetic responses of mouse embryonic somites to notochord and ventral spinal cord. *Devel. Biol.*, 1967, **15**, 193–205.

16. Garber B., Kollar E. J. and Moscona A. A.   Aggregation *in vivo* of dissociated cells. III. Effect of state of differentiation of cells on feather development in hybrid aggregates of embryonic mouse and chick skin cells. *J. exp. Zool.*, 1968, **168**, 455–472.

17. Golosow N. and Grobstein C.   Epitheliomesenchymal interaction in pancreatic mor-phogenesis. *Devel. Biol.*, 1962, **4**, 242–255.

456 PHILIPPE SENGEL

18. Grobstein C. Mechanisms of organogenetic tissue interaction. *Nat. Cancer Inst. Monogr.*, 1967, **26**, 279–299.
19. Grobstein C. Developmental significance of interface materials in epitheliomesenchymal interaction. *In* "Epithelial-Mesenchymal Interactions" (R. Fleischmajer and R. E. Billingham, eds.), pp. 173–176. Williams & Wilkins, Baltimore, Maryland, 1968.
20. Grobstein C. and Cohen J. Collagenase: effect on the morphogenesis of embryonic salivary epithelium *in vitro*. *Science*, 1965, **150**, 626–628.
21. Hilfer S. R. The stability of embryonic chick thyroid cells *in vitro* as judged by morphological and physiological criteria. *Devel. Biol.*, 1962, **4**, 1–21.
22. Hilfer S. R. Cellular interactions in the genesis and maintenance of thyroid characteristics. *In* "Epithelial-Mesenchymal Interactions" (R. Fleischmajer and R. E. Billingham, eds.), pp. 177–199. Williams & Wilkins, Baltimore, Maryland, 1968.
23. Holtzer H. Induction of chondrogenesis: a concept in quest of mechanisms. *In* "Epithelial-Mesenchymal Interactions" (R. Fleischmajer and R. E. Billingham, eds.), pp. 152–164. Williams & Wilkins, Baltimore, Maryland, 1968.
24. Houssaint E. and Le Douarin N. La différenciation de l'endoderme hépatique de poulet associé au mésenchyme métanéphrétique de l'embryon de souris. *C. r. Acad. Sci.*, 1968, **267**, 201–202.
25. Kallman F. and Grobstein C. Source of collagen at epitheliomesenchymal interfaces during inductive interaction. *Devel. Biol.*, 1965, **11**, 169–183.
25a. Kallman F. and Grobstein C. Localization of glucosamine-incorporating materials at epithelial surfaces during salivary epithelio-mesenchymal interaction *in vitro*. *Devel. Biol.*, 1966, **14**, 52–67.
26. Koch W. E. *In vitro* differentiation of tooth rudiments of embryonic mice. I. Transfilter interaction of embryonic incisor tissues. *J. exp. Zool.*, 1967, **165**, 155–170.
27. Kollar E. J. An *in vitro* study of hair and vibrissae development in embryonic mouse skin. *J. invest. Dermatol.*, 1966, **46**, 254–262.
28. Kollar E. J. and Baird G. R. The influence of the dental papilla on the development of the tooth shape in embryonic mouse tooth germs. *J. Embryol. exp. Morphol.*, 1969, **21**, 131–148.
29. Lash J. W. Chondrogenesis: genotypic and phenotypic expression. *J. cell. Physiol.*, 1968, **72**, *Suppl.* 1, 35–46.
30. Lash J. W., Holtzer S. and Holtzer H. An experimental analysis of the development of the spinal column. *Exp. Cell Res.*, 1957, **13**, 292–303.
31. Le Douarin N. Induction de l'endoderme préhépatique par le mésoderme de l'aire cardiaque chez l'embryon de poulet. *J. Embryol. exp. Morphol.*, 1964, **12**, 651–661.
32. Le Douarin N. La différenciation de l'endoderme hépatique étudiée en culture *in vitro*. *C. r. Soc. Biol.*, 1965, **159**, 90–96.
33. Le Douarin N. Perte du pouvoir de synthétiser du glycogène par des hépatocytes mis en contact avec du mésenchyme métanéphrétique. *C. r. Acad. Sci.*, 1967, **265**, 698–700.
34. Le Douarin N. Détermination précoce des ébauches de la thyroïde et du thymus chez l'embryon de poulet. *C. r. Acad. Sci.*, 1967, **264**, 940–942.
35. Le Douarin N. Étude ultrastructurale du foie sans glycogène résultant de l'association d'hépatocytes avec le mésenchyme métanéphrétique de l'embryon de poulet. *C. r. Acad. Sci.*, 1968, **267**, 886–888.
36. Le Douarin N. Synthèse du glycogène dans les hépatocytes en voie de différenciation: rôle des mésenchymes homologues et hétérologues. *Devel. Biol.*, 1968, **17**, 101–114.
37. Le Douarin N. Modifications morphologiques et fonctionnelles des hépatocytes

d'Oiseaux adultes associés au mésenchyme métanéphrétique d'embryons de poulet. *C. r. Acad. Sci.*, 1968, **266**, 2283–2286.

38. Le Douarin N. and Bussonet C. Détermination précoce et rôle inducteur de l'endoderme pharyngien chez l'embryon de poulet. *C. r. Acad. Sci.*, 1966, **263**, 1241–1243.

39. Le Douarin N., Bussonet C. and Chaumont F. Étude des capacités de différenciation et du rôle morphogène de l'endoderme pharyngien chez l'embryon d'Oiseau. *Ann. Embryol. Morphol.*, 1968, **1**, 29–39.

40. Le Douarin N. and Chaumont F. La différenciation morphologique et fonctionnelle de l'endoderme hépatique en présence de mésenchymes hétérologues. *C. r. Soc. Biol.*, 1966, **160**, 1868–1871.

41. Le Douarin N., Ferrand R. and Le Douarin G. La différenciation de l'ébauche épithéliale de l'hypophyse séparée du plancher encéphalique et placée dans des mésenchymes hétérologues. *C. r. Acad. Sci.*, 1967, **264**, 3027–3029.

42. Le Douarin N. and Houssaint E. Rôle du mésoderme dans l'induction de la synthèse du glycogène lors de la différenciation de l'endoderme hépatique. *C. r. Acad. Sci.*, 1967, **264**, 1872–1874.

43. Le Lièvre C. and Le Douarin N. Évolution des capacités de différenciation de l'endoderme thyroïdien de l'embryon de poulet après le stade de la détermination. *C. r. Acad. Sci.*, 1968, **267**, 2174–2177.

44. Mc Loughlin C. B. The importance of mesenchymal factors in the differentiation of chick epidermis. I. The differentiation in culture of the isolated epidermis of the embryonic chick and its response to excess vitamin A. *J. Embryol. exp. Morphol.*, 1961, **9**, 370–384.

45. Mordoh P. R. and Lustig E. S. Dermoepidermal interactions in tissue culture between heterologous species. *Exp. Cell Res.*, 1966, **42**, 384–386.

46. Muthukkaruppan V. Inductive tissue interaction in the development of the mouse lens *in vitro*. *J. exp. Zool.*, 1965, **159**, 269–287.

47. Propper A. Relations épidermo-mésodermiques dans la différenciation de l'ébauche mammaire d'embryon de lapin. *Ann. Embryol. Morphol.*, 1968, **1**, 151–160.

48. Redler P. and Lustig E. S. Differences in the growth promoting effect of normal and peritumoral dermis on epidermis *in vitro*. *Devel. Biol.*, 1968, **17**, 679–691.

49. Renaud D. and Le Douarin G. Influence de l'environnement tissulaire et des conditions de culture sur l'évolution du mésoderme précardiaque de l'embryon de poulet. *C. r. Acad. Sci.*, 1968, **267**, 431–434.

50. Rutter W. J., Wessells N. K. and Grobstein C. Control of specific synthesis in the developing pancreas. *In* "Molecular and Cellular Aspects of Development" (E. Bell, ed.), pp. 381–391. Harper & Row, New York, 1965.

51. Sengel P. Recherches expérimentales sur la différenciation des germes plumaires et du pigment de la peau de l'embryon de poulet en culture *in vitro*. *Ann. Sci. Nat. Zool.*, 1958, **11**, 430–514.

52. Sengel P. "La morphogenèse de la peau et des phanères chez les Oiseaux." Dunod, Paris, 1969.

53. Sengel P., Dhouailly D. and Kieny M. Aptitude des constituants cutanés de l'aptérie médio-ventrale du poulet à former des plumes. *Devel. Biol.*, 1969, **19**, 436–446.

54. Sengel P. and Pautou M. P. Experimental conditions in which feather morphogenesis predominates over scale morphogenesis in the chick and duck embryos. *Nature*, 1969, **222**, 693–694.

55. Soriano L. Différenciation des épithéliums du tube digestif *in vitro*. *J. Embryol. exp. Morphol.*, 1965, **14**, 119–128.

56. Taderera J. V. Control of lung differentiation *in vitro*. *Devel. Biol.*, 1967, **16**, 489–512.

57. Wessells N. K.   Tissue interaction during skin histodifferentiation. *Devel. Biol.*, 1962, **4**, 87–107.
58. Wessells N. K.   Effects of extra-epithelial factors on the incorporation of thymidine by embryonic epidermis. *Exp. Cell Res.*, 1963, **30**, 36–55.
59. Wessells N. K. and Cohen J. H.   The influence of collagen and embryo extract on the development of pancreatic epithelium. *Exp. Cell Res.*, 1966, **43**, 680–683.
60. Wessells N. K. and Cohen J. H.   Early pancreas organogenesis: morphogenesis, tissue interactions and mass effects. *Devel. Biol.*, 1967, **15**, 237–270.
61. Wessells N. K. and Cohen J. H.   Effects of collagenase on developing epithelia *in vitro:* lung, ureteric bud, and pancreas. *Devel. Biol.*, 1968, **18**, 294–309.

CHAPTER X

ORGAN CHIMERAS AND ORGAN CULTURE
OF MALIGNANT TUMORS

Emilienne Wolff

INSTITUT D'EMBRYOLOGIE DU C.N.R.S. ET DU COLLÈGE DE FRANCE
PARIS, FRANCE

I. INTRODUCTION

This chapter is concerned with "organ chimeras" and with heterologous associations between avian embryonic organs and mammalian tumors. The connection between these two topics will soon become apparent: in both cases we are dealing with heterologous associations, that is, with combinations of tissues from different species.

Parabiosis between two organs from the same species can be used to study the correlations between them and the interactions that occur between them under both normal and abnormal conditions. Organs that are normally never associated together may be associated *in vitro*, for example, two gonads of different sexes or an embryonic organ with an adult organ.

The limits to which such disparate associations can be carried and the possibilities for association and collaboration have been studied by Wolff and his school (28, 29) working with organs and organ fragments, and by Moscona (10) working with organs previously dissociated into their constituent cells. Avian and mammalian tissues were placed in contact with one another. While such associations between adult tissues are doomed to failure, embryonic cells of widely divergent species have been shown to be markedly tolerant of one another. They have also shown affinities to one another and have shared in the composition of communal structure. The cells of homologous tissues group together, whatever their origin. These affinities demonstrate better than any theoretical argument the idea of homology as suggested by comparative anatomy.

The association between chick embryo organs and human tumors marks a bold stage in the journey into experimental paradox. Combinations between unrelated species have been made, and postulate an analogy between the properties of embryonic tissues and malignant tumors. These associations first behave like chimeras of normal embryonic organs. The two tissues are tolerant of one another and interpenetrate, but soon this is no longer parabiosis or symbiosis; equilibrium becomes disturbed in favor of the tumor cells, which behave as parasites on the normal cells.

II. ORGAN CHIMERAS

The method of culturing embryonic organs *in vitro*, as described by Et. Wolff and his school, has made possible the culture of many organs from birds, mammals, other vertebrates, and invertebrates.

The first idea was to associate different organs from the same species; and second, to associate homologous organs from different species. Experiments were carried out to determine the results of associating these embryonic organs and to discover if they showed intolerance, indifference, or cooperation.

A. Association between Pieces of Different Organs from the Same Species

Such combinations, explanted on the standard culture medium, showed that tissues from different sources but with a similar structure exhibited affinities for one another. Epithelia from mesonephros and lung, from mesonephros and thyroid, and from lung and thyroid, unite and form continuous tubes, thus forming true histological chimeras (2, 12, 22).

Liver parenchyma and the cell cords of the immature thyroid become organized near the lung or mesonephros into tubules that closely resemble and prolong those of the associated tissue.

B. Association between Homologous Organs from Different Species

Even more instructive are associations between homologous organs derived from different species, such the duck, chicken, and mouse. What is the behavior of such mosaics that never occur under normal conditions? Several types of results can be expected.

1. The cells of the two species may show serious incompatibility and may destroy one another, as happens in the case of heterologous grafts in the adult.

2. Smaller incompatibility may result in repulsion between the cells of the two species with movement away from one another followed by regrouping into two distinctly separate explants. The two cell types may ignore one another and there may be no contact between them.

3. A third possibility is that the tissues from the two species may show affinities for one another so that exchanges and regrouping the cells from the different sources will take place.

It was the last possibility that was achieved with unexpected success. Close affinities were demonstrated between the different tissues of the associated organs, with connective tissue and epithelia, for instance. The connective tissue cells could migrate considerable distances into the middle of the foreign tissue. Epithelia from two sources fused to build or reconstitute communal structures forming true tissue chimeras where the cells from the two species joined together with no discontinuity.

1. Parabiosis between Duck and Mouse Embryo Gonads

Pieces of 7–9 day duck embryo testes were associated with fragments of the testis or ovary from 13–14 day mouse embryos. The connective tissue elements of the two tissues fused together and then penetrated into the opposite tissue (Fig. 1). Fibroblasts migrated a long way from their point of origin. In this way, long trails of mouse connective tissue followed the basal membranes of the epithelia (remainder of germinal epithelium, external border of the Sertoli epithelium).

Mixed cords or ampullae were formed in the areas where the germinal cell cords of the two species were in contact. In these cases the epithelial duck and mouse cells contributed toward one Sertoli epithelium, where the germinal cells of both species were contained together in the lumen of the ampullae (28, 29).

2. Parabiosis between Mouse and Duck Ovaries

If pieces of mouse and duck ovaries are associated together, several kinds of union between the tissues of the two species can be seen. In particular, the somatic and germinal cells intermingle and the mouse ovary becomes covered by the duck ovarian cortex (Figs. 1e–f).

3. Parabiosis between Mouse and Chicken Lungs

Fragments of embryonic lung from 8–10 day chickens and 12–16 day mice were associated together as a mosaic on the medium.

Two essential phenomena occurred (14). The terminal buds of the mouse bronchi ramified and proliferated into the chicken mesenchyme. The epithelial cells multiplied actively, as they would in their normal environment. Then the bronchi of the two species became closely associated. The walls of some bronchi were covered on one side by mouse epithelium and on the other side by chicken epithelium (Fig. 2a,b). This combination was seen even in the smallest branches and some inductor influence of one epithelium on the other was shown.

Tissues with a different function but similar structure and taken from two different species may combine when associated together. Thus, epithelium

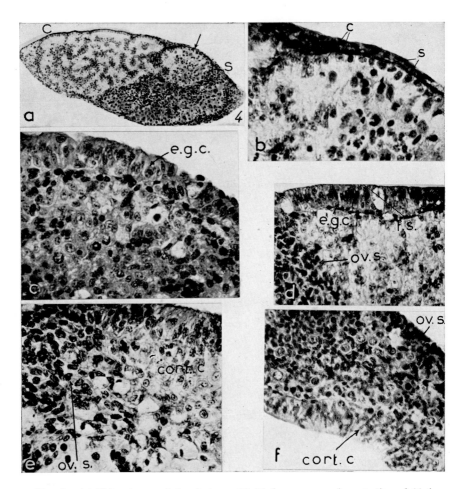

FIG. 1.   (a) Chimeric association between 13–14 day mouse embryo testis and 11-day duck embryo testis, after culture for 5 days. On the right can be seen the convoluted tubules of the duck testis, and on the left the ampullae of the mouse testis. In the region of contact a duck tubule communicates with a mouse tubule. The arrow indicates a mixed testicular tubule. × 96.   (b) Detail of a mixed testicular tubule of a mouse-duck chimera. The Sertoli epithelium is composed of mouse cells above and of duck cells below. In the transitional zone the mouse cells (S) alternate with duck cells (C). Many mouse spermatogonia can be seen in the lumen of the tube. × 320.   (c) Combination between a duck embryo testis (8 days) and a mouse embryo ovary (13 days) after 6 days of culture. A thick germinal epithelium (e.g.c.) has developed over the duck testis. It is the rudiment of an ovarian cortex. Some mouse connective tissue cells with dark elongated nuclei can be seen creeping under this epithelium. In the area underlying the testicular cords, the mouse and duck tissues intermingle. Many mouse connective tissue cells lie between the cell cords, inside which duck spermatogonia with large clear nuclei lie close to mouse oocytes, with chromatin clumped at the edges of the nuclei. × 336.   (d) Another chimera between

from the seminiferous tubules of the mouse combines easily with epithelium from chicken mesonephros (Bermann, 1960).

Chimeras between tissues or organs show that homologous tissues have marked affinities even though they come from widely divergent species. It is as though homologous cells "recognize" one another as belonging to the same family. On the other hand, connective tissue cells show the same attractions and the same affinities whatever their origin and whatever species they are derived from. This appearance is evidence of a chemical or antigenic relationship between the homologous tissues of different species. Later experiments will no doubt deal with the idea of homology from the biochemical aspect (18).

The extraordinary tolerance that exists between tissues from such different origins is astonishing, but it must be remembered that these experiments were carried out using embryonic organs taken at stages before the individuals had formed antibodies. In addition, the explants were removed from all circulatory connections and from all connections with other organs. Thus, throughout the culture period they escaped the effects of antibodies formed in other parts of the organism.

III. THE PROBLEM OF HETEROPLASTIC ASSOCIATIONS BETWEEN EMBRYONIC AVIAN ORGANS, MAMMALIAN MALIGNANT TUMORS, AND HUMAN MALIGNANT TUMORS

The success of heteroplastic chimeras in embryonic organs encouraged Et. Wolff and his colleagues to associate *in vitro* embryonic avian organs with mammalian tumors, just as organs from these two groups had been associated. Malignant tumors have certain features in common with embryonic tissues. In the first place, they both possess a considerable capacity for multiplication. Secondly, there is poor differentiation in one and incomplete differentiation in the other.

Results of research *in vivo* suggested that the two types of tissues would be tolerant of one another. Experiments carried out by Bueker (3) followed by the work of Levi-Montalcini and Hamburger (9), Kautz (5), and Karnofski

---

mouse embryo ovary (15–16 days) and duck embryo testis (8 days) after 6 days of culture. The zone of contact between the two gonads is shown. × 225. (e) Chimera formed between mouse embryo ovary and duck embryo ovary. The somatic tissues have intermingled. The follicular and connective tissue cells of the mouse (ov. S.), with dark nuclei, have penetrated in large numbers into the vacuolated medulla and cortex of the duck ovary (cort. C.) (× 320). (f) Another chimera between mouse and duck embryo ovaries. The epithelium of the duck ovary is covering the mouse ovary (ov. S.) (× 225). After Wolff and Weniger.

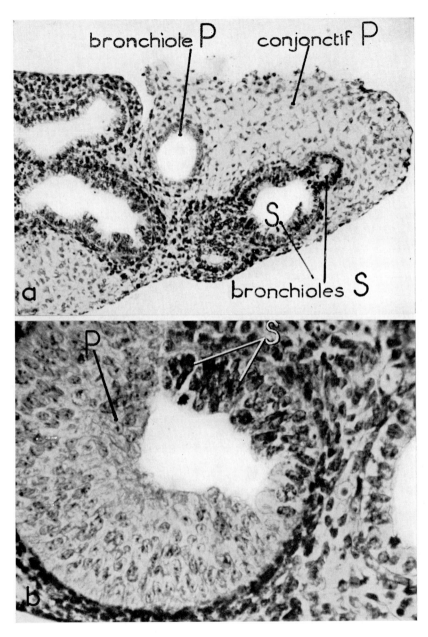

FIG. 2. (a) Heteroplastic association between pieces of chick and mouse embryonic lung. The bronchioles of the mouse are penetrating and developing within the chicken mesenchyme. × 160. (b) Transverse section of a bronchiole in a chimera of mouse and chicken lung. The bronchiole is formed by combination between chicken epithelium (P) (thick epithelium with clear nuclei) and mouse epithelium (S) (dark nuclei) (× 540). After Wolff.

464

et al. (4) showed that mouse sarcoma (S 180) could be explanted *in vivo*, either onto the membranes of a chick embryo or onto the body itself. This method was later extended to the study of certain human tumors.

Leighton and his school (6–8) had shown that organized structures could be obtained when pieces of animal tumors were cultured using the "cellulose sponge" technique. Small pieces of mouse or rat tumors were explanted onto the meshes of this sponge matrix which was moistened with plasma and thus gave the explants a solid coagulum. Cells from a tissue culture strain of connective tissue from a 4-year old child were also cultured in the sponge matrix and were later associated with a culture of HeLa cells. In this way small aggregates of cancer cells replaced the connective tissue. These cultures were of short duration.

Experiments using organ culture of tumors were carried out by Et. Wolff and his school (1956–1964) in successive stages. In a first attempt, malignant tumors from small rodents (mice, rats) were cultured. In the second stage, cell strains from human tumors were cultured *in vitro* using the classical techniques of cell culture. These cells were cultured on organs from chick embryos. In the third stage, fragments of human tumors were taken from biopsies and surgical operations and were associated directly with chick embryo organs that had been explanted onto the medium.

A. *In Vitro* Association between Malignant Mammalian Tumors and Chick Embryo Mesonephros

1. *In Vitro* Association between Mouse Sarcoma S 180 from
   the C 57 Black Strain and Chicken Mesonephros (Et. Wolff, 1956;
   Et. Wolff and Schneider, 1956, 1957, 1958; Schneider, 1957)

Sarcoma S 180 was maintained in the laboratory by repeated transplantation into the C 57 black strain of mice. If pieces of tumor were explanted onto the standard medium for organ culture, they became dissociated and necrotic after a few days. Thus, this medium was unsuitable for the culture of malignant tumors.

However, if the explants were associated on the same medium with fragments of mesonephros from $8\frac{1}{2}$-day chick embryos, they proliferated actively and invaded the embryonic kidney. The cultures were carried out in parallelepiped culture glasses with a square cross section, with sides 4 cm long and 1.2–1.5 cm high. The upper part was hollowed into a spherical cup whose depth was about a quarter of the diameter of the sphere. The cup was filled with 7 parts of 1% agar in Gey's solution, 3 parts of Tyrode's solution and 3 parts of 9-day chick embryo extract diluted to 50% with Tyrode's solution. A hundred pieces of mesonephros, 0.1–0.3 mm in diameter, were scattered in a flat layer on the semisolid surface, and pieces of malignant tumor were placed on the mesonephros forming with it a plane mosaic. The culture chamber was closed by a 4×4 cm square cover glass. The edges were sealed with a mixture of liquid paraffin and wax. After 20–24 hours all of the explants had fused into a lens-shaped mass of varying thickness. Histological sectioning of 3–5 day culture showed that the malignant cells had migrated from the site of implantation and invaded the pieces of embryonic kidney. They did not just mix with the chicken cells but destroyed the mesonephros and often replaced it completely. The presence of many mitotic figures indicated active proliferation of the malignant cells. Only the mesonephros lived at the expense of the culture medium—the tumor cells lived at the expense of the mesonephros and showed a great affinity for it. This was second-degree culture (Fig. 3a) (15, 23, 24, 25, 11).

The tumor culture could be transplanted every 3–5 days onto a fresh medium with explanted pieces of mesonephros. Sarcoma S 180 was thus maintained in culture for 157 days. When a tumor that had been transferred onto a chick embryo organ cultured *in vitro* was regrafted into an adult C 57 Black mouse, it reproduced the initial sarcoma, even after 30 transplants.

Other chick embryo organs were found to be suitable for culturing sarcoma S 180. These were the metanephros, liver, gonads, lung and periosteum, and could be taken at different stages of development (Fig. 3b–d). The mesonephros was shown to be most favorable for cultures of long duration.

2. Behavior of Other Malignant Mouse and Rat Tumors Associated *in Vitro* with Chick Embryo Organs (Et. Wolff and M. F. Sigot, 1961)

Four other types of tumor were associated *in vitro* with pieces of $8\frac{1}{2}$-day mesonephros.

1. Myelosarcoma of the rat, T 58.
2. Uterine epithelioma of the rat, T 8 (Fig. 4c).
3. Mammary epithelioma of the rat, G 6.
4. Mammary adenocarcinoma of the mouse, R 2633 (Fig. 4a,b).

The four cell types proliferated and invaded the mesonephros. The degree of invasion varied according to the type of tumor, each type having its own mode of invasion. Transplants were carried out every 7 days. It was possible to maintain the three rat tumors for 30 days and the mouse tumor for 50 days. The latter was also associated successfully with the skin, liver, and gonads of 8-day chick embryos. The structure and behavior of the tumor varied with the nature of the associated organ (26, 27).

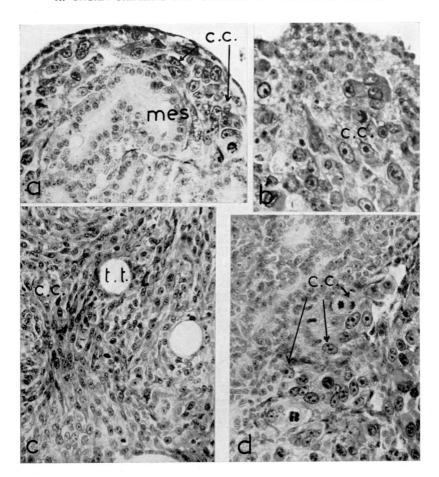

Fɪɢ. 3.   (a) Association between the tumor S 180 and chick embryo mesonephros cultured *in vitro*. c.c. = S 180 tumor cells, mes. = mesonephric tubules. (× 240).   (b) Cross section of 15-day chick embryo liver, cultured *in vitro* and invaded by the sarcoma S 180. c.c. = S 180 cells. (×320).   (c) Cross section of 15-day chick embryo metanephros cultured *in vitro* and invaded by S 180 sarcoma cells. c.c. = S 180 cells, t.t. = metanephric tubles. (× 213).   (d) 10-day chick embryo ovary cultured *in vitro* and invaded by S 180. The presence of many mitotic figures in the tumor tissue demonstrates the vitality of the sarcoma associated with the ovary. (× 320).   After Wolff and Schneider.

3. *In Vitro* Association between Zajdela's Hepatoma and Chick Embryo Mesonephros (Et. Wolff, M. F. Sigot, and F. Zajdela, 1963)

Zajdela's hepatoma is a malignant ascites tumor of the rat. The cells are very similar to liver cells and form small colonies which float in the ascitic

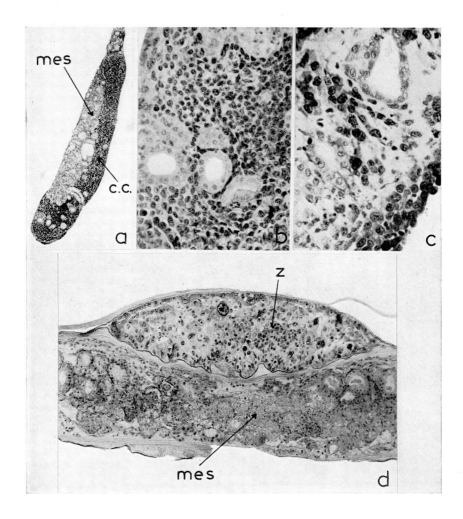

FIG. 4. (a) Association between mouse mammary adenocarcinoma T 2633 and chick embryo mesonephros cultured *in vitro*. mes., Mesonephros; c.c., tumor cells (× 40). (b) Section of the tumor in Fig. 4a at a higher magnification. × 253. (c) *In vitro* association between rat uterine epithelium T 8 and 8½-day chick embryo mesonephros (× 308). After Wolff and Sigot. (d) *In vitro* association between Zajdela's hepatoma of the rat with chick embryo mesonephros after 5 months of culture. Culture was carried out by the double folded membrane technique. (× 330). After Wolff, Zajdela and Sigot.

Translator's note: The magnifications in this figure are wrong. Fig. d is not × 330. If a is × 40, d is roughly × 70.

fluid. When these cells were cultured alone on the standard medium they became necrotic within 5 days.

Associated *in vitro* with mesonephros, the cells multiplied, infiltrated the loose mesenchyme, and then penetrated the mesonephric tubules and gradually destroyed them. These cultures could be maintained for 7 months by repeated transplantation (Fig. 4d) (48).

When these cultures were reinjected into mice of the same strain the tumor was reproduced.

Thus, it has been shown that mammalian tumors can be associated in chimeras with embryonic chicken tissues on which they live as parasites.

4. *IN VITRO* ASSOCIATION BETWEEN SEVERAL MALIGNANT CELL STRAINS OF MICE AND CHICK EMBRYO MESONEPHROS (Et. Wolff, G. Barski, and Em. Wolff, 1961 (21); Barski and Em. Wolff, 1964, in press)

Three highly malignant cell lines from mice, cultured *in vitro* by cell culture, were associated *in vitro* with chick embryo mesonephros. Two of these cell lines were derived from fibroblasts of C 3 H mice. These were the NCTC 2472 strain of Sanford and Earle (this will be referred to as N1) and Barski's hybrid strain M1. Cell strain PTT 12 was derived by Barski from C 57 Black mice. All these cell lines proliferated actively in the mesonephros, which they invaded more or less completely. They were transplanted many times and did not lose their ability to multiply and invade over periods of up to 300 days. When these tumors, which had been maintained *in vitro* for a prolonged period, were regrafted into mice of the same strain from which the tumor was derived, they reproduced the initial malignant tumor. (Fig. 5a–d). Thus, cultures of N1 and Barski's hybrid strain M1 were cultured for 263 days in association with chick embryo mesonephros. When they were injected or grafted into mice of the same type as they were derived from, they reproduced the same malignant tumor.

B. *In Vitro* Organ Culture of Human Malignant Tumors
(Et Wolff and Em. Wolff, 1958-1964) (30-48)

The incompatibility of human cells has been demonstrated using both homologous and heterologous grafting. To investigate whether this incompatibility of human tissues with tissue from another individual or species extended also to tumor cells, human tumors were cultured at the expense of chick embryo tissues.

It is known that young embryonic tissues do not produce antibodies—these appear only later in embryonic development. Consequently, these embryonic tissues should show great tolerance to the antigens brought by the human

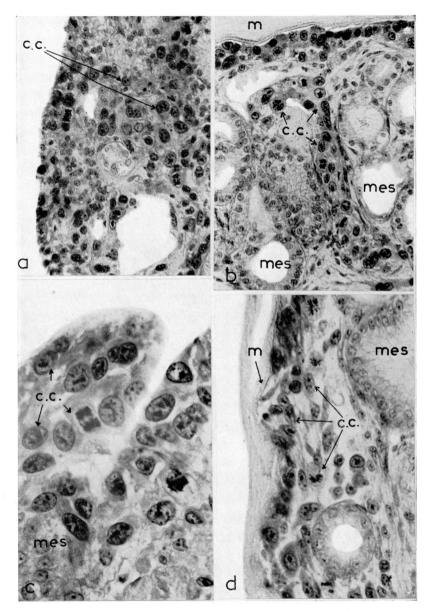

FIG. 5.   (a) *In vitro* association between the very malignant cell strain N1 (c.c.) and
8½-day chick embryo mesonephros (mes). This section was made after 35 transplants and
263 days of culture *in vitro*. The tumor cells are dividing rapidly, are characteristically
polymorphic, and show many mitotic figures. ($\times$ 300).   (b) N1 cells were cultured for
263 days in association with chick embryo mesonephros and were then reimplanted into

tumor tissue. The specificity of the antibodies for these antigens is very restricted.

A similarity that exists between the embryonic and cancerous tissues is the extraordinary capacity for rapid proliferation that they both possess.

Use was made of a new technique with a modified medium. The experiments were done in stages, since it was doubtful that human tumors could immediately adapt to such a different medium as chick embryo tissues. Thus, the first experiments were carried out using human tumor cells cultured for years in liquid media, such as Gey's HeLa or Eagle's KB strain. Following these experiments, an attempt was made to culture under the same conditions pieces of malignant tumor taken directly from the patient.

1. CULTURE OF HUMAN MALIGNANT CELL STRAINS

a. Parasitic Nutrition of the Cell Strains. Human tumor cells have been successfully grown in culture in association with pieces of mesonephros. When small pieces of the sheet of tumor cells were cultured alone on the culture medium, the cells did not proliferate and soon died. The cells were derived from such strains as KB, isolated by Eagle (epithelioma of the buccal surface of the tongue), HeLa, isolated by Gey (tumor of uterine cervical epithelium), HEp-2, isolated by Toolan (epidermoid carcinoma of the layrnx), Oregon J 111, isolated by Osgood (monocytic leukemia), Detroit 116P, isolated by Berman and Stulberg (pleural fluid from a patient with lymphosarcoma), Detroit 6, isolated by Berman and Stulberg (sternal marrow from a patient with carcinoma of the lung), and F1, isolated by Fogh and Lund (human amnion transformed *in vitro*).

In classical cell culture, the cells of these malignant strains appear undifferentiated and only develop in a monocellular layer on the glass walls of the culture flasks.

To set up a culture, fragments of the cellular layer were obtained by scratching the cell sheet from the walls of the culture flask. The cells were then washed several times and associated in a flat mosaic with pieces of

---

isologous mice, where tumors occurred. These tumors were then reassociated with chick embryo mesonephros *in vitro*. They invaded the mesonephros and again multiplied in organ culture. This section was made from one of these cultures taken after the 9th transfer, that is, after about 75 days of culture. There are many mitoses among the N1 cells. ($\times$ 300). (c) Higher magnification to show the very malignant cells of Barski's hybrid clone M1 (c.c.) cultured in association with $8\frac{1}{2}$-day chick embryo mesonephros. After 7 days of culture; the mesonephros has been totally invaded. ($\times$ 750). (d) *In vitro* culture of cells from the very malignant cell line PTT 12 (c.c.) in association with $8\frac{1}{2}$-day chick embryo mesonephros (mes). The PTT 12 cells are very invasive and are multiplying actively in the mesonephros; there are many mitotic figures. This section was made from a 70-day-old culture that had already been transferred 8 times. ($\times$ 450). After Barski and Wolff.

$8\frac{1}{2}$-day chick embryo mesonephros on Wolff and Wolff's culture medium. This medium is composed of 10 parts of 1% agar-agar in Gey's solution, 4 parts 50% embryo extract in Tyrode's solution, and 4 parts of horse serum. A few hours after explantation, the pieces of embryonic tissue and the tumor cells had completely fused. Histological sectioning of a culture after a few days showed that the tumor cells had migrated from the sites of proliferation into the middle of the mesonephros, which they had invaded more or less completely.

Each strain showed certain individual characteristics in organ culture, such as the shape of the cells, their capacity for penetration, and their mode of grouping. All cells lost the fusiform or star-shaped appearance (that is, became dedifferentiated) that they had acquired in cell culture, returning to a form analogous to that in the original living state (Fig. 6a–c).

The cultures could be transferred from one lot of mesonephric tissue to another on fresh culture medium every 7–14 days. Some cultures could be transplanted for varying periods up to 300 days. It is probable that they could have been transferred indefinitely without losing their capacity for proliferation (Et. Wolff, 1956; Et. and Em. Wolff, 1958 (30, 31), 1959, 1960 (33, 34), 1961 (35–37, 39); Em. Wolff, 1962).

b. Nutrition by Dialysis. A new improvement was achieved by placing a filtering membrane, namely the vitelline membrane from a hen's egg, between the mesonephros and the mass of tumor cells. The latter could no longer receive their nutrients by direct parasitism of the embryonic cells. The nutrients to be derived from substances produced by the mesonephros could pass by osmosis across the membrane. It was mainly this second method of culture that allowed the cells of each strain to group and swarm in their own particular way. The cells reconstituted nodules of varying size and varying degrees of organization, and some gave rise to multilayered epithelia. The characters of the initial tumor were reproduced. In all cases the masses were formed of many layers of cells, which contrasted with the tissue cultures where the undifferentiated cells formed only a single layer (Figs. 7a–d).

The liver and the gonads were also suitable for the culture of these cell strains, but 8–9 day chick embryo mesonephros was the most suitable organ for prolonged culture of the tumors by repeated transplantation.

c. Nutrition from Extracts of Mesonephros. Paired mesonephric kidneys from 100 $8\frac{1}{2}$-day embryos were finely homogenized in a microhomogenizer. A few drops of Tyrode's solution were added to the homogenate, which was then centrifuged for 10 minutes at 16,000 rpm at $0°C$. The supernatant liquid was used at various dilutions.

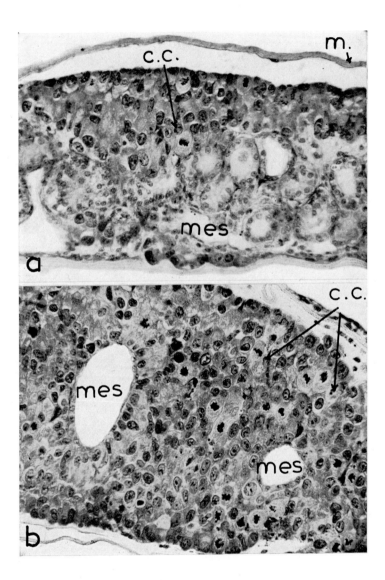

FIG. 6.   (a) Vertical section of a nodule of KB tumor cells (c.c.) parasitizing 8½-day chick embryo mesonephros (mes.) with which they are associated *in vitro*. The vitelline membrane (m) which envelopes the combination and which adheres to the inferior surface of the explants during culture is often displaced during the histological procedures. (× 246). (b) Invasion of the whole thickness of the mesonephros by HeLa cells. The urinary tubules (mes) are still lined by a very reduced epithelium and have been totally surrounded by the tumor cells (c.c.). Many mitotic figures are seen. (× 262). After Wolff and Wolff.

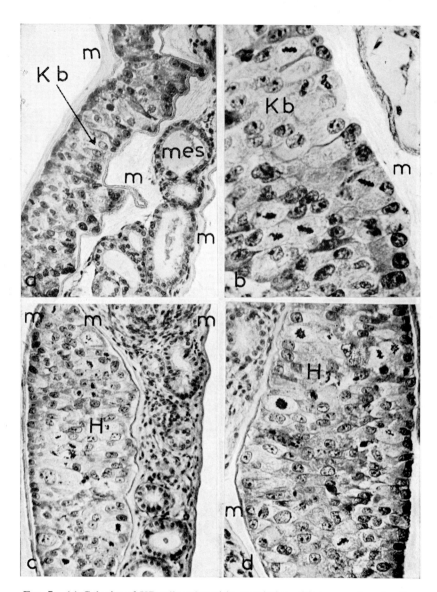

Fɪɢ. 7. (a) Colonies of KB cells cultured in association with mesonephros by the so-called double membrane method. The KB cells are in an envelope of vitelline membrane and are not in contact with the mesonephros from which they derive their nutrients by dialysis. Note the adhesion of the cells to the membranes that limit them, and their regular epithelial arrangement. (× 227). (b) Detail of a colony of KB cells in close contact with the fibrous side of the vitelline membrane. Note the epithelial arrangement of the cells and the great mitotic activity of the KB cells. (× 453). (c) Colony of cells from the tumor cell line Fogh F1 (Fogh's amnion cells). These have been transformed *in vitro* and show intense mitotic activity with a palisade-type epithelial arrangement. (× 213). (d) High power view of another Fl Fogh-mesonephros culture, showing the numerous mitotic figures. (× 266). After Wolff and Wolff.

474

The colonies of tumor cells were contained in small pockets of vitelline membrane which had been spread over the culture medium. A drop of the extract was placed on the upper surface of the pocket at intervals of 1, 2, or 3 days. The explants were fixed and studied after 5–7 days of culture.

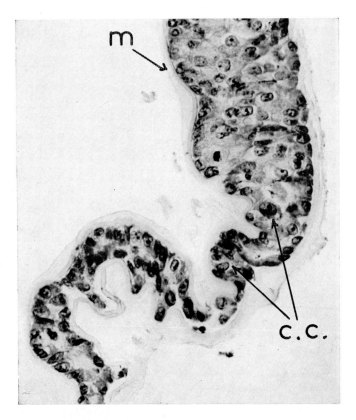

Fig. 8.   HeLa cells (c.c.) cultured *in vitro* on an extract of mesonephros. The cells have divided and formed nodules within an envelope of vitelline membrane (m) placed on the culture medium to which the extract was added (× 375). After Wolff and Wolff.

The supernatant liquid obtained after centrifuging the mesonephric extract retained its nutrient or stimulant properties for the following cells: KB, HeLa, HEp 2, Osgood J111, Detroit 6, and Detroit 116 P.

The results with other cell strains studied were more or less satisfactory (Fig. 8).

It is possible that the extract contained toxic compounds to which some tumors were more sensitive than others.

This extract is being studied and an attempt is being made to find the favorable compounds contained in it.

d. Media "Conditioned" by the Mesonephros. The method of "conditioned" media was used to avoid the probable toxic effects of crude mesonephros extracts.

Pieces of mesonephros were cultured for 2–4 days on the usual culture medium. The pieces fused together into a single flat mass which was carefully removed. A shred of vitelline membrane was placed over the same area and the small masses of tumor cells were then explanted onto the vitelline membrane. In all cases the explants proliferated, and considerable cell migration took place. These experiments show that compounds necessary for the proliferation of the tumor cells had been liberated into the medium and had retained their activity in the absence of the mesonephros from which they were derived.

Several problems arise from these experiments, which are now being investigated.

Is the stimulatory substance a compound formed from common constituents such as amino acids or peptides? Is one of these substances clearly specific? Is the stimulatory substance a common catalyst, a widely distributed enzyme, or a specific compound?

2. Organ Culture of Malignant Human Tumors Taken Directly from the Patient (Et. Wolff and Em. Wolff, 1958–1964)

The human cell strains cultured in liquid media for several years were cultures that had long been adapted to media very different from that of the human organism. These cell strains were the starting point for research into human tumors. It has been shown that they possess high tolerance to varied conditions and have a considerable capacity for adaptation to new media.

Experiments were carried out to see if it would be possible to culture pieces of fresh human tumors on embryonic explants without first passing them through intermediate cell culture in a liquid medium. It was also necessary to investigate whether the cells had to be progressively adapted to the very different conditions of life, such as those provided by avian kidney, and whether the specificity of such demanding tissues, with such strict requirements, would have to be reduced.

Success was eventually achieved after modification of the technique. Judicious choice of the origin of the explant from the tumor (young region, not necrotic, not infected, and proliferating) yielded tissue that could be cultured. The pieces had to be taken quickly from the patient in the operating theater to the laboratory, and placed immediately on the culture medium.

3. DIFFERENT TYPES OF CULTURE AND NUTRITION

a. Parasitic Nutrition by Contact. Et. Wolff and Em. Wolff managed to culture many human tumors taken directly from the patient either by surgical operation or biopsy. The tumors were cultured *in vitro*, on pieces of chick embryo mesonephros.

The following tumors were cultured: gastric epitheliomas of glandular origin and gastric adenocarcinomas of various types; liver neoplasm of gastric origin; many tumors of the colon; epidermoid bronchopulmonary cancers; primary bronchial tumors; small-celled anaplastic carcinoma of the lung; pulmonary adenocarcinoma; epitheliomas of the bladder; epidermoid carcinoma of the tongue; glandular epithelioma of the body of the uterus and a small-celled cervical carcinoma; epitheliomas of the breast; carcinomas of the pancreas; lymph-node metastases from these tumors; lymphomas and lymphoblastic granulomas; lymph nodes from Hodgkin's disease.

Culture was carried out by associating the tumor fragments with fragments of $8\frac{1}{2}$-day embryonic kidney explanted onto a sheet of nonincubated hen's egg vitelline membrane spread out on the medium. The membrane itself was washed very carefully several times in Tyrode's solution to remove from it all yolk and albumin. The albuminous side was placed on the medium. The membrane was folded over the top of the tissue mosaic being cultured. Wolff and Wolff's medium was used, composed of 10 parts agar-agar solution in Gey's fluid, 4 parts of horse serum and 4 parts of $8\frac{1}{2}$-day chick embryo extract.

The associated tissues fused after a few hours, increasing in size and extending in all directions. Histological sections of the tumors after 7–10 days showed that the tumor cells proliferated actively. Many mitotic figures were present, and the mesonephros was invaded by cells from the initial explants. The cells retained their differentiation and were organized in well-defined structures characteristic of the histopathological structure of the parent tumor.

It must be remembered that these cancer cells were as easily distinguished as labeled cells since there was a striking difference between them and the chick embryo cells. They were distinguished by their large size and the strong basophilia of their nuclei.

Earlier experiments had shown that of adult mammalian cells under these conditions of culture, only the tumor cells could multiply and be transferred several times; normal cells died after a few days. Tumor explants lived as parasites of the embryonic tissue that was deriving its own nutrients from the medium. This was still second-degree culture. The malignant tumor grew and obtained its nutrients in a living medium and it was really a miniature tumor independent of the organism from which it had been taken.

It should be noted that the nutrient medium used was inadequate for supporting tumor cells explanted alone, with or without membranes.

These cultures could be transferred every 7–12 days onto fresh media with fresh vitelline membrane and mesonephros.

A few examples of culture of malignant human tumors derived directly from the patient will now be given.

Typical glandular epithelioma of the stomach from a 49-year-old man.   This was a lymph node metastasis that was the source of many thriving and invasive cultures. The mesonephros was substantially invaded. The nodules (Fig. 9a) were epithelial in appearance. There were well-developed cell masses with palisade formation and many mitotic figures, and tubules with regular multilayered walls, often with collapsed lumina (Fig. 9b). Despite the variation in structure, the epithelial appearance was predominant. The developed structures retained the original pathological anatomical structure of the parent tumor (38, 41).

Glandular epithelioma of the body of the uterus from a 54-year-old woman. When associated *in vitro* in organ culture in direct contact with the mesonephros, the explants showed considerable proliferation, and invasion of the mesonephros was severe. Large pieces of epithelium with large cells, often in the process of division, lined the ducts (Fig. 10c), ampullae, and pouches, or folded up to form piled-up layers (Figs. 10a–c) (40).

Epithelioma of the bladder (Z 237).   This was cultured in direct association with $8\frac{1}{2}$-day chick embryo mesonephros (Fig. 11a).

Liver metastasis from a malignant pancreatic tumor.   This was cultured in direct association with the mesonephros (Fig. 11b).

Anaplastic bronchial carcinoma from a 66-year-old man.   This was a very malignant primary "oat-celled" tumor of the bronchus. The biopsy showed a uniform appearance, and there was rapid multiplication of cells in dense infiltrating sheets.

This tumor was very invasive when in contact with the mesonephros, and formed dense, actively proliferating masses of cells. The cells infiltrated into all the tissues of the mesonephros (Fig. 12a,b). The tumor retained in culture the dynamic and structural properties that it showed in the original patient (45).

b. Nutrition by Dialysis across a Separating Membrane (19).   In the mosaic cultures described on the preceding pages the tumor nodules lived at the expense of the embryonic kidney, which they progressively destroyed and replaced. It was necessary to investigate if such contact was indispensable and if the special texture of the kidney was necessary for the cells to proliferate and invade the organ.

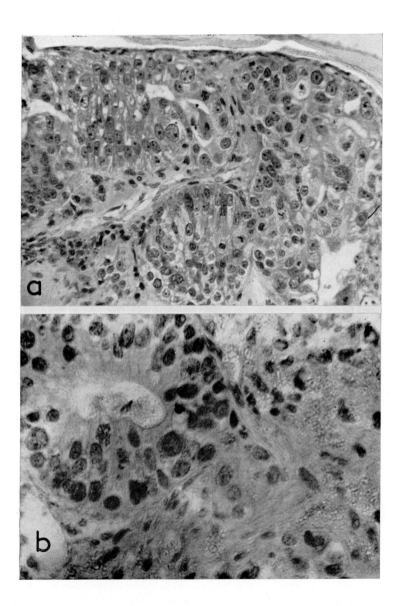

FIG. 9. (a) Lymphatic metastasis from a glandular epithelioma of the stomach, associated *in vitro* with 8½-day chick mesonephros. The section shows extreme proliferation of nodules, cavities with only a potential lumen, and epithelial bands from the metastasis. A few remnants of the mesonephric tubules are seen on the right (× 298).   (b) In other explants, the same association showed epithelial tubules in which the cells were arranged radially (× 500). After Wolff and Wolff.

A vitelline membrane was placed between the fragments of embryonic
kidney and the tumor nodules, so that there was no direct contact between
the tissues. The tumor grew considerably and formed raised plates and
thick transparent or milky disks. In the case of tumor Z 200 (liver metastasis
from a primary gastric tumor), the tumor had increased in diameter by a
factor of 2–4 within 7–10 days of each transfer. After 110 transfers and
after 33 months of culture under these conditions, the tumor always grew

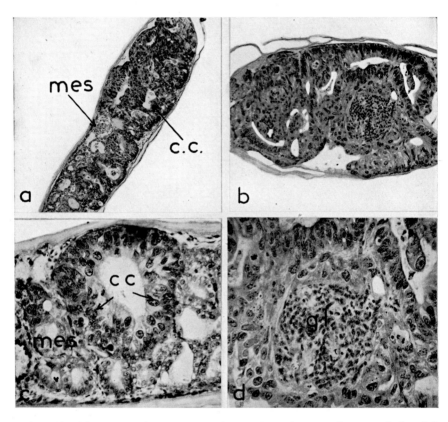

FIG. 10. (a) Macroscopic appearance of an explant of mesonephros grossly invaded
by the cells of a glandular epithelioma of the body of uterus. Well-developed invasive
epithelial ducts are seen in the upper part of the figure. Some healthy mesonephric tissue
is being invaded in the lower half of the specimen ($\times$ 53). (b) Part of a tumor mass from
the same uterine tumor. It has completely surrounded and isolated a glomerulus which is
reduced to a group of small dense cells ($\times$ 95). (c) An epithelial tube from the tumor of
the body of the uterus, in contact with mesonephric tubules. Note, on the left, the invasion
of two tubules by the tumor cells ($\times$ 212). (d) Detail of Fig. 10b at a higher magnification.
The glomerulus (gl.) is completely encircled by the tumor tissue ($\times$ 212). After Wolff and
Wolff.

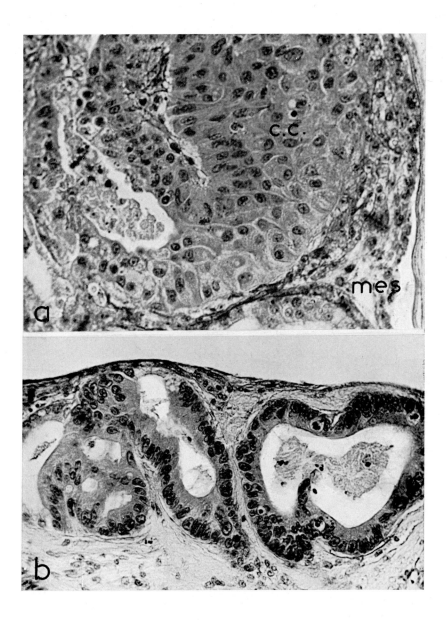

FIG. 11.   (a) Malignant tumor from human bladder (c.c.) cultured in association with mesonephros (mes.). Appearance after 7 days of culture ($\times$ 375).   (b) Hepatic metastasis of a tumor of human pancreas cultured in association with chick embryo mesonephros ($\times$ 400). After Wolff and Wolff.

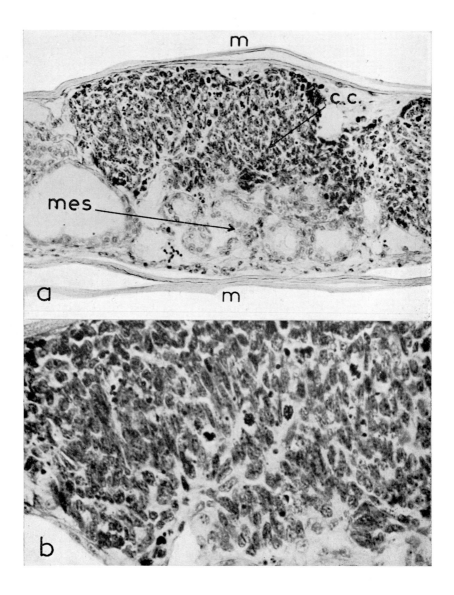

FIG. 12.   (a) General appearance (as seen in vertical section) of an anaplastic bronchial carcinoma, small cell type cultured *in vitro* on chick embryo mesonephros (mes). The whole explant was cultured within an envelope of vitelline membrane from a hen's egg (m) (× 270).   (b) Detail of the nodule at a higher magnification. The tumor cells ("oat cells") are arranged in parallel fashion. Mitotic figures are common (× 560) (Wolff, Wolff, and Renault).

at the same rate. It often covered the whole area of the underlying kidney, from which it was separated by the membrane. Histological sections showed that the explants always retained their organized structure. Thus a human malignant tumor could be cultured in a pure state, obtaining its nutrients from compounds developed by the mesonephros and able to cross the membrane. Further experiments should show if these substances are the only source of nutrients for the tumor nodules, or if they only supply an essential component needed to complement the nutrients present in the medium.

In all the cases it was shown that the mesonephros is an eminently suitable medium for the growth of tumor tissue.

The problem of the size of the molecules that can pass across the membrane is now under investigation. Work is now in progress on the fine structure of the membrane and its capacity for dialysis. Other membranes, such as Millipore filters and cellophane, have been studied. The activity is certainly due to relatively small molecules.

c. Culture on "Conditioned" Media.   Tumors Z 200 (derived from a liver metastasis from a gastric primary) and Z 516 (derived from a cylindrical epithelioma of the descending colon) were also cultured on "conditioned" media. This was carried out in two stages.   (a) $8\frac{1}{2}$-day chick embryo mesonephros was grown on the medium.   (b) The mesonephros was removed after 48 hours and a piece of freshly obtained vitelline membrane was placed on the medium. Tumor explants were then placed on the membrane over the area on which the mesonephros was cultured.

Controls consisted of pieces of tumor explanted in an identical fashion onto media where the mesonephros had not previously been cultured. Under these conditions the control explants degenerated whereas the explants cultured on "conditioned" media remained alive and proliferated. In the course of several trials the culture was maintained for 117 days and 15 transplants. The explants had been previously cultured for 21 months on the mesonephros. Substances liberated into the medium by the mesonephros were thus able to maintain the tumor cultures for a significant period but it is not yet known for how long they can survive in this way.

C. Long-Term Culture by Successive Transfers

The first tumors used were exhausted after 3–7 transplants, probably because of defects in the technique. Transplants were carried out every 7–10 days. Since then many tumors have been cultured in this way, for periods of one to several years.

a. Pulmonary Adenocarcinoma Ra 90.   A pulmonary carcinoma was taken from a 63-year-old woman and was explanted in association with $8\frac{1}{2}$-day mesonephros. It was composed of small compact masses of cells, in which cylindrical or polygonal cells were crowded together. Eosinophilic cytoplasm was abundant, and the cells were clearly outlined. These characteristics had led to the diagnosis of cylindrical cell adenocarcinoma.

From the first culture the same characteristics were observed. The tumor explants appeared as compact masses or islets, epithelioid in appearance. Sometimes the cells formed large plates and sometimes they were grouped in palisade layers. This culture was maintained through 42 transplants over a period of $15\frac{1}{2}$ months. It was then abandoned, although still healthy. Many mitotic figures were seen after each passage (Fig. 13) (44).

b. Cylindrical Epithelioma of the Colon Z 516.   Pieces of a tumor from the descending colon were taken from an 80-year-old woman and were explanted *in vitro* with $8\frac{1}{2}$-day mesonephros. This tumor had the structure of a cylindrical mucous epithelioma of the colon, characterized by the presence of tubules composed of one or many layers of tall cylindrical cells, which were arranged around large mucus-containing cavities. In other cases they formed a discontinuous lining around large cavities filled with mucus.

These structures were preserved as an integral feature in the initial culture and throughout successive transplants. The tumor proliferated rapidly, forming cystic nodules, 2–5 mm in diameter. These nodules were transparent, subdivided, and visible macroscopically. They were distended with mucus and lined with an often discontinuous epithelium. This epithelium was composed of several layers of very elongated cylindrical cells (Fig. 14).

Rapid proliferation of these tumors permitted a multiplication of the number of explants in the ratio of 1 to 700 in the space of 12 months. Equally good results were obtained when the tumor explants were cultured in direct contact with the mesonephros and when they were separated from it by a vitelline membrane (Fig. 15). After a long period of culture it was shown that the explants separated from the mesonephros by a membrane were more vigorous and proliferated more actively than the others.

Previous experience indicates that this culture could continue to proliferate for a long time, and perhaps even indefinitely (44).

FIG. 13.   (a) Human pulmonary adenocarcinoma cultured *in vitro* on chick embryo mesonephros (mes). The culture lived for 15 months and was transplanted 42 times onto fresh mesonephros each time ($\times$ 300). (b) Detail of the same section at a higher magnification ($\times$ 500). (c) Section of the original tumor as taken from the patient. The section was fixed at the time of the first explantation ($\times$ 300). After Wolff, Wolff, and Renault.

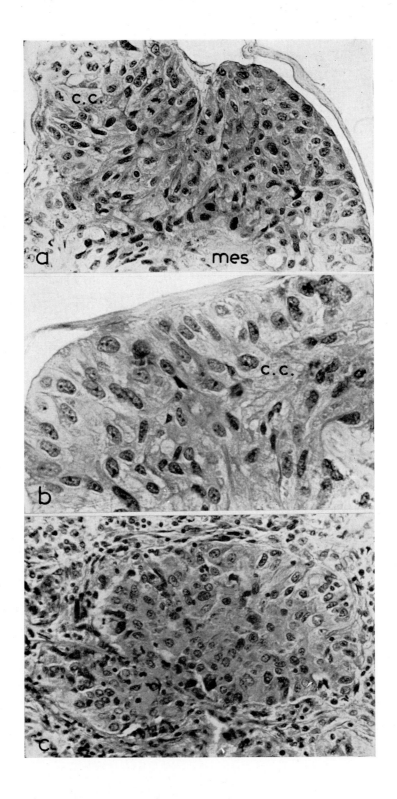

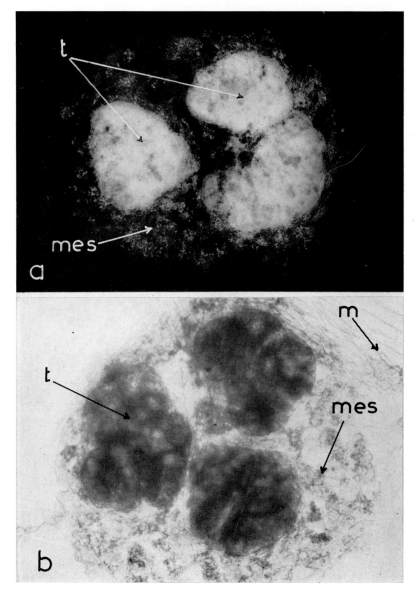

FIG. 14. (a) A group of explants of the epithelioma of the colon (Z 516) as seen by reflected light. Note the cystic appearance of the surface of the explant, due to the vesicles within the tumor. The explants are clearly distinguishable from the underlying mesonephros (mes) on which they have been cultured *in vitro* (× 16). (b) Three other explants of the same epithelioma (t) cultured *in vitro* on the mesonephros. Transmitted light (× 20). After Wolff and Wolff.

c. Liver Metastasis from a Primary Tumor of Gastric Origin, Z 200. This tumor was first explanted on January 10, 1962. After 110 transplants and 33 months of culture *in vitro* it was still surviving and retained its initial structure, being composed of epithelial cords surrounding mucus-containing cavities. The cells were more or less regularly oriented on the edges of these cavities.

Two types of explantation have been used:

1. The explants were associated directly with chick embryo mesonephros following the usual technique. These were the cultures that were transplanted continuously for 33 months (Fig. 16a,b, p. 357).

2. The tumor was separated from the mesonephros using the vitelline membrane from a nonincubated hen's egg, and following the modified technique (Fig. 16c). Under these conditions the tumor explants derived their nutrients only from substances that passed across the membrane. Seventy passages were carried out in 21 months, the explants having been previously cultured for 12 months on a simple membrane. After 33 months of culture *in vitro* the explants still retained their original structure. This method of culture seems to be more satisfactory than the first (Figs. 17 and 18, pp. 358 and 360) (40–44).

IV. CONCLUSIONS

From these experiments it may be concluded that it is possible to culture malignant human tumors of many types for a long time or perhaps indefinitely. The case of tumor Z 200 was not exceptional. The results show the possibility that culture of tumors will become a general method of investigation.

They are associated with chick embryo mesonephros (Et. Wolff, G. Barski, and Em. Wolff (21); G. Barski and Em. Wolff, in press).

Some cells occasionally become malignant in cell lines cultured for a long time *in vitro* in a liquid medium, and tumors develop when animals of the same strain as that from which the cell line was originally derived are inoculated with these malignant cells. Production of a tumor that results in the death of the animal is a proof of malignancy.

Interpretation of these results is often complicated, as unforeseeable variations in the organism's defence mechanisms may prevent the graft from taking, even if the animal has been previously irradiated or has been treated with cortisone.

Using the mesonephros of chick embryos for culture makes it possible to determine the malignancy of the associated cells.

Three cell lines, derived from the pulmonary tissue of a normal C 57 Bl. adult mouse have been studied. These were cell lines PG, PT, and PTT 12.

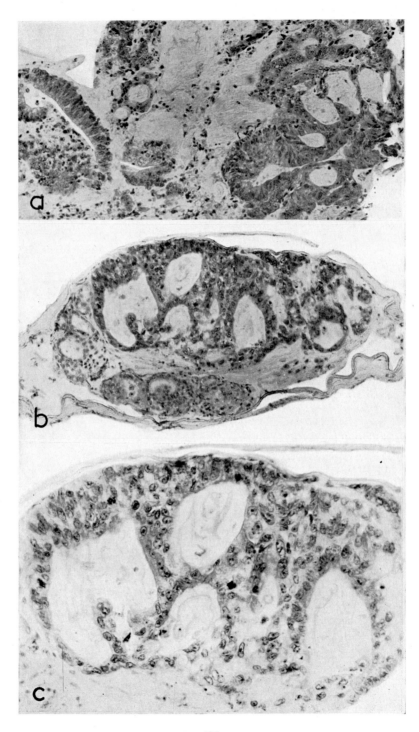

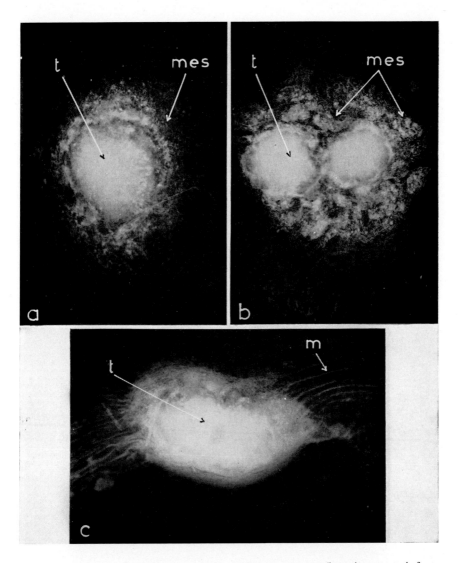

FIG. 16. (a, b) Living appearance of two Z 200 tumor masses (hepatic metastasis from a tumor of the stomach) (t) cultured in direct contact with the mesonephros (mes). The latter forms the background of the image (× 15). (c) Mass from the same tumor (t) photographed in the living state. In this culture, the tumor explants were separated from the mesonephros by the vitelline membrane of a hen's egg. The folds of the membrane can be seen (m). The masses have become confluent during growth and now cover almost all of the mesonephros. This culture had been transferred 31 times and was 237 days old at the time of photographing (× 15). After Wolff and Wolff.

FIG. 15. Opposite. (a) Biopsy of the epithelioma of human colon (Z 516). (× 166). (b, c) Histological sections of the same epithelioma after the 10th transfer and 78 days in culture on chick embryo mesonephros. Many mucus-filled vesicles are seen. In Fig. 15b, the chick mesonephros used for culturing can be seen below and on the left. (× 166) and (× 332). After Wolff and Wolff.

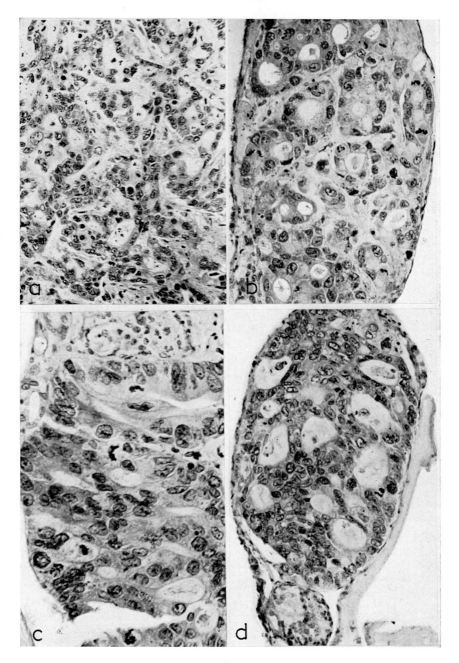

Fig. 17. (a) Biopsy of tumor Z 200. This was a hepatic metastasis of a stomach tumor. The characteristic appearance of the tumor was recognized after organ culture (× 190).

The line PG was found to be very weakly malignant, PT weakly malignant, and PTT 12 very highly malignant. When 3×10^6 to 5×10^6 cells from the so-called weakly malignant cell lines were inoculated into isologous mice, only a very small percentage of these mice produced malignant tumors.

When 10^4 to 10^5 cells from the highly malignant cell lines were inoculated into isologous mice, malignant tumors developed in 100% of the cases and the tumors developed finally resulted in the death of the injected animals.

Three other cell lines were derived from normal fibroblasts of normal adult C 3 H mice. The clone NCTC no. 2472 of Sanford and Earle (designated here as N1) was highly malignant. The clone NCTC no. 2555 (designated by N2) was malignant in only 2–3% of the cases when it was inoculated into C3H mice. Barski's clone M1, a hybrid of N1 and N2 possessing a karyotype intermediate between N1 and N2, is highly malignant.

Pieces of cell sheet from these different cell lines were associated separately *in vitro* with chick embryo mesonephros. Their degree of adaptation to the living medium as provided by the embryonic kidney, and their ability to multiply and penetrate into the embryonic tissues in the absence of immunological reactions are as good a measure of malignancy in culture as they are in animals inoculated with these strains.

All cells of the highly malignant cell lines such as N1, PTT 12, and M1 invaded the mesonephros in the first culture and could be transferred through many transplants for almost 300 days without losing their capacity to proliferate and invade. The cultures were discontinued while still healthy (Fig. 5a–d).

Cells from weakly malignant or normal cell lines, such as PG, PT, and N2, died after the second or third transfer.

This method may thus serve as a test of malignancy, especially for human cells, where grafts are impossible.

V. GENERAL CONCLUSIONS

The work described in this chapter will now be summarized, and the new problems that may be investigated by using this fruitful method will be generally discussed.

Embryonic tissues from very different groups have been associated.

(b) Histological appearance of tumor Z 200 after 7 days of growth on the mesonephros. ($\times$ 330). (c) Structure of the tumor after the 3rd transplantation onto the mesonephros. The same structure of epithelial cords surrounding the alveoli is seen. Some mesonephros is seen in the upper part of the photograph. Many mitotic figures are present ($\times$ 366). (d) Structure of an explant after the 4th transfer and 35 days of culture in association with mesonephros ($\times$ 240). After Wolff and Wolff.

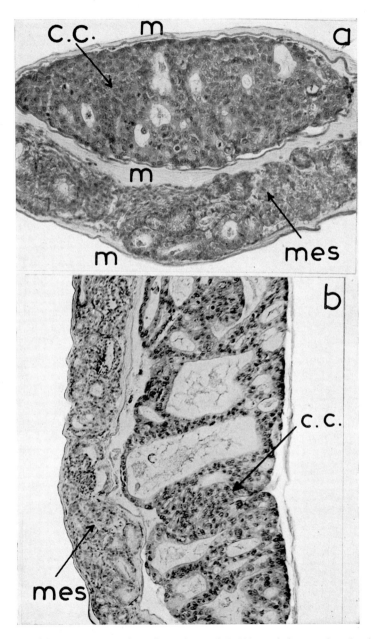

FIG. 18. (a) Transverse section of a culture of Z 200 carried out using the double membrane technique. The tumor is separated from the mesonephros by the vitelline membrane of an unincubated hen's egg, which acts as a dialyzing membrane. Section taken after the 72nd transfer and 514 days of culture ($\times$ 15.5). (b) Culture Z 200. Section made from an explant after the 91st transfer and 644 days of culture. ($\times$ 120). Unpublished.

They meet and intimately mix together. They become regrouped in harmonious fashion, family by family, as though they could recognize one another. Epithelial cells from mouse and chicken became arranged side by side to form a mixed testicular tubule or communal bronchus. Cartilage cells from the two species agglomerate and show more affinity for one another than would two different types of cells from the same animal. The connective tissue cells of birds constitute the medium for the organization and ramification of mammalian epithelial tubules. What is the reason for these affinities and these combinations? The problem, first encountered on the morphological level, must be explained at the molecular level. What are the forces of attraction or cohesion that make these cells interdependent and what are the substances that cement them together and maintain them? These problems have now been posed, and many workers are trying to answer them at the moment.

Heterogeneous associations between embryonic organs led to the association of avian embryonic organs with malignant mammalian tumors. The problem of how malignant mammalian cells would behave in the presence of avian embryonic tissues arose from the time when it became possible to associate tissues as different as those of the chicken and the mouse. Mouse and rat tumors, human cell lines, and malignant tumors taken from patients gave positive results, when cultured in contact with chicken mesonephros. The results of these experiments quickly led to the following important conclusions.

Pieces of tumor which cannot survive alone on the culture medium can be cultured in the presence of fragments of embryonic organs, particularly the mesonephros. Thus substances that favor the survival and growth of malignant cells must be present in these tissues.

It is remarkable that the pieces of tumor retain their specific structure of the parent tumor, as do the embryonic organs. Are there in the medium, or in the associated organ, physical or chemical factors essential for the maintenance of tissue organization?

Another very important point is the potential immortality of the tumor cell cultures. While no embryonic organ has been maintained in culture for more than a few weeks, and the growth of these stops even sooner, malignant tumors of animal or human origin have retained their structure and shown unlimited growth. They provide a unique example of organized tissues capable of multiplying in an unlimited fashion. These cultures demonstrate in an even more striking way than they do in the intact organism the character that distinguishes them from normal tissues, that is, their lack of growth limitation.

Lastly, even though the presence of embryonic tissues is necessary for organ culture of malignant tumors, direct contact between the two explants is not necessary. A filtering membrane placed between them does not prevent the tumor from thriving. The tumor uses the substances secreted by the embryonic tissues, which pass across the membrane. It is interesting to note that in the first case the malignant cells grow as parasites on the embryonic tissues, which they destroy. In the second case, however, the tumor cells make use only of the secretions of the embryonic cells. There is no doubt that such results can contribute to the elucidation of the mode of nutrition of cancer cells and the factors favorable for their multiplication. This is one of the principal aims of future reasearch.

These are some of the problems to which we have been led by organ culture. Advance has been made in progressive stages; some of the attempts were timid, some bold, but the final results of the successful experiments could not have been forecast at the very beginning.

BIBLIOGRAPHY

1. Bermann F.   Associations xénoplastiques d'organes embryonnaires: étude de quelques structures mixtes obtenues *in vitro* et *in vivo*. *C. R. Soc. Biol.*, 1960, **154**, 911–914.
2. Bresch D.   Recherches préliminaires sur les associations d'organes embryonnaires de Poulet en culture *in vitro*. *Bull. Biol.*, 1955, **89**, 179–188.
3. Bueker E. D.   Implantation of tumors in the hind-limb field of the embryonic chick, and the developmental response of the lumbosacral system. *Anat. Rec.*, 1948, **102**, 369–390.
4. Karnofsky D. A., Leavitt C. G. W. and Ridgway L. P.   Effects of Boric acid on the Developing chick embryo and on tumors explanted to the chorio-allantoic membrane. *Proc. Am. Assoc. Cancer Res.*, 1953, **1**, 218.
5. Kautz J.   Differential invasion of embryonic chick tissues by sarcomas 180 and 37. *Cancer Res.*, 1952, **12**, 180–187.
6. Leighton J.   The growth patterns of some transplantable animal tumors in sponge matrix tissue culture. *Jour. of Nat. Cancer Inst.*, 1954, **15**, 275–293.
7. Leighton J. and Kline I.   Studies on Human Cancer using sponge matrix tissue culture. II: Invasion of connective tissue by carcinoma (Strain HeLa). *Texas Rep. Biol. Med.*, 1954, **12**, 865–873.
8. Leighton J., Kline I., Belkin M. and Tetenbaum Z.   Studies on Human Cancer using sponge matrix Tissue Culture. III: The invasive properties of a carcinoma (Strain HeLa) as influenced by conditionned media, and in contact with rapidly growing chick embryonic tissue. *J. Nat. Cancer Inst.*, 1956, **16**, 1353–1373.
9. Levi-Montalcini R. and Hamburger V.   Selective growth stimulating effects of mouse sarcoma on the sensory and sympathetic nervous system of the chick embryo. *J. exp. Zool.*, 1951, **116**, 321–362.
10. Moscona A.   The development in vitro of chimeric aggregates of dissociated embryonic chick and mouse cells. *Nat. Ac. Sc. N. J.*, 1957, **43**, 184–194.
11. Schneider N.   Sur les possibilités de propagation d'un sarcome de Souris sur des organes embryonnaires de Poulet à différents stades du développement. *Arch. Anat. Micr. Morph. exp.*, 1958, **47**, 573–604.

12. Vakaet L.   L'étude expérimentale par la méthode des cultures d'organes des réactions de l'épithélium bronchial de l'embryon de Poulet. *Arch. Anat. Micr. Morph. Exp.*, 1956, **245**, 48–64.
13. Wolff Em.   Adaptation de quatre nouvelles souches cancéreuses humaines à la culture organotypique *in vitro*. *C. R. Soc. Biol.*, 1962, **156**, 1217–1219.
14. Wolff Et.   Potentialités et affinités des tissus révélées par la culture *in vitro* d'organes en associations hétérogènes et xénoplastiques. *Bull. Soc. Zool. Fr.*, 1954, **79**, 357–368.
15. Wolff Et.   Essais de culture d'une tumeur de Souris sur des organes embryonnaires de Poulet cultivés *in vitro*. *C. R. Acad. Sc.*, 1956, **242**, 1537–1538.
16. Wolff Et.   La culture des cellules tumorales sur des explants d'organes *in vitro*. *Expérientia*, 1956, **12**, 321–322.
17. Wolff Et.   La culture de tumeurs sur des organes embryonnaires explantés *in vitro*. *Rev. Méd. Bruxelles*, 1956, **36**, 2235–2243.
18. Wolff Et.   Les parabioses d'organes embryonnaires *in vitro*. *C. R. Colloque sur l'Homogreffe*, 1957.
19. Wolff Et.   Utilisation de la membrane vitelline de l'œuf de Poule en culture organotypique. I: Technique et possibilités. *Dévelop. Biol.*, 1961, **3**, 767–786.
20. Wolff Et.   Long-term organotypic cultures of human surgical tumors at the expense of substances elaborated by the mesonephros of the chick embryo. *In* "Discussion of J. Leighton's report". Symposium on Organ Culture. 13th Annual Meeting of the Tissue Culture Association, Washington D.C., May 29–31. 1962. *National Cancer Institute Monograph*, No. 11, 180–195.
21. Wolff Et., Barski G. and Wolff Em.   Mise en évidence de différents degrés de malignité de souches cellulaires de Souris en Culture d'organes embryonnaires de Poulet. *C. R. Acad. Sc.*, 1960, **251**, 479–481.
22. Wolff Et. and Bresch D.   Sur les parabioses hétérogènes d'organes embryonnaires en culture *in vitro*. *C. R. Acad. Sc.*, 1955, **240**, 1014–1016.
23. Wolff Et. and Schneider N.   Sur l'association d'une tumeur de Souris et d'organes embryonnaires de Poulet en culture *in vitro*. *C. R. Soc. Biol.*, 1956, **150**, 845–846.
24. Wolff Et. and Schneider N.   La culture d'un sarcome de Souris sur des organes de Poulet explantés *in vitro*. *Arch. Anat. Micr. Morph. exp.*, 1957, **46**, 173–197.
25. Wolff Et. and Schneider N.   La transplantation prolongée d'un sarcome de Souris sur des organes embryonnaires de Poulet cultivés *in vitro*. *C. R. Soc. Biol.*, 1957, **151**, 1291–1292.
26. Wolff Et. and Sigot M. F.   Comportement de différents types de tumeurs de Rongeurs associés à du rein embryonnaire de Poulet en culture *in vitro*. *C. R. Soc. Biol.*, 1961, **155**, 265–267.
27. Wolff Et. and Sigot M. F.   Les divers aspects d'une tumeur mammaire de Souris, associée à différents organes embryonnaires de Poulet en culture *in vitro*. *C. R. Soc. Biol.*, 1961, **155**, 960–962.
28. Wolff Et. and Weniger J. P.   Sur les associations xénoplastiques de gonades embryonnaires de Canard et de Souris en culture *in vitro*. *C. R. Acad. Sc.*, 1953, **237**, 936–938.
29. Wolff Et. and Weniger J. P.   Recherches préliminaires sur les chimères d'organes embryonnaires d'Oiseaux et de Mammifères en culture *in vitro*. *J. Embr. Exp. Morph.*, 1954, **2**, 161–171.
30. Wolff Et. and Wolff Em.   La propagation d'une souche de cancer humain sur des organes embryonnaires de Poulet cultivés *in vitro*. *C. R. Acad. Sc.*, 1958, **246**, 1116–1118.
31. Wolff Et. and Wolff Em.   Les résultats d'une nouvelle méthode de culture de cellules cancéreuses *in vitro*. *Revue Fr. d'Etudes Clin. et Biol.*, 1958, **3**, 945–951.

32. Wolff Et. and Wolff Em. Sur le comportement de souches cancéreuses humaines en association avec des organes embryonnaires de Poulet cultivés *in vitro*. *C. R. Soc. Biol.*, 1959, **153**, 1898–1900.

33. Wolff Et. and Wolff Em. Comment un sarcome de Souris se nourrit-il des tissus du rein embryonnaire de Poulet. *C. R. Soc. Biol.*, 1960, **154**, 2182–2184.

34. Wolff Et. and Wolff Em. Mise en évidence de substances favorables à la prolifération de cellules cancéreuses dans le rein embryonnaire de Poulet. *C. R. Acad. Sc.*, 1960, **250**, 4076–4077.

35. Wolff Et. and Wolff Em. Cultures de cellules cancéreuses humaines sur des organes embryonnaires de Poulet explantés *in vitro*. *Coll. Intern. C.N.R.S.*, Nogent, 1961, 199–208.

36. Wolff Et. and Wolff Em. Le rôle du mesonephros de l'embryon de Poulet dans la nutrition de cellules cancéreuses. II: Étude par la méthode de la membrane vitelline. *J. Embryol. exp. Morph.*, 1961, **9**, 678–690.

37. Wolff Et. and Wolff Em. Culture de cancers humains sur du rein embryonnaire de Poulet explanté *in vitro*. *Presse Médic.*, 1961, **69**, 1123–1126.

38. Wolff Et. and Wolff Em. Le comportement, en culture *in vitro*, de cancers humains associés à des explants de rein embryonnaire de Poulet. *C. R. Soc. Biol.*, 1961, **155**, 441–443.

39. Wolff Et. and Wolff Em. Peut-on associer, en culture organotypique, des cancers humains fraîchement prélevés à des tissus embryonnaires de Poulet? *C. R. Acad. Sc.*, 1961, **252**, 1873–1875.

40. Wolff Et. and Wolff Em. La culture prolongée de cancers humains sur le mesonephros de l'embryon de Poulet explanté *in vitro*. *C. R. Soc. Biol.*, 1962, **156**, 240–241.

41. Wolff Et. and Wolff Em. Sur la culture pure organotypique de nodules cancéreux humains *in vitro*. *C. R. Acad. Sc.*, 1962, **254**, 3452–3453.

42. Wolff Et. and Wolff Em. Sur la culture de longue durée d'un cancer humain *in vitro*. *C. R. Acad. Sc.*, 1963, **256**, 1173–1174.

43. Wolff Et. and Wolff Em. Les facteurs de la croissance de tumeurs associées à des organes embryonnaires de Poulet. Dans *International Society for Cell Biology*, vol. II, Academic Press, Inc., New York, N. Y., 1963, 179–198.

44. Wolff Et. and Wolff Em. Nouveaux résultats de la culture organotypique de cancers humains. *C. R. Acad. Sc.*, 1964, **258**, 2439–2441.

45. Wolff Et., Wolff Em. and Renault P. Sur la culture organotypique de carcinomes humains très proliférants, en présence de mesonephros d'embryons de Poulet. *Path. Biol.*, 1962, 1161–1169.

46. Wolff Et., Wolff Em., Zagury D. and Leger L. Recherches sur les conditions de la culture organotypique des cancers humains. I: Possibilités de la méthode. *Presse Médicale*, 1962a, **70**, 2387–2389.

47. Wolff Et., Wolff Em., Zagury D. and Leger L. Recherches sur les conditions de la culture organotypique de cancers humains. II: Étude au microscope électronique. *Presse Médicale*, 1962b, **70**, 2759–2762.

48. Wolff Et., Zajdela Fr. and Sigot M. F. Sur la culture organotypique d'une nouvelle tumeur de Rat *in vitro*. *C. R. Acad. Sc.*, 1964, **258**, 4633–4634.

ADDENDUM

I. ORGAN CULTURE OF MALIGNANT HUMAN TUMORS

The two long-term organ cultures Z 200 (hepatic metastasis of a gastric adenocarcinoma) and Z 516 (coelomic epithelioma of the colon) are still being cultured on various media. They now constitute stable strains that have been maintained for 7 and 6 years, respectively (8)*.

A. Growth Factors for Malignant Tumors *in Vitro*

The authors' main work has been concerned with the biochemical analysis of factors permitting tumor growth. After it had been shown that "parasitic" nutrition at the expense of the mesonephros was not essential, and that membranes could be interposed between the tumor and the organ allowing only filtrates to pass through, there was some conjecture about the size of molecules capable of passing through the filter without losing their activity. The dialyzing membranes, Visking cellulose and cellophane, interposed between the mesonephros and the tumor allowed the passage of substances favorable to tumor growth. This result indicates that the molecular weight of these substances is less than 15,000 (8).

PREPARATION OF ACTIVE EXTRACTS

Tumor explants thus derive their nourishment partly from nutrients contained in the medium and partly from growth substances exuded by the mesonephros.

The nature of these substances must be determined. Crude extracts of mesonephros and embryonic liver were shown to be toxic, and the authors therefore used a fat-free yeast extract treated with acetone, the residue being redissolved in Tyrode's solution and incubated for 3 hours at 37°. The supernatant fluid remaining after centrifugation of this extract proved to be extremely favorable for tumor growth, and it was thus possible, in the absence of living tissue, to culture organized explants of the Z 200 and Z 516 strains (3, 9).

The explants of these two tumors, subcultured every 7 days, showed a 4- to 8-fold increase in size during the time intervening between two subcultures. The tumors Z 200 and Z 516 each acquired a highly characteristic and specific morphology and structure. The explants of Z 200 appeared as spherical or oval nodules with a smooth surface (Fig. A-1), with dense contents

* Translator's note: These figures are later given in reverse order.

497

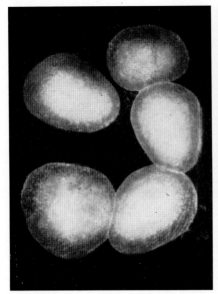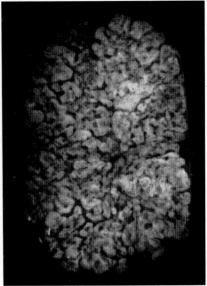

Fig. A-1.   Explant of Z 200.   Fig. A-2.   Explant of Z 516.
(See text for description.)   (See text for description.)

of epitheloid structure and some mucous-secreting alveoli. The explants of
Z 516 had an irregular outline and were marked by deep furrows, giving the
whole a brainlike appearance (Fig. A-2). Histological examination showed
a cortex of epithelial cells projecting inward as sinuous and ramified cords.
Within the nodules, and between the cords, there was a considerable mass
of mucus that was constantly being secreted within the explants. The chemical
characteristics of this mucus have been defined in detail (1, 2).

Thus, organ-type human tumors cultured in the absence of any living tissue
tend to develop a specific morphology and structure which is much more
clearly characteristic than in the primary tumor. This is especially true when
they are completely freed from both the initial human stroma and the normal
embryonic cells on which they had first been cultured.

Yeast extract has the same essential role as the mesonephros for growth of
organized tumors *in vitro*.

Activity of Dialyzates

Dialyzates of yeast extracts have been shown to have the same activity as
the extracts themselves. While crude extracts of liver and mesonephros were
toxic, their dialyzates were as active as those of yeast.

The crude extracts were dialyzed at 4° for 18 hours in tubes of Visking
cellulose against deionized water. A solution of substances of known mole-

cular weight was used to determine the approximate pore diameters of these tubes. Cytochrome of mol wt 16,500 did not pass through the pores of these tubes, ribonuclease of mol wt 12,700 did so easily, and lysozyme of mol wt 14,380 could barely pass through. From this it can be stated that the molecular weight of the substances contained in the dialyzates of liver, mesonephros, and brewers' yeast was less than 15,000. This result is in accord with the conclusions drawn from experiments in which interposing membranes were placed between the two explants. Further evidence for the relatively simple composition of the active factors was provided by the fact that boiling the extracts for 1 hour at pH 7.2. did not decrease their activity.

FRACTIONATION OF DIALYZATES

In an attempt to define the nature of the active substances more precisely, the authors fractionated the dialyzates by various methods: filtration on Sephadex gel, ion-exchange chromatography on Amberlite columns, and fractional dissolutions.

As it is difficult to obtain sufficiently large quantities of embryonic liver and mesonephros extracts, the authors used yeast extracts and dialyzates of 3-month-old chick liver, which were also shown to be favorable for tumor proliferation (7).

The yeast dialyzate was first fractionated by filtration on Sephadex gel G 25 (60 × 2.5 cm). Absorption studies at 260 mμ enabled four fractions to be defined: A, B, C, D. When introduced separately into the culture media they were inactive. Only the mixture (A + B) termed "Sep X" was active and permitted proliferation of the organ strains for more than 35 weeks. Both the Sep X mixture, and the liver dialyzate were subsequently subjected to ion-exchange separation. The passage of either through a column of Amberlite I.R. 120 (cation exchanger in the H$^+$ form) gave separation of an inactive fraction Cat. A (eluted with H$_2$O) from a highly active fraction Cat. B (eluted with NH$_4$OH).

In addition, the passage of either through a column of Amberlite I.R. A400 (anion exchanger in the OH$^-$ form) permitted separation of an inactive fraction, Ano B (eluted with H$_2$0) from a highly active fraction Ano A (eluted with CH$_3$COOH). Both Cat. B and Ano A, whether obtained from brewers' yeast or 3-month-old chick liver produced intensive growth of tumor nodules in both human organ strains; the growth periods were 46 weeks for strain Z 200 and 35 weeks for Z 516. The cultures were arrested while still flourishing.

In the next step, the liver or yeast fractions Cat. B and Cat. A were each adsorbed on to columns of Amberlite I.R.A. Four new fractions were obtained in this way: one "neutral" and one "acidic" from Cat. A, and one "basic" and the other "amphoteric" from Cat. B. Only the amphoteric fraction was shown to be active, whether it came from chick liver or brewers' yeast.

For purification, this amphoteric fraction was subjected to filtration on a 60 × 2.5 cm column of Sephadex G 10, which enabled separation of an active fraction Dis A from an inactive fraction Dis B. Figures A-3, A-4 and A-5 show the various steps in fractionation.

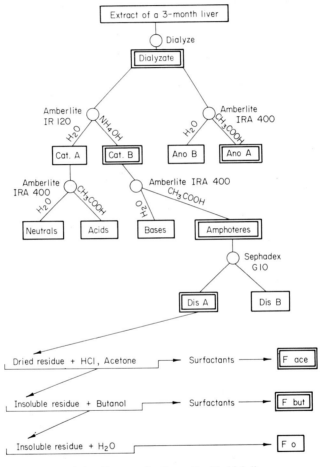

FIG. A-3.   Extract of a 3-month-old chick liver.

Using paper and thin-layer chromatography, it was possible to check that all the active fractions contained a large number of ninhydrin-positive substances, among which were numerous amino acids.

The biuret reaction confirmed the presence of numerous polypetides. There

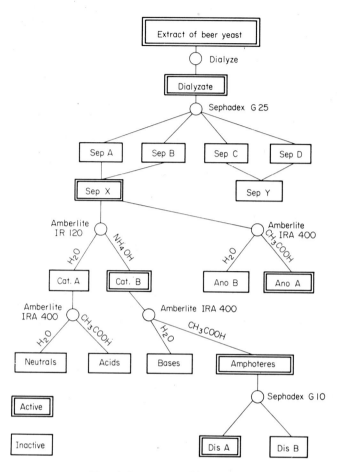

FIG. A-4. Extract of beer yeast.

were, in addition, substances absorbing in ultraviolet light, substances that fluoresced in the UV, and chromogenic substances.

It can be seen that there is an excellent agreement between the results of fractionations of yeast and chick liver dialyzates.

Continuing the analysis, Mason *et al.* (4) used a technique of fractional dissolution. The fraction Dis A, dried under reduced pressure, was recovered in the form of a highly disperse film on the walls of the container. This deposit was extracted at 55° with acetone and concentrated HCl, and then with pure acetone. The residue was treated with butanol at 70°. Two fractions were obtained in this way, one soluble in acetone and the other in butanol. Both were shown to be active, and allowed maintenance of the cultures for more

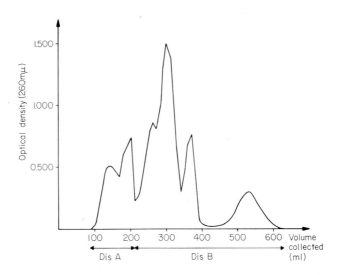

F IG . A-5   Purification of amphoteric fraction provides reparation Dis A from Dis B.

than 17 weeks. Thin-layer and paper chromatography have shown that the acetone-soluble fraction contained the major portion of the amino acids, lysine being the only amino acid present in any significant amount in the butanol-soluble fraction.

Addition of lysine to the basic nutrient medium did not permit growth of tumor explants to be maintained. Lysine is, therefore, not the substance that gives the extract its activity.

To define more precisely the chemical nature of the active principles, the authors prepared a hydrolyzate of the amphoteric fraction. This fraction was heated in presence of 6 N HCl for 24 hours in sealed tubes. After the HCl had been removed, the residue was redissolved in water and the pH was adjusted to 7.2. The resulting fraction was very active. The cultures flourished for 28 weeks and were arrested while still in full growth. The hypothesis that the active fraction is a protein or a polypeptide can thus be eliminated.

Chromatographic analysis of the hydrolyzate revealed the presence of 18 common amino acids and no unusual ninhydrin-positive compound. A synthetic medium containing the same amino acids at the same concentrations as in the hydrolyzate was prepared. Recent results have shown the addition of the synthetic medium to the basic medium to be highly favorable for proliferation of the cultures.

The following conclusions can now be drawn from these experiments:

1. A certain number of compounds can be considered inactive as growth substances. These are the proteins, nucleic acids, nucleotides, nucleosides,

free bases, thiamine, riboflavin, pyridoxine, folic acid. The active substances must, therefore, be sought among the relatively simple molecules resistant to hydrolysis at 105°.

2. Although the amphoteric fraction and the Dis A and acetone-soluble subfractions Dis A and acetone-soluble contain other still unidentified substances in addition to amino acids, there is a strong likelihood that the growth factors studied consist of one or more amino acids. Such a conclusion may seem surprising, as all the common amino acids are present in the basic medium both in the embryonic extracts and in the serum. However, attention is drawn to the concentrations that must be attained for them to be active and to the possible role of amino acid groups in high concentrations.

These questions are now under investigation.

B. Experiments with Substances Inhibiting the Growth of Malignant Tumors in Culture

Using organotypic strains of human tumors, it is possible to test the action of various substances known or suspected of having anticancerous properties. For the experiments to be valid, both normal and cancerous tissue explants have to be cultured on identical media. Pageot-Simpson (5) attempted this using chick embryo gonads as controls.

p-Di(2-chloroethyl)amino-L-phenylalanine (Melphalan) belongs to a group of alkylating agents used in cancer chemotherapy. The effects of Melphalan were compared on chick embryo gonads and human cancers in organ culture. The tumors used were the organotypic strains Z 200 and Z 516, maintained by Wolff and Wolff for 6 and 7 years, respectively.

The gonadal somatic tissues proved to be the most resistant to Melphalan. They exhibited growth inhibition and a reduction in the number of mitoses, but no necrosis. The human cancer cells and the chick embryo gonocytes both showed high sensitivity. One week's treatment produced abundant necroses in the tumors and a total absence of gonocytes in the gonads. The female germinal cells treated after 10–17 days of incubation were more sensitive than the male germinal cells.

Mention should be made here of the great difference in sensitivity between normal tissues and the cancerous strains utilized, and of the same type of sensitivity shown by both the germinal cells and the cancer cells toward an alkylating substance of known cancer-inhibiting properties.

II. CULTURE OF EXPERIMENTAL HEPATOMAS AT DIFFERENT STAGES OF CARCINOGENESIS

Sigot (6) took liver fragments from rats fed on carcinogenic azo dyes.

Various stages could be distinguished in the development of the cancers. The first stage was termed the "precancerous "phase, being characterized by an increased cell proliferation in the bile canaliculi and then in the parenchyma, although as yet no malignant cell characteristics were discernible. Major degeneration phenomena of the cells appeared in subsequent stages, giving rise to regeneration nodules and then to tumor islets increasing in size and number.

Five successive stages have been described by Lacassagne and Hurst, corresponding to fixed times after the start of administration of the toxic substance. Stages 1 and 2 correspond to the precancerous condition, and stages 3 and 5 to the appearance and development of tumors.

Sigot attempted to culture the hepatic tissues removed at these different stages in presence of chick embryo mesonephros and demonstrated that at all stages cancerous nodules were obtained in culture, and that these could be subcultured for 77 days. After a variable time, the precancerous tissues acquire the histological appearance and behavior of tumor nodules. The tissues removed between stages 3 and 5 developed more rapidly and abundantly than the precancerous tissues.

It can be concluded from these results that transformation from the precancerous to the cancerous state can be obtained *in vitro*. Evidence for the latter is provided by the histological appearance of the explants and by the fact that long-term proliferating cultures can be obtained only from these tissues, whereas fragments of healthy liver can never be cultured *in vitro* under the conditions of these experiments.

BIBLIOGRAPHY

1. Beaupain R.   Histochimie du mucus sécrété par une tumeur du côlon humain (la tumeur Z 516) en culture organotypique de longue durée. *Ann. Histochim.*, 1968, **13**, 89–96.
2. Beaupain R. and Wolff Em.   Étude histochimique du mucus sécrété par une tumeur maligne du côlon cultivé *in vitro*. *C. R. Acad. Sc.*, 1967, **264**, 1953–1956.
3. Croisille Y., Mason J., Wolff Em. and Wolff Et.   Analyse biochimique des facteurs déterminant la croissance de tumeurs cancéreuses humaines en culture d'organes *in vitro*. *Europ. J. Cancer*, 1967, **3**, 371–379.
4. Mason J., Wolff Em. and Wolff Et.   Analyse biochimique des facteurs conditionnant la croissance organotypique d'une tumeur humaine cultivée *in vitro*. *Ciba Found. Symp.*, 1969.
5. Pageot-Simpson P. A.   La sensibilité différentielle d'une tumeur humaine et des tissus somatiques et germinaux des gonades embryonnaires en culture organotypique *in vitro*. *Europ. J. Cancer*, 1969.
6. Sigot M. F.   Études sur la culture organotypique de tumeurs animales associées à des organes embryonnaires de poulet et ses applications. Thèse, 1969.

7. Wolff Em., Croisille Y., Mason J. and Wolff Et.   Sur le fractionnement des substances favorables à la croissance de nodules cancéreux humains cultivés *in vitro*. *C. R. Acad. Sc.*, 1967, **265**, 2157–2160.

8. Wolff Et. and Wolff Em.   Cultures organotypiques de longue durée de deux tumeurs humaines du tube digestif. *Europ. J. Cancer*, 1966, **2**, 93–103.

9. Wolff Et., Wolff Em. and Croisille Y.   Culture organotypique de deux épithéliomas humains en l'absence de substratum vivant. *C. R. Acad. Sc.*, 1965, **260**, 2359–2363.

SUBJECT INDEX

A

Adenocarcinoma, culture of, 494

Adhesion phenomenon, in *in vitro* reassociation of cells, 359–367

Adrenal gland, differentiation studies on, 26, 220

Alimentary canal, differentiation studies on, 29–31

Amino acids, in synthetic media for organ culture, 72–75

Amphibians
  in vitro gonad culture of, 155–157
  organ differentiation studies on, 57–58
  organogenesis studies on, 380–384

Appendages, differentiation studies on, 18–22

Auto differentiation
  in vitro characteristics, 33–39
  proof by organ culture, 4–5

B

Birds
  blastoderm culture of, 234–266
  embryo skin culture of, differentiation in, 391–410
  heteroplastic association between organs of and malignant tumors, 473–497
  organogenesis studies on, 385–386
  sexual differentiation *in vitro*, 121–141, 163–169
  hormone secretion and, 166–168

Blastoderm culture and parabiosis, 233–281, 283–295
  of birds, 234–266
  inhibitory factors, 289–291
  metabolic and enzymic activities in, 259–261
  methods of, 234–235
  morphogenesis problems in, 235–254, 283
  nutritional requirements, 254–259, 289
  teratogenic effects on, 261–266

Bones
  of embryos, culture of, 103–106
  corticosteroid effects on, 220
  parathyroid and parathormone effects on, 183–186
  insulin effects on, 188–189
  papain effects on, 189–192
  pituitary growth hormone effects on, 138
  thyroxine and triiodothyroxine effects on, 186–188
  vitamin A effects on, 189–192

C

Calcitonin, effect on bone development, 217–218

Chick embryo, differentiation studies on, 58–67

Chimeras of organs, *see* Organ chimeras

Chimney swift, salivary gland development in, 226

Colchicine, effect on gonad development *in vitro*, 134

Collagen
  effects on epithelial differentiation, 451–454
  formation in bone culture, 111–115

Collagenase, effect on collagen in bone culture, 113–115

Corticosteroids, effects on cultivated organs, 220–222

Creeper factor, in bone culture, 192–196

Crustaceans, organ culture in, 302–305

D

Diethylstilbestrol, hormonal action of male gonads feminized by, 163

Differention of organs in natural media, 13–51
  analysis of the characteristics of, 32–45
  autodifferentiation, 33–39

507

PRINTED IN BELGIUM BY THE ST. CATHERINE PRESS, LTD, TEMPELHOF, 37, BRUGES.